A Century of Homeopaths

Jonathan Davidson

A Century of Homeopaths

Their Influence on Medicine and Health

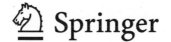 Springer

Jonathan Davidson, MD
Department of Psychiatry
Duke University Medical Center
Durham, NC
USA

ISBN 978-1-4939-0526-3   ISBN 978-1-4939-0527-0   (eBook)
DOI 10.1007/978-1-4939-0527-0
Springer New York Heidelberg Dordrecht London

Library of Congress Control Number: 2014934676

Printed on acid-free paper

Springer is part of Springer Science+Business Media (www.springer.com)

Preface

My first encounter with homeopathy was involuntary and almost disastrous. It occurred in 1947 when, at the age of 3, I became sick and was the subject of an unintended de facto experiment in which homeopathy and a new antibiotic were compared. In this contest of therapeutic philosophies, homeopathy nearly proved fatal, whereas the antibiotic produced full recovery.

The circumstances were as follows. In the summer of 1947, while my recently widowed mother was recuperating on a brief vacation, I was left under the care of my late father's family. During that time, I developed pneumonia and was seen by the Davidson family's primary doctor, Ernest Hawkes, a well-respected Liverpool homeopath. An anxious parent might have drawn succor from knowing that a physician of illustrious pedigree and long experience was looking after her tender child, for Ernest Hawkes and his brother James were prominent homeopathic physicians in Liverpool and their father Alfred had been a nationally renowned and influential homeopath in Victorian Britain. Unfortunately, things went badly for the young patient, who was deteriorating rapidly on homeopathic treatment. Upon returning home, my mother was alarmed to see how ill her son had become and insisted against family resistance that I be taken to a family doctor of her choice who, without hesitation, determined that the patient needed a newly introduced drug, penicillin, which was then called "M & B," after the pharmaceutical manufacturer May and Baker. Recovery was rapid, and I lived to write this book almost seven decades later. But apparently it was a close call. Besides serving as a personal introduction, this anecdote is useful in that it illustrates why and when homeopathy went into nearly terminal decline in many parts of the world. From its position as a well-endowed, securely established, lively medical minority, homeopathy was rapidly dying out of medicine in the United Kingdom and the United States by 1950. One of the main reasons was the introduction into medicine of life-saving drugs such as penicillin. This era of revolutionary pharmacology took place chiefly in the 1930s and 1940s and led to the view that homeopathy was no more than an anachronistic irrelevance.

So how could a psychiatrist become sufficiently interested to write a book about homeopathy? In subsequent years, as my career developed along "orthodox" lines, for a long time, I paid almost no attention to homeopathy, although as a medical student at University College Hospital, I once attended a case conference at the nearby Royal London Homeopathic Hospital, which was presided over by an aging Sir John Weir, who was personal physician to King George VI and Queen Elizabeth II. But apart from the pomp and Weir's plethoric complexion, I recall little about the actual conference. Although psychiatry became my specialty of choice, I have always retained curiosity about what was in the 1960s called, somewhat disparagingly, *fringe* medicine, then later *alternative* medicine, *complementary* medicine, *complementary and alternative* medicine (CAM), and, now, *integrative* or *integrated* medicine. The CAM movement has grown into a visible and quite well-funded constituency, which is represented in the United States as a separate institute within the National Institutes of Health. Thus, as the CAM road show became increasingly popular in the 1990s and opportunities presented themselves, it made sense to pursue research in CAM. Better yet, why not be among the first to put a stake in the ground as there was more territory to claim and less competition in those early days? Of considerable influence in kick-starting my new career direction was a critical review of homeopathy which appeared in the *British Medical Journal* in 1991. This review found that homeopathy seemed to be more than a mere placebo effect, even though no plausible mechanism of action declared itself. It was a good time to investigate homeopathy, which meant embarking on a quest for funding and training, both of which I was fortunate enough to obtain. As it turned out, a greater part of my energies were directed into the study of herbal and dietary supplements, but homeopathy was where a 15-year CAM trek began, and it has provided an information base that I have used to tell a story about homeopathy that is hopefully new. Added to the above, it may be said that, to this author at least, homeopathy is appealingly similar to psychiatry, yet these two ships of the line have rarely recognized themselves as belonging to the same fleet.

Seabrook Island, SC   Jonathan Davidson, MD

Acknowledgments

The following individuals have given generously of their time and been most helpful in providing materials and source documentation and graciously answering many questions: at Boston University, A'Llyn Ettien, head of Technical Services, Boston University Alumni Medical Library, Peter Reich, Aram Chobanian, MD, Judy Watkins, and Claire Grimble; at the Bentley Historical Library, University of Michigan, Karen Jania and Anthony Timek; Barbara Shipman, at the Alfred Taubman Health Sciences Library, University of Michigan; at the Michigan State University Archives and Historical Collections, Ed Busch; at the History of Medicine Division, National Library of Medicine, Leona Hammond and Stephen Greenberg, PhD; at the Wood Library-Museum of Anesthesiology, Judith Robins and Teresa Jimenez; at the Rochester Medical Museum and Archives, Robert Dickson and Kathleen Britton and at the Central Library of Rochester and Monroe County, New York, Christine Ridarsky; at the Institut für Geschichte der Medizin der Robert Bosch Stiftung Stuttgart, Germany, Robert Juette, PhD, MD, and Martin Dinges, PhD; at the New York Medical College, Shawn Manning; Jenny Benjamin, director of the Museum of Vision, and Stanley M. Truhlsen, MD, director of Ophthalmic Heritage; at the Lloyd Library and Museum, Devhra Bennett Jones; Johanna Goldberg, at the Center for the History of Medicine and Public Health, New York Academy of Medicine; former archivist at Hahnemann Medical College, Barbara Williams; archivist at the American College of Surgeons, Susan Rishworth; Debbie Lancaster, managing editor, *The Pharos*; and at the Cleveland Clinic, Jay Persaud.

For information about Conrad Wesselhoeft and the Wesselhoeft family, I am indebted to Caroline Williams, Anne Smalley, Dianne Wesselhoeft, Conrad Wesselhoeft (grandson), and Walter Johannes Wesselhoeft; for Solomon Carter Fuller, Mary Kaplan, MSW, University of South Florida and author of *Where My Caravan Has Rested*, a biography of Fuller; Mott R. Linn, head of Collections Department, Robert Hutchings Goddard Library, Clark University; and Jack Eckert, public service librarian, Harvard Medical School.

For Otto Guttentag, the following individuals provided information: Christoph Guttentag, PhD, Duke University; Nicholas Nossaman, MD; and Josue Hurtado, University of California San Francisco Library.

My gratitude goes to the following: Walter Munz, MD, former medical director, Albert Schweitzer Hospital at Lambaréné, Gabon; Ralph G. Hirschowitz, MD; Harry Kerr, MD; Jay Yasgur, R.Ph; Jeffrey Baker, MD, Duke University; Eric J. Engstrom, PhD, Humboldt University; Francis Treuherz, FSHom; Martin Lengwiler, PhD, University of Basel; George Guess, MD; Peter Morrell, Staffordshire University; Franco Carli, MD, McGill University; Ludwig Deppisch, MD; Flavio Dantas, MD, University of Sao Paulo; Rt. Hon Lord David Owen, CH, PC, FRCP, MB, BCh; Reverend Josh Thomas; Larry Kiroff; Renee Glaim; Matthias Goerig, MD; Volney Steele, MD; Sarah Hartwell; Harald Hamre, MD; Steven L. Danver; and Thierry Montfort; Susan Hoffius, Ph.D, Medical University of south Carolina; Roy W. Menninger, MD., Past President, Menninger Foundation.

Special thanks are due to the following for their review of book content: Jerry Reves, MD, Medical University of South Carolina; Ira Rutkow, MD; Jon van Heerden, MD, Medical University of South Carolina; Charles Bensonhaver, MD; Iris Bell, MD, PhD, University of

Arizona; Bernardo Merizalde, MD, Thomas Jefferson University Medical School; and David Hay-Edie.

Turning closer to home, my sister, Naomi Davidson, reminded me of those early experiences with homeopathy, adding that she used to raid the family homeopathic medicine cupboard and sample the available remedies at hand because, as she put it, they tasted more like candy than medicine! Others doubtless share her opinion, but I remain unsure.

Special thanks are due to Ben, my son and expert "in-house" editor, whose discerning eye has helped in many ways and whose comments and suggestions gave better voice and greater polish to what is in this book.

The enthusiastic encouragement of my wife and best cheerleader, Meg, has been ever present, and her zest for life continues to inspire.

Contents

1 Introduction... 1
A Brief History of Homeopathy 1
Defining a Homeopath 2
Synopsis 3
References.. 4

2 Samuel Hahnemann: Rebarbative Genius 5
Personality and Relationships... 5
Hahnemann as Medical Pioneer 7
References.. 8

3 Women, Reform, and Medical Leadership........................... 9
Professional Barriers, Social Reform, and the Role of Women
in Homeopathy 9
New York Medical College and Hospital for Women 10
    Clemence Lozier.. 10
    Elizabeth Blackwell 11
    Harriet Clisby 12
    Emily Stowe 12
    Mary Safford Blake.. 14
    Alice Boole Campbell.. 15
    Susan Smith McKinney Steward (Also Known as
    Susan Smith McKinney).. 15
    Florence Nightingale Ward.. 16
    Maria Augusta Generoso Estrella..................................... 17
    Geraldine Burton-Branch 17
New Boston Graduates and Students 18
    Mercy B. Jackson 18
    Mary H. Thompson.. 18
    Lucy Waite 19
    Rebecca Lee Crumpler 19
    Esther Hill Hawks... 19
    Julia Holmes Smith.. 20
    Leila Gertrude Bedell 20
    Martha George Ripley... 21
    Anna Howard Shaw 22
    Rebecca Lee Dorsey 22
    Clara Barrus 23
    Eliza Taylor Ransom... 25
Cleveland Graduates 25
    Caroline Brown Winslow 25
    Susan Edson 26

    Others 26
       Laura Matilda Towne 26
    References 27

4 The Homeopathic Scalpel: Contributions to Surgery
   from the World of Homeopathy 29
    Dental Surgery 30
       Josiah Foster Flagg 30
    Gynecology and Obstetrics 32
       George Taylor 32
       Rebecca Lee Dorsey 32
       George Southwick 32
       James Wood 32
       James Ward and Florence Nightingale Ward 32
       Lucy Waite 33
       Walter Crump 33
       Geraldine Burton-Branch 34
    Urology 35
       Bukk Carleton 35
       Sprague Carleton 35
       George Nagamatsu 35
       Leonard P. Wershub 35
    General Surgery 35
       Edward C. Franklin 35
       William Tod Helmuth 37
       Israel Tisdale Talbot 37
       John Mallory Lee 40
    Ophthalmology and Otolaryngology 40
       Edwin Sterling Munson 40
       L. Grant Selfridge 43
    Cardiac Surgery 43
       Charles Bailey 43
    Others 44
    References 44

5 Homeopaths and the Dawning of Anesthesiology 47
    Herbert Leo Northrop 48
    Thomas Drysdale Buchanan 49
    Walter M. Boothby 50
    Everett A. Tyler 50
    Henry Ruth 51
    Harold Randall Griffith 52
    Rolland Whitacre 54
    William Neff 55
    Brant Burdell ("BB") Sankey 56
    Kenneth K. Keown 56
    Caleb Matthews 57
    Thomas Skinner 58
    August Bier 59
    Summary 60
    References 61

6   Homeopathy and the Mind: From Alienists to Neuroscientists   63
   Hahnemann's Attitude Towards Mental Illness   63
   Kinship of Homeopathy and Psychiatry   63
   Influential Individuals   65
      Charles Frederick Menninger: An Ambassador-at-Large
      from the Court of Nature   65
      Rudolf Arndt   66
      Selden Talcott   66
      Samuel Worcester   69
      Bayard Holmes   70
      Emmons Paine   72
      Frank C. Richardson   72
      Henry M. Pollock   73
      Clara Barrus   74
      Henry I. Klopp   74
      Psychiatrists at Fergus Falls State Hospital   76
      The Life and Career of Solomon Carter Fuller: America's First
      African-American Psychiatrist   77
      Winfred Overholser: The Dean of Forensic Psychiatry   82
      Oswald Boltz: From Psychiatry to Homeopathy   84
      James Cocke   85
   References   85

7   Public Health   89
   Tullio S. Verdi   89
   Charles Sumner   91
   Eugene Porter   91
   Charles V. Chapin   93
   Rebecca Lee Dorsey   93
   Hills Cole   94
   James W. Ward   94
   Royal Copeland   94
   Pedro Ortiz   94
   Marcus Kogel   95
   Geraldine Burton-Branch   97
   The Domestic Sanitation Movement   97
      John James Drysdale and John William Hayward   97
   References   97

8   The Early Days of Radiation: Homeopathic Shadows   99
   Emil Grubbé: First to Use X-Rays in Medicine or Teller of Tall Tales?   99
   The Discovery of X-Rays and Its Impact on Grubbé   100
   Francis Benson   101
   William Dieffenbach   102
      Other Activities   103
   John Mallory Lee   104
   References   105

9   Heartbeat, Heart Failure, and Homeopathy   107
   Constantine Hering and His Contributions   107
      Nitroglycerin   107

Snake Venoms. 108
Hering's Law of Cure 109
The Cardiovascular Institute (CVI) at Hahnemann Medical College. 109
Other Contributors to Cardiology. 110
Milton Raisbeck 110
Measuring Cardiovascular Physiology: Nineteenth-Century British Studies. 111
Robert Dudgeon and the Dudgeon Sphygmograph 111
The Sphygmograph. 112
Experimental Physiology at Boston University School of Medicine (BUSM). 112
Arthur Weysse. 112
References. 112

10 **Allergy and Allergic Disorders: Homeopathic Leaders** 115
Introduction. 115
Charles Blackley. 115
Grant L. Selfridge. 118
Homeopathy, Immunology, and Allergy: Other Considerations. 119
Charles Frederick Millspaugh. 120
References. 121

11 **Academic Homeopaths Reinvented**. 123
Roy Upham: Promoter of International Homeopathy. 123
Conrad Wesselhoeft: Physician in Search of an Identity 123
Homeopathic Career. 125
Career in Regular Medicine 128
Linn J. Boyd: From Homeopathic Philosophy to Cardiology 130
Thomas H. McGavack: Embracing Homeopathy, Endocrinology,
and Gerontology 132
References. 133

12 **Oncology** 137
Oscar Auerbach. 137
Charles Cameron. 138
Howard W. Nowell 140
Ita Wegman 141
Edward Cronin Lowe 141
References. 142

13 **Other Stars in the Sky** 143
Gymnastics, Education, Temperance, and Social Reform 143
Diocletian Lewis. 143
Swedish Massage 146
Matthias Roth, George Taylor, and Charles Taylor. 146
Chemistry and Administration 147
Ira Remsen 147
Pediatrics. 148
Carl Fischer. 148
The First Native American Indian in Modern Medicine. 149
Charles Eastman 149
Pathology 150
Edward Cronin Lowe 150
References. 151

14 **Congress, Parliament, Presidents, and Monarchs**. 153
Charles E. Sawyer. 153
Joel Boone. 154

Willis Danforth 157
John Weir: The Monarch's Doctor 157
Homeopaths in Elected Office 158
   Jacob H. Gallinger 158
   Royal S. Copeland 159
   J. Dickson Mabon 161
The Royal London Homeopathic Hospital 162
References 162

15 Bioethics and the Contributions of Otto Guttentag 165
Personal Background and Training 165
Academic Career 166
Guttentag as Homeopath 166
Contributions to Bioethics and Medical Humanities 167
References 168

16 Less Is More: Finding the Right Dose 169
Rudolf Arndt 170
Hugo Schulz 171
Hormesis 173
Limitations of the Arndt-Schulz Law 174
Drugs: To Be Given Every Day or Intermittently? 175
Time-Dependent Sensitization 176
Does the Label Tell the Truth? How Much Medicine Is Really There? 177
References 177

17 A Homeopathic Rogues' Gallery 179
Three Charlatans 179
   Edwin Hartley Pratt 179
   Albert Abrams 180
   William Koch 184
License Fraud 184
   Robert Reddick 184
   Gregory Miller 186
Power and Betrayal: George Simmons 186
Homeopaths in Nazi Germany 188
   Karl Koetschau 189
   Other Transgressors: Hans Wapler and Gerhard Madaus 190
   Other Events Relevant to Homeopathy in Nazi Germany 191
Homeopathy and Murder 191
   Hawley Crippen and James Munyon 191
   Luc Jouret 194
References 195

18 Concluding Thoughts 197
Persecution Against Homeopaths 198
The Evidence for Efficacy: Does Homeopathy Work? 199
   Basic Rules of Medical Evidence: Some Brief Considerations 199
   Major Reviews of Homeopathy 199
   How Might Homeopathy Work? 201
References 202

Index 203

Introduction

Any discussion about homeopathy is bound to evoke passionate feelings, feelings that can interfere with our capacity for scientific objectivity. Fisher has accurately described much of the discourse as a "dialogue of the deaf" [1]. The divide does not just apply to the believers and skeptics in homeopathy – it is endemic within the homeopathy community, too. Homeopathy has polarized opinions almost since the beginning for two main reasons (other than that of professional rivalry). First, the visionary who introduced homeopathy to the world, Samuel Hahnemann, was a prickly character who antagonized friend and foe alike. Second, some homeopaths maintain the belief (some might say "dogma") that drugs become more potent as the dilution increases, even to amounts that contain no original substance – an absurd assumption to the majority of scientists. It is not the purpose of this book to enter into this particular discussion in any depth, although I will address it periodically. The reason for drawing attention to these two points is to recognize how profoundly they have determined the discourse on homeopathy, which has largely revolved around this limited agenda. Opponents of homeopathy have constantly attacked Hahnemann's teachings and scorned the remedies, while homeopathy's proponents have been forced to go on the defensive over these same issues. Far less attention has been paid to other aspects of homeopathy, including the possibility that, as a system of health, it has influenced conventional medicine to a greater extent than is realized. If any credit has been given by those in the larger medical community, it has usually been a grudging admission that homeopathy hastened the demise of traditional medicine's more deadly treatments like bleeding, blistering, purging, and toxic drug doses. However, the profession has been more inclined to see homeopathy as a tiresome absurdity which would best be eradicated. The possibility that homeopathy may have had more extensive positive effects has rarely been considered. Furthermore, in most discourse, the word "homeopathy" has been taken only in the narrow sense to refer to small doses and the *simile* principle of "let like be cured with like."

Many questions can legitimately be asked of homeopathy. Does it work? How does it work? Is there a difference between low dilutions, which contain measurable amounts of drug, and higher dilutions, which contain no original substance? Does the *simile* principle have any validity? Do the medicines produce side effects? All of these are fair questions that relate to the remedies themselves, and many are now the focus of research. It is also possible to frame different, broader, questions about homeopathy, ones which expand the horizon beyond remedies. It is the purpose of this book to investigate one of these, the question of how homeopathically trained physicians have influenced medical progress, health, and culture.

A Brief History of Homeopathy

Homeopathy was introduced in Germany circa 1796. It spread throughout the world over the next 50 years, reaching Russia by 1823, the United States by 1825, England by 1827, France by 1830, India by 1839, and Brazil by 1840. As such, homeopathy is a global form of medicine, with each country having evolved its own way of teaching, practicing, and regulating homeopathy. In India, as of the early twenty-first century, there are over 100 homeopathic medical schools and 100,000 licensed homeopaths. In Great Britain, homeopathy has never been part of the medical school curriculum, and the discipline is taught as a postgraduate course at a few centers. In the United States, from the late 1830 s until the mid-twentieth century, there were homeopathic medical schools that numbered over 20 at their peak and trained 10 % of all physicians. For a time, American homeopathy maintained a vigorous presence in the nation's medical culture, with its own subspecialties, journals, regulations, and local and national societies. By the 1960s however, it had almost completely died out. In Brazil, at least one university medical school boasts a homeopathy department, and homeopathic treatment is covered under many public and private insurance plans; as a medical specialty, in terms of number of doctors, it was ranked 16th out of 60 in 2007 [2].

J. Davidson, *A Century of Homeopaths*,
DOI 10.1007/978-1-4939-0527-0_1, © Springer Science+Business Media New York 2014

Thus, it is reasonable to view homeopathy as more than a matter of small doses and the dogmas of its founding guru. Homeopathy can also be seen as a system, that is, a method of training, practice, and research, which, depending on the country and period in history, has played a significant role in medical practice. This book examines the extent to which homeopathically trained doctors have contributed to medical progress, public health, and culture. It also examines the manner in which their labors have borne fruit. It does so by investigating the influence of homeopathy in different medical specialties, as well as the social and political change that some homeopathic practitioners have achieved throughout history. During the course of writing this book, the author was struck by the number of times that subjects had been acclaimed by observers as being "ahead of their time." Because these practitioners belonged to a marginalized community, it usually took generations for the true impact of their work to be recognized, and in some cases, it has remained unrecognized.

Defining a Homeopath

Since this is a book about homeopaths, it is well to consider what the term "homeopathy" means. A homeopath can be defined in various ways, and homeopaths themselves have disagreed on what constitutes homeopathy. For example, homeopaths hold different views about the place of high and low potencies in defining whether a medicine is homeopathic. By the early twentieth century, training, diagnostic practices, and treatments in US homeopathic medical schools closely resembled those of orthodox medical schools, with the chief difference being the inclusion of courses on homeopathic *materia medica* and their use in everyday practice. Some might ask if that was the only difference, and the answer to that question is perhaps more complex. It is possible that subtle differences existed between homeopathic and allopathic medical training, differences concerning homeopathy's holistic commitment to treating the "patient who has the disease" rather than focusing on the "disease." Homeopathy may have been the first form of "personalized" medicine, which strove to identify what was unique to the patient with the illness as a way of tailoring treatment accordingly. One sees constant acknowledgement by homeopaths of the importance of a healthy lifestyle, attention to diet, exercise, stress management, and the like. This holistic attitude could have characterized the way in which homeopaths viewed their patients, in comparison to the allopathic view. Well-trained homeopaths may have been more attuned to nonverbal signals in the patient, as well as preferences and idiosyncrasies which, to most physicians, seemed of little consequence. Their training may have led to more developed listening skills, and it could be said that there is more of the

psychotherapist about the homeopath than other types of doctor, with the obvious exception of psychiatrists (see Chap. 6 for a more in-depth discussion). That an individualized homeopathic assessment confers meaningful therapeutic benefit over and above regular treatment is suggested in a study of rheumatoid arthritis described in Chap. 18. It therefore bears considering whether the curriculum of homeopathic medical schools included more of these personalized elements. If this was to have been the case, and it is not implausible to make the argument, then there were greater differences between homeopathic and allopathic medical schools than appear at first glance.

The personalities in this book cover the spectrum of allegiance to homeopathy. I chose them not simply as upholders of the faith but instead because they contributed tangibly to the betterment (or detriment) of general medicine, public health, or culture. To merit inclusion, subjects were required to have either graduated from a homeopathic medical school or received specialty training. Some qualified for inclusion if, as regular (allopathic) physicians, they embraced homeopathy later in life. Inclusion does not necessarily imply that the subject practiced or overtly believed in homeopathy – in some cases, they did so (e.g., Griffith); in other cases, there was continuing but unpublicized loyalty (e.g., Fuller, Guttentag); some were conflicted and later abandoned homeopathy (e.g., Wesselhoeft, Boyd, McGavack), while others professed no allegiance (e.g., Bailey) or sought to argue away their contact with homeopathy (e.g., Remsen). Regarding the last two groups, one might ask why I included them. The answer is that they were products of the homeopathic culture, which served as their gateway into medicine. The system can thus "take some credit" as it were for their later achievements. A small number of individuals have been included by virtue of their faculty service in a homeopathic medical school, even though they were neither trained in, nor practitioners of, homeopathy. Technically, they were not homeopaths but were part of the homeopathic culture at the time, and their work reflects to some extent what homeopathy had to offer. Homeopathy is not without its share of villains, and they too will be discussed.

While homeopaths from various countries are included, the great majority here hail from the United States and Canada. This is not to diminish homeopaths elsewhere, but reflects several factors. First, easily accessible records exist of American homeopathy and the activities of its medical schools. Secondly, homeopathy arguably penetrated more extensively into US healthcare than in other English-speaking countries like Great Britain, so there is simply more material to work with. Homeopathy plays a notable role in French and central European medicine, but, without being fluent in the relevant languages, it would be a daunting task for this author to tackle such literature. Along with France, other countries may well have their own stories to tell. Hopefully, similar accounts will one day be forthcoming. Even weighting this book with material from North America, there is much to say.

Synopsis

This book describes how homeopaths and allopaths who were supportive of homeopathy have influenced medicine in several notable ways.

In the area of allergic disease, the homeopath Charles Blackley discovered that grass pollen is the etiological agent of hay fever in susceptible people. Grant Selfridge was pivotal in establishing allergic disease as a medical specialty.

Anesthesiology illustrates par excellence the formative role of homeopaths in establishing a medical specialty. Active in this regard were Henry Ruth, Harold Griffith, and Rolland Whitacre (who also founded one of the nation's first anesthesiology residency programs). Harold Griffith revolutionized surgical practice with the muscle relaxant drug curare. Kenneth Keown opened up new possibilities for cardiac surgery by introducing lidocaine for anesthesia.

Bioethics was placed on the national political agenda by Senator Jacob Gallinger and became an academic-clinical concern owing to the efforts of Otto Guttentag, who is now hailed as a key twentieth-century figure in this specialty.

Cardiology has been well represented by Constantine Hering, who introduced nitroglycerin; by George Geckeler, a famous teacher in the mid-twentieth century; and by Linn Boyd, author of a textbook and of many peer-reviewed publications. Hahnemann Medical College, Philadelphia, became internationally renowned in the 1940s and 1950s for its innovations in cardiac surgery, under the leadership of Charles Bailey, assisted by Kenneth Keown, William Likoff, and George Geckeler.

Thomas McGavack was an early leader in gerontology and earned fame for his expertise in treating obesity, as well as for treating metabolic and thyroid disease. At one point, McGavack served as president of the American Institute of Homeopathy, but later resigned from the organization over its lack of commitment to a research agenda. McGavack went on to become a distinguished gerontologist and endocrinologist.

Knowledge of infectious disease was advanced by the work of Conrad Wesselhoeft, professor at Harvard and Boston Universities in the mid-twentieth century. An endowed chair in his name at Boston University has been held by some of medicine's most distinguished figures.

Pharmacology has engaged the attention of several researchers sympathetic to homeopathy. In particular, their work demonstrated the stimulating effects of some drugs at low doses and suppressive effects at higher doses – the so-called biphasic or hormetic properties of drugs. The two individuals most associated with this work were not homeopaths, but were, respectively, a psychiatrist (Rudolf Arndt) and a pharmacologist (Hugo Schulz). Both were positively inclined towards homeopathy and willing to understand how homeopathic remedies could work.

In the world of politics, three homeopaths have been singled out for their achievements. In the United States, Senators Gallinger and Copeland long campaigned for causes such as ethical research and drug safety. Copeland's 1938 bill has had far-reaching effects on drug and food safety. In Britain, Dickson Mabon performed useful work that helped sustain a major center of complementary and alternative medicine (CAM) in London when this important arm of the National Health Service was threatened with closure. Homeopaths have held a prominent role in caring for political leaders and monarchs, including Susan Edson (President Garfield), Charles Sawyer (President Harding), Joel Boone (Presidents Harding, Coolidge, and Hoover), Tullio Verdi (Secretary Seward), Thomas McGavack (Ronald Reagan, before he became president), and Sir John Weir (at least nine European kings and queens over a nearly 60-year period).

For almost 100 years, homeopathic physicians were active in public health and the domestic sanitation movement and took initiatives to improve healthcare and minority training in various communities. Royal Copeland, Tullio Verdi, Solomon Carter Fuller, Charles Eastman, James Ward, and many women homeopaths were among such advocates during the late nineteenth and early twentieth centuries.

Psychiatry perhaps competes with anesthesia for being the specialty where homeopaths have made the most notable contributions. Indeed, a national system of homeopathic asylums existed for about 70 years in which psychiatric inpatients received treatment according to homeopathic principles. Included in the chapter on psychiatry are Solomon Carter Fuller for his pioneering work in Alzheimer's disease and neuropathology, Winfred Overholser for his administrative and forensic work, and Harold Klopp for his innovations in child psychiatry. Bayard Holmes is an unusual case: he was trained as a homeopath and practiced as a surgeon, but for personal reasons became preoccupied with finding a cure for schizophrenia, and did much to advocate for social reform and better treatment of the mentally ill.

From the mid-1800s to mid-1900s, homeopaths distinguished themselves in the field of surgery, and around 20 are discussed in this book. Some of the more famous include Ralph Lloyd and Royal Copeland (ophthalmology), Charles Bailey (thoracic surgery), Edward Franklin and William Tod Helmuth (early pioneers, teachers, and prolific writers), and Israel Talbot (early US tracheostomy pioneer). Surgeon George Taylor introduced Swedish massage to North America and homeopath Matthias Roth introduced it into the United Kingdom.

Perhaps most conspicuous is the large number of women who graduated from homeopathic medical schools, mostly at a time when conventional medical schools forbade the entry of women into their programs. Their groundbreaking work created opportunities for other women to enter the medicinal field, and they provided services for the disadvantaged in society and for ethnic minorities. Moreover, they loomed large as agents of social change beyond medicine. It is here that the legacy of homeopathy is possibly strongest. Among the group are founders of colleges, hospitals, and unions: Clemence Lozier founded the New York Homeopathic Women's College; Emily Stowe founded Canada's first medical school for women and the Toronto Women's College Hospital; Harriet Clisby, an Australian, founded the Women's Educational and Industrial Union (WEIU); Maria Estrella pioneered greater opportunities for women in Brazilian higher education; Anna Howard Shaw chaired the women's section of Woodrow Wilson's Council for National Defense in World War I and campaigned for women's suffrage and acceptance of women for ordination in the church; and Laura Towne established the Penn Center in South Carolina as a place where freed slaves could receive healthcare and education and learn job skills.

Other distinguished figures include Dioclesian Lewis, who has been described as a "harvesting machine" of causes, including temperance and women's suffrage, but who is best known for introducing a system of gymnastics that educators incorporated into many American school systems. Ira Remsen, who downplayed his homeopathic training, became a world famous chemist, inventor of saccharin, and president of Johns Hopkins University. Emil Grubbé claimed to have been the first to use radiation in medical treatment and was an early leader in the field of radiology. Edward Cronin Lowe was recognized for his inoculation program for New Zealand servicemen in World War I.

Not all contributions are positive, however. Among the handful who brought disrepute on themselves are George Simmons, the power behind the growth of the American Medical Association, who left behind a trail of scandal; Hawley Crippen and Luc Jouret, murderers of one (Crippen) and many (Jouret); Robert Reddick, who organized a license scam; and Edward Pratt, Albert Abrams, and William Koch, commercial promoters of unproven treatments. Others (Karl Koetschau and Hans Wapler) became closely aligned with Nazi politics in the 1930s.

Rounding out the presentation are two chapters: an introductory essay about Samuel Hahnemann and a closing account that considers the legacy of homeopathy and the evidence of whether it works. A number of extensive reviews have been conducted on human and animal studies, and some conclusions from these will be drawn by the author, who is personally familiar with clinical research, having spent 40 years conducting trials and evaluating treatments in psychiatry and complementary and alternative medicine. All but two of the chapters chronicle the deeds of individuals, but two chapters (Chap. 16 on pharmacology and the concluding Chap. 18) journey more into published literature on scientific work about the mechanism of action and therapeutic efficacy of homeopathy.

Over 100 homeopaths are presented, who largely circumscribe two symbolically important events in the life of American homeopathy. In 1848, Constantine Hering and his colleagues opened the doors of Hahnemann Medical College in Philadelphia, with the first lecture being given in October of that year. Hahnemann was America's first enduring homeopathic medical school, its flagship institution. One hundred years later, 1948 marked the first full year in which that same institution, by then the last remaining US homeopathic medical school, no longer required its students to attend lectures on homeopathy as it let go of its past for a new post-homeopathic identity. One might think of these years as emblematic of the birth and death of homeopathy as a significant force in American healthcare. Nearly all that is told in the following chapters took place during this 100-year period.

References

1. Fisher P. Homeopathy and mainstream medicine: a dialogue of the deaf? Wien Med Wochenschr. 2005;155:474–8.
2. Teixeira MZ. Brief homeopathic pathogenetic experimentation: a unique educational tool in Brazil. Evid Based Complement Alternat Med. 2009;6:407–14.

Samuel Hahnemann (Fig. 2.1) is an acknowledged pathfinder for his contributions to medicine, although recognition is usually muted, except by Hahnemann's more adulatory supporters who sometimes view his pronouncements as infallible.

Hahnemann was born in 1755, in the town of Meissen, Germany, where his father was employed in the porcelain industry. Overcoming paternal resistance, Hahnemann determined to become a physician and entered medical school, first in Leipzig, then later in Erlangen, where he received his degree in 1779. He practiced medicine for 2 years but grew disillusioned and abandoned it to pursue work as a translator and library director. He later returned to medicine and led an extremely peripatetic life, moving a total of 22 times. In 1830, Hahnemann's first wife died, and in 1835, he met and married a French women 50 years his junior; they moved to Paris, where Hahnemann continued to practice medicine until his death in 1843 at the age of 88. Before appraising Hahnemann's successes and failures, his personality and psychological makeup will be reviewed. This side of Hahnemann is important because it played a significant part in determining the relationships that developed between homeopathy and regular medicine, or *allopathy*, to use the name given by Hahnemann. (The word *homeopathy* means "equal suffering," in contrast to *allopathy*, a word coined by Hahnemann as a derogatory term which meant "opposite suffering," in reference to the effects of each treatment.)

Personality and Relationships

At an early stage in his career, Hahnemann undertook to reform the practice of medicine, seeing the damaging effects of what has been referred to by Boyd as the "tripod of cure-alls," namely, bloodletting, emetics, and purgatives [1], in addition to widespread polypharmacy (i.e., the use of multiple drugs). In setting this course, Hahnemann quickly alienated himself from his medical and apothecary colleagues, and even from his own friends. Such alienation was not simply due to differences in philosophy, but had roots in his

personality and confrontational manner. There are reasons to suspect that Hahnemann had either a variant of bipolar ("manic-depressive") disorder or at least a personality characterized by unusual levels of grandiosity, paranoia, abrasiveness, confrontational behavior, and interpersonal sensitivity, flavored with mood swings and a degree of misrepresentation, even dishonesty. If any of this holds true, it could well explain why he kept wandering from town to town, no doubt at great cost to his wife and large family of 11 children. It would also account for Hahnemann's poor

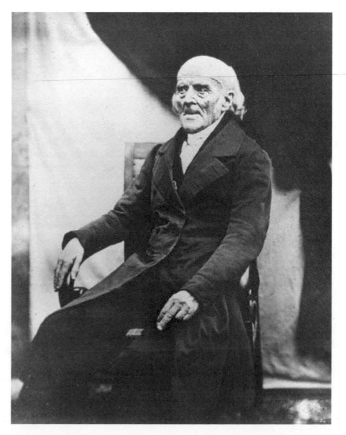

Fig. 2.1 Samuel Hahnemann 1841. Founder of homeopathy. In the public domain

relations with the medical profession, as he attempted to introduce a system of medicine that threatened the prosperity of doctors and apothecaries and went against their beliefs.

Evidence for possible psychopathology comes from at least three sources: Cameron, Wesselhoeft, and Boyd [2–6]. Cameron, a nonpsychiatrist, raises the possibility of Hahnemann's psychopathology being manifested by his countless moves, restlessness, and swings in mood from dejected frustration to messianic militancy, which, in Cameron's words, amounted to "probably a symptomatic record." Wesselhoeft presents evidence of dishonesty, or at least misrepresentation by Hahnemann of his own achievements between 1791 and 1795. For example, Hahnemann referred to his wide experience in treating mental illness and to setting up a mental asylum, whereas he treated only one patient in the asylum. He further claimed to have seen cases of malaria in Hungary, even though he never practiced there. To quote Wesselhoeft, Hahnemann "was given to extravagant claims as to his experience." He noted that, far from gaining wide experience in general practice, Hahnemann saw a restricted kind of ambulatory care patient in the course of a carriage trade practice, yet this was not how Hahnemann presented himself in his writings. Wesselhoeft refers to the fierce fights that Hahnemann picked with the apothecaries and doctors while he lived in Königslutter, where he accused the pharmacists of unreliable compounding of prescriptions. The pharmacists took him to court and won their case. As to the doctors, he denounced their allopathic practices in harsh language, which understandably drew a similar response. After having started and lost both these fights, the unpopular Hahnemann left Königslutter.

Wesselhoeft alludes to Hahnemann's Calvinistic denouncements as an apostate of anyone who did not walk on exactly the same path with him; it was this religious bent in Hahnemann which led others to see homeopathy as a sect. He was a suspicious and inflexible leader who readily adopted the role of martyr. In his preface to the *Organon* (first edition), Hahnemann grandiosely and solely assumed the mantle of discovering truth in medicine, in words that amount to an assertion that he is God's mouthpiece. The following description by Wesselhoeft captures some of Hahnemann's more troublesome attributes: "… an extreme fundamentalist in his belief in his own doctrines. He was as extravagant in his speculative claims as our evangelists, as vindictive as a politician the day before election, and as inconsistent as most human beings who persuade themselves that because they know a lot about one thing their opinions on other matters are invaluable and final." Wesselhoeft illustrates some of Hahnemann's more improbable claims, made later in life, such as embracing mesmerism and his assertion that by stroking one's hand across the body of a patient in a purposeful manner, certain ailments will be dispelled when the hand moves in one direction and other ailments

will be removed if the hand moves in the opposite direction. Wesselhoeft believed that the author of the *Organon* did not always practice what he preached in his canon. He was also struck by Hahnemann's tendency to only accept data which favored his preconceptions, while ignoring contradictory evidence.

Like Wesselhoeft, Boyd was a dedicated homeopath, so his critical comments about Hahnemann deserve to be taken seriously, since he would have no desire to hurl brickbats at the founder of homeopathy without good reason. In his book, *A Study of the Simile in Medicine*, Boyd refers to Hahnemann's careless approach in the later drug provings (an experimental method of testing the effects of drugs in healthy volunteers) and to poor referencing in his *materia medica*. He notes that Hahnemann departed from his own protocol criteria when conducting provings on patients rather than healthy volunteers, some of who were taking multiple medicines. As a result, it is almost certainly the case that Hahnemann's original proving experiments were a *mélange* of low and high doses, healthy volunteers and sick patients, those taking no other drugs, and those taking many.

Richard Haehl has written a two-volume biography of Hahnemann. While stopping short of asserting that Hahnemann manifested clear mental illness, he refers several times to Hahnemann's peregrinations, feistiness, and poor relations with the medical community. On the other hand, Haehl stresses the stable supportive relationships that Hahnemann had with his immediate family, who provided him with much comfort. In this respect, Hahnemann's family life presented a striking contrast to the instability of his professional life [7, 8]. Another source, Sir John Weir [9], noted that, constitutionally, Hahnemann needed little sleep and was a "prodigious worker." With regard to sleep, it is recorded that for 40 years, he customarily stayed up every fourth night studying. His "prodigious" output included 116 publications and 120 pamphlets, as well as all his clinical and didactic work. It is most probably the case that Hahnemann shared with the composer George Frederick Handel a state of chronic hypomania, which fuelled his amazing creativity. But it is always possible in people of hyperthymic ("elevated mood") temperament that mental balance can be tipped either upwards into mania, with its frenzy, grandiosity, irritability, and hostility, or that it tips the other way into depression and withdrawal. Given that Hahnemann has been identified as a "fussy pedant" by Morrell [10], one might expect that he would be a tenacious stickler for detail, perfectionism, and rigorous method, so the fact that at times he was careless, dissembling, and extravagant in self-attribution suggests there were occasions when his bipolar tendencies were poorly regulated.

Lest there be any doubt about Hahnemann's genetic predisposition, it is impossible to ignore the serial misfortunes that struck many of his children. His son Friedrich was a "lunatic" according to Haehl, who moved around, first to England, then to the United States, where he practiced homeopathy before disappearing; Haehl is in no doubt that Friedrich was a victim of insanity, showing many of his father's features. Two daughters developed "morbid anxiety," which today might be considered to reflect an anxiety disorder; two other daughters were murdered and three divorced. Clear evidence of instability existed in his children, and the likelihood is that this predisposition came from Hahnemann's side of the family.

Hahnemann as Medical Pioneer

We can now turn to Hahnemann's contributions, as well as to some of the inconsistencies and speculations that have burdened homeopathy.

Boyd has suggested that Hahnemann was one of the first observers of his time to grasp (1) the concept of stimulation and reaction, (2) the notion of hypersensitivity in the diseased organism, (3) the value of the diluted medicine, (4) the biphasic response to a drug at low and high doses, (5) the importance of the single drug, and (6) the *similia* principle as foundation of a therapeutic system. Additionally, Hahnemann introduced (7) the decimal system into pharmacology, (8) the need to consider the subjective in pathology, (9) a method for making insoluble drugs useful, and (10) an experimental method to test the effects of drugs in healthy volunteers, which he referred to by the German word "Prüfung" and which has been anglicized to "proving." Other accomplishments of this polymath include his mastery of eight languages (including Arabic): at 12 years of age, he was teaching Greek. He became a renowned chemist, a good musician, and a knowledgeable astronomer and devised a test to detect adulteration of wine, which was officially adopted by the Prussian state in 1791. Boyd notes that if Hahnemann had done no more than compel medicine to abandon excessive polypharmacy, he would have earned greatness. Today, it is easy to overlook the toxicity of some eighteenth-century concoctions, such as "Venice treacle," which contained 65 ingredients, and "mithridate," which contained 50 ingredients. The famous physician Sir William Osler said that "No one individual has done more good to the medical profession than Hahnemann." Voltaire's quip that "medicine is an art founded on conjecture and improved by murder" was more than likely a fair characterization of medical practice in Hahnemann's time and was something Hahnemann set out to change. In 1852, William Alison, the famous Edinburgh professor of medicine, president of the Royal College of Physicians, and vice-president of the British Medical Association, confessed that he had undergone a radical reconception of inflammatory disease and its treatment, being led to adopt a new treatment approach

from the reports of doctors who had "witnessed the practice of homoeopathic hospitals on the Continent" [9]. Unfortunately for Hahnemann and homeopathy, recognition of his achievements by the medical community has fallen casualty to fighting between the advocates of homeopathy and allopathy. Some of his wilder speculations about the potency of infinitesimal dilutions have not helped homeopathy's cause.

Other insights for which Hahnemann deserves credit include (1) enlightened attitude to managing patients with mental illness; (2) emphasis on the individual (i.e., the person with the disease, as contrasted with the disease alone), which today has been reborn in the practice of personalized medicine; (3) stressing the importance of a whole person approach by means of a detailed and individualized history; (4) grasping the idea of the minimal dose; and (5) introducing a fundamental reform of medical thought – the idea of arousing the body's natural resisting force – with the notion of host reactivity. Additionally, Hahnemann's approach was revolutionary in that the medicine of his day was largely hypothesis driven and stood or fell on logic, rather than being related to clinical results; Hahnemann tried to change this approach by studying the actual effects of treatments in various diseases and in his proving experiments.

While Hahnemann's provings added much information, experiments of this kind generate huge numbers of symptoms in small samples where the role of expectancy is a determinant of outcome. Typically, they were (and often still are) poorly controlled for possible placebo effects. How to understand this avalanche of information is no easy task. Also, with the caveats mentioned above by Wesselhoeft, caution should be applied in accepting the findings of Hahnemann's provings. Nevertheless, some have been more carefully repeated and confirmed by later generations of homeopaths and valuable medicines have been introduced by the proving route, for example, nitroglycerin and snake venoms. A final point on provings is that, for all their deficiencies, they were medicine's first attempt to systematically study new drugs in healthy subjects, a stage that is now essential to the testing process before drugs can be approved for marketing. A significant difference between provings and today's trials is that the former are designed to elicit a profile of effects in healthy subjects that can inform doctors on the diseases which would respond, whereas phase I trials today are geared only to establish safety prior to larger clinical tests for efficacy and dosing in populations with disease.

Many consider that the one core feature of homeopathy centers on the *simile* principle. This in itself was not first discovered by Hahnemann, as he readily acknowledged, but he was perhaps the first to construct an entire therapeutic system around the principle. Interestingly, Hahnemann formulated the principle in the following words: "similia similibus curentur," in which the last word is expressed in the subjunctive as "let likes be cured by likes." Others have subsequently introduced a subtle but important change in which "curentur" has become the indicative "curantur," asserting that likes *are* cured by likes. The original phrase is more qualified and leaves room for the use of other therapeutic approaches, while the latter imparts greater and, many may think, unwarranted certainty. The simile principle is of undoubted value but does not deserve to be held up as the only approach to treatment.

Sapere Aude. These two words from the Roman poet, Horace, became a kind of mantra for Hahnemann, who used them to introduce later editions of his *Organon*. Immanuel Kant had already popularized the term as a guiding principle for the Enlightenment, and Hahnemann first included the quotation in 1806 [7, p. 76] at the end of a paragraph about remedies as poison or cure, in which he wrote about how the majority might find offensive something that to the wise man was a clear truth: he concluded those words with the injunction *sapere aude*! Dare to be wise, or dare to know – Hahnemann was certainly not guilty of any feebleness in this respect; *sapere aude* became his motto. Despite Hahnemann's many achievements, the seeds of homeopathy's problems and its later demise from the US medical scene in the 1930s have been ascribed by Cameron to Hahnemann having "reached too far," but, as Cameron wrote, "yet had he not, he probably would not have reached at all." Hahnemann was a risk taker, as pioneers must be. His theories gave rise to a system of medicine that has spread across the world. Today, homeopathy is very healthy in some countries, is moderately healthy in others, has no more than a trace in others, and has to fight a constant battle for survival in many countries. As noted, some of Hahnemann's insights have been adopted by con-ventional medicine, yet homeopathy continues to be a practice situated at the outer margins of medicine. Nevertheless, there have been many homeopaths, and other physicians with homeopathic sympathies, whose work has left a significant impact on medicine from the nineteenth century up to the present day, and it is these men and women with whom this book is concerned. Without the fruit of Hahnemann's labors, it is not possible to know whether some of these men and women would have been able to enter medical school or, if they had done so under different circumstances, what paths their careers might have taken.

References

1. Boyd LJ. Principles of homeopathy. J Am Inst Homeopath. 1924; 17:593–602.
2. Cameron CS. Homeopathy in retrospect. Trans Stud Coll Physicians Phila. 1959;27:28–33.
3. Boyd LJ. A study of the simile in medicine. Philadelphia: Boericke and Tafel; 1936.
4. Wesselhoeft C. Hahnemann's place in "the dawn of modern medicine". J Am Inst Homeopath. 1920;13:712–6.
5. Wesselhoeft C. Hahnemann's Organon in the light of the twentieth century. J Am Inst Homeopath. 1925;18:669–80.
6. Wesselhoeft C. Elementary homeopathy. J Am Inst Homeopath. 1927;20:99–121.
7. Haehl R. Samuel Hahnemann: his life and work, vol. I. New Delhi: B. Jain Publishers Pvt Ltd; 2006. p. 133.
8. Haehl R. Samuel Hahnemann: his life and work, vol. II. New Delhi: B. Jain Publishers Pvt Ltd; 2006.
9. Sir Weir J. Samuel Hahnemann and his influence on medical thought. Proc R Soc Med. 1933;26:668–76.
10. Morrell P. The character of Hahnemann and the nature of homeopathy [Internet] [Cited 2011 Dec 12]. Available from: www.homeoint. org/morrell/articles/pm_chara.htm.

3

Women, Reform, and Medical Leadership

Professional Barriers, Social Reform, and the Role of Women in Homeopathy

Throughout most of the nineteenth century, orthodox medicine was a male monopoly in which women were seen as "the weaker sex" and almost entirely excluded from the academic and political power structures. Traditional stereotypes held them to be "delicate" and therefore unsuitable for the stressful demands of a physician's life. Women, it was thought, were better suited to nursing, midwifery, or other roles which kept them subordinate to (male) doctors. To break down these barriers would prove to be a struggle in which homeopathy gave conspicuous leadership, as described by Kirschmann in her book *A Vital Force* [1]. An affinity had existed between women and homeopathy in the United States since the 1850s, when "ladies' physiological societies" sprang up for the purpose of raising women's consciousness about their bodies and the use of natural healing methods [2, p. 214]. Allied to this was an eagerness of women to proselytize on behalf of homeopathy. Winston has observed how some women successfully converted whole communities to homeopathy. It was no surprise that women who were attracted to these societies were often supporters of liberal causes like temperance, suffrage, and abolition of slavery. The first homeopathic medical colleges emerged from these physiological societies, a move which provoked criticism from Alfred Stillé, a founder of the American Medical Association, who opined that "women lacked rational judgment and were unfit to be scientific physicians."

Homeopaths played a conspicuous part in breaking down the barriers against women in American medicine. Much of this was due to the establishment of women's medical colleges in Boston and New York. The Boston Female Medical College was founded in 1848 as the first medical school for women in the world. The college changed its name in 1851 to the New England Female Medical College (NEFMC), which functioned autonomously for 23 years until it encountered serious financial problems. At its inception, the NEFMC was an eclectic school [3], teaching a mix of eclectic (herbal) and allopathic medicine, but like most eclectic schools, however, its students may have been exposed to some homeopathy. Among the school's backers was at least one ardent homeopath, Harriet Beecher Stowe. According to some sources, the prominent Boston homeopath, Israel Tisdale Talbot, was a cofounder of the college [4, 5], but this appears unlikely since he would have only been 19 years old at the time, and Waite does not mention this in his comprehensive history of the institution [6]. It has been said that the school's orientation became increasingly homeopathic, and it was thus classified by the American Medical Directory [7]. The school's identity was confusing, however, with eclectics coming and going on the faculty throughout the 1850s: was it eclectic, allopathic, or some kind of hybrid [6, p. 33, 37]? In its later years, and prior to the takeover by Boston University, at least one homeopath, David Thayer, was on the NEFMC faculty. Thayer opened the first free homeopathic dispensary in Massachusetts, was president of the American Institute of Homeopathy, and served in the state legislature. It may be these considerations that led some to assert that important medical pioneers like Mary Thompson and Rebecca Crumpler, who graduated from NEFMC, were "homeopathically trained" when history does not record them as homeopathic practitioners. While some NEFMC graduates became apostles of homeopathy, a greater number maintained allegiance to allopathic medicine. In a survey of its graduates, 10 of 54 were practicing homeopathy, 41 allopathy, and 3 both [6, p. 87]. Waite states that nearly all faculty between 1852 and 1872 were from allopathic schools (page 72), yet the college was long considered by some to be sectarian (page 34). The school's identity was decided in 1874 when, owing to financial straits, it merged with Boston University to form the Boston University School of Medicine (BUSM) and adopted an exclusively homeopathic allegiance, being staffed with an influx of 26 new homeopathic faculty members.

While credit must be given to the NEFMC for enabling women to enter medicine, the college had a poor reputation among many women physicians on account of its lackluster training program and the reactionary attitudes of its director, Samuel Gregory: on one occasion when a faculty member requested the purchase of a microscope, Gregory refused on the grounds that such a piece of equipment was a "new fangled European notion" [8, pp. 83–85]. A number of prominent female doctors grew concerned that conditions in the NEFMC were below accepted standards and posed a threat to the cause of women in medicine. Many kept their distance from the institution, and the college lost one of its most effective voices when, after 3 years on the faculty, Marie Zakrzewska left to create the New England Hospital for Women and Children [8, p. 82]. These negative perceptions were less related to the hybrid philosophy of the NEFMC and more to Gregory's difficult, antagonistic personality. Notable FMC/BUSM graduates included Rebecca Lee Crumpler, Julia Holmes Smith, Esther Hawks, Clara Barrus, Martha George Ripley, Eliza Taylor Ransom, Leila Gertrude Bedell, and Mary Harris Thompson. Considering only 98 women graduated from the college, its influence on American medicine has been out of all proportion.

In New York, the New York Medical College and Hospital for Women (NYMCHW) was founded in 1863/1864 by Clemence Lozier (Fig. 3.1), who served as president and dean until her death in 1888. Among its notable graduates

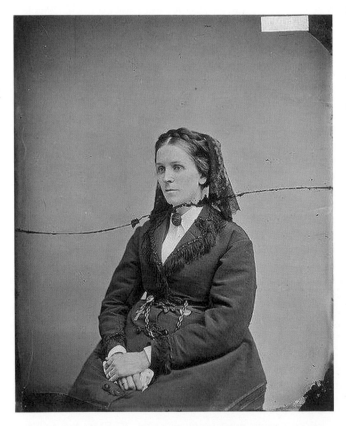

Fig. 3.1 Mrs. Dr. Clemence Lozier, founder New York Medical College for Women, taken c. 1863. In the public domain, courtesy National Archives. Photo no. 111-B-1691 (Brady Collection)

were Maria Estrella, Emily Stowe, Susan Smith McKinney Steward, Mary Jane Safford Blake, and Florence Nightingale Ward, who later became a professor at Hahnemann Medical College in San Francisco and was one of the earliest women to be elected Fellow of the American College of Surgeons. Two generations later, after the institution had become part of the New York Homeopathic Medical College, Geraldine Burton-Branch also graduated. In addition to these graduates from Boston and New York, other women warrant inclusion: the Cleveland graduates Susan Edson and Caroline Brown Winslow, Lucy Waite from Chicago, and Laura Towne from Philadelphia.

Medical progress is measured by different yardsticks. It is not merely by scientific advances, although they are important; progress includes the extent to which medicine addresses "social and economic determinants [of poor health, which is] … often rooted in inequality, conflict, overcrowding, lack of rights, lack of financial security, and poor living" [9]. As a result, it reflects poorly on the medical profession that physicians have been "gross underachievers on a social scale," according to Senator William Frist, the one-time Republican leader of the Senate and himself a medical doctor [10]. By this standard, homeopathy has spoken loudly, considering the size of its community. The women who appear in the following pages have all advanced the cause of medicine over the last 150 years.

For convenience, subjects are grouped chronologically, according to their places of training.

New York Medical College and Hospital for Women

Clemence Lozier

Pride of place goes to the doyenne, Clemence Lozier (1813–1888), for her foundational work in establishing the New York Medical College for Women (NYMCW) (Fig. 3.2). Lozier showed an early interest in teaching when she opened a school at the age of 19. Colleagues were impressed by her desire to benefit humanity, which she originally intended to direct into education but later expressed itself in the field of medicine. She trained as a doctor, graduating from the Syracuse Eclectic College in 1853. Lozier prospered but remained unfulfilled solely in clinical practice. She therefore relentlessly pursued state legislation to authorize a women's medical school. After overcoming considerable opposition, with the assistance of Elizabeth Cady Stanton, she succeeded in her quest and, on November 1, 1863, opened the NYMCW. In 1864, the state legislature approved the establishment of an affiliated teaching hospital. Lozier served as dean of the renamed New York Medical College and Hospital for Women (NYMCHW) for 25 years and saw the school grew in stature

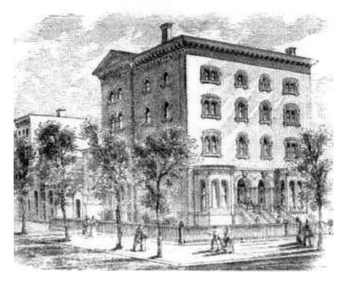

Fig. 3.2 Image of New York Medical College for Women, 1873. In the public domain

and in size, from 7 students in its initial class to a total of 219 graduates at the time of her death in 1888. A number of women graduates went on to make their mark in medicine and society as will follow.

The NYMCHW was a trailblazer in several ways. Besides being one of the few schools founded by and for women, it set a new national standard for medical training in 1869 by requiring a 3- and, later, a 4-year curriculum, as well as creating the first public health course for medical students. In respect of these two innovations, the school was two decades ahead of the major orthodox medical schools like Harvard and Penn. Lozier enjoyed the respect of her homeopathic colleagues and many leading allopathic doctors in New York, including the famous surgeons James Marion Sims and Valentine Mott, who consulted with her about their patients.

Although graduating from a non-homeopathic institution, Lozier specialized in homeopathy early in her career and held an appointment as professor of gynecology and obstetrics at the Homeopathic College of Physicians and Surgeons. Her booklet Child Birth Made Easy was widely read.

In addition to her medical activities, Lozier welcomed to her home many reformers, including Elizabeth Cady Stanton, Susan B. Anthony, and Wendell Phillips; she was friendly with Frederick Douglass. Lozier was generous in the degree to which she gave financial support from her own earnings, to the college, to Cady Stanton, and to her various social causes. At one point, she was forced to declare bankruptcy because of the financial plight into which NYMCWH had fallen after a stock market crash, which left it unable to repay its debts; in 1878, a large number of bonds had unexpectedly been called in, which the college and Lozier were unable to pay. She helped as far as she could, but it depleted her life savings. Nevertheless, after this setback, the college obtained

further support from an alumnae fund and flourished for many more years. Among the organizations with which Lozier was associated were the Women's Christian Temperance Union, the New York Moral Reform Society, and SOROSIS, an influential women's society. She was active in the antislavery movement, in prison reform, and in Indian reform. She served as president of the New York City Women's Suffrage Society for 13 years and as president of the National Woman Suffrage Association for 2 years.

Lozier combined great charm, tact, and modesty with determination and refusal to back down in the face of opposition; she was an inspirational speaker. On one occasion, when her students had visited Bellevue Hospital for clinical instruction, they were greeted with verbal abuse from the all-male class and pelted with chewed paper balls, while the faculty sat by and took no action. Soon afterwards, Lozier called a "public indignation meeting" to condemn this outrage, calling on support from speakers like Horace Greeley, Henry Ward Beecher, and other reformers. As a result of this event, the New York press weighed in on her side, and the mayor of New York agreed to send a marshal and police force to the Bellevue clinics to protect Lozier's students in the future [1, p. 59].

Lozier, the great teacher and reformer, died in 1888. She bequeathed to medicine and society a legacy comparable to that of her better-known rival Elizabeth Blackwell and inspired many of her students to achieve their own greatness.

Elizabeth Blackwell

Despite Lozier's substantial contributions to the cause of women in medicine, the name of Elizabeth Blackwell is far better known; Blackwell is generally acclaimed as the first and greatest to advance the interests of women in medicine. Blackwell (1821–1910) was born in England, came to the United States, and graduated as the first female doctor in 1849; she later qualified as the first British female doctor after returning to her home country. Like Lozier, Blackwell was an ardent campaigner against slavery and for the rights of women, but had no truck with sectarian medicine, and an "icy gulf" forever existed between the two [1, p. 61]. It is likely that the relationship between Lozier and Blackwell was competitive in nature, and, although Blackwell waited 5 years longer than Lozier in opening her allopathic Women's College in New York, the curriculum reforms at NYMCHW described above were paralleled by similar changes at Blackwell's college. The two institutions competed for medical students, and it is of interest that Blackwell's college came into existence as the reaction of several prominent New York male doctors who were upset that a homeopathic school had been established [8, p. 74]. Morantz-Sanchez [8, p. 75] is of the opinion that Blackwell's hostility derived in part from being upstaged by Lozier, and it is interesting that Susan B. Anthony worked hard, but largely without success, at bringing the two pioneers closer together.

Harriet Clisby

Harriet Clisby (1830–1931) was born in London in 1830 and moved with her parents to Australia when she was 8 years old. After completing her education, Clisby took up work as a journalist, edited a women's periodical *The Southern Phonographic Harmonia*, and copublished another, but short-lived, magazine called *The Interpreter. The Interpreter* was Australia's first magazine published by women and contained a medical section which provided practical advice for its readers on the prevention and cure of disease, almost certainly an indication of Clisby's early interest in medicine and the promotion of health awareness. As a young woman on the Australian frontier, Clisby's social activism led her to organize a community rehabilitation home for female prisoners.

Clisby read Elizabeth Blackwell's 1852 book on health for women, and she consulted with a medical friend how she could train as a doctor. He advised her of the pitfalls which lay ahead, but she pursued her goals nonetheless and travelled to England, where she met a prominent female doctor, Elizabeth Garrett Anderson, who suggested that it would be easier if Clisby went to the United States for her training. After receiving some financial support from a friend, she was able to make her way to Clemence Lozier's college. She graduated in 1865 and moved to Boston to practice homeopathy. Clisby believed that many psychiatric problems in women stemmed from social causes such as lack of education and fulfilling work.

Clisby is best remembered for founding the Women's Educational and Industrial Union (WEIU). Having been moved by the exploitation of women and children in America's growing urban population, Clisby created the WEIU in 1877 to address their social problems. The WEIU reflected the view of many social activists that individual capitalism fostered inequality, particularly affecting women; it was a main goal of the union to serve those who suffered from the conflicts in society caused by racial, gender, and class divisions. Joining Clisby were other prominent Boston homeopaths like Arvilla Haynes, Mary Safford Blake, and Mercy Jackson, and for the first 10 years of the WEIU's existence, all its associated doctors were homeopaths who positioned themselves as directors of "hygiene and physical culture" and of "moral and spiritual development" [1, p. 43]. The WEIU grew into one of Boston's major advocacy organizations, expanding to Buffalo, Washington, and Rochester. Many prominent women actively supported the WEIU, such as Mrs. Louis Brandeis, Josephine Ruffin (an African-American reformer), Mary Kenney O'Sullivan (Irish Catholic labor organizer), Louisa May Alcott, and Julia Ward Howe. One client to benefit from the organization was Amelia Earhart, who in 1926 asked for assistance with employment and was placed as a social worker in a community settlement for immigrants. Earhart was at the time preparing for her career as an aviatrix and 2 years later became the first woman to fly across the Atlantic. In 1982, the WEIU established the annual Amelia Earhart Award to honor a person who made a significant contribution to expanding opportunities for women.

The WEIU has had a far-reaching impact and can take credit for a number of important innovations. Among these was successful lobbying to create the Massachusetts Commission for the Blind (1899), the nation's first hot lunch program for public schools (1907), the country's first credit union (1913), Massachusetts' first transitional housing program for homeless or battered women and children (1985), and a Woman to Woman program which offered professional development to low-income families (2001). Over the course of its 130-year existence, the WEIU is estimated to have provided career and employment assistance to hundreds of thousands of women. In 2006, the WEIU joined with Crittenton Inc. to become the Crittenton Women's Union. Clisby's reach has been a long one indeed as far the WEIU is concerned.

Clisby herself lived almost as long as her offspring organization. She passed away in 1931 at the age of 100, her life having been one of unremitting activity even into old age. Among her friends, she counted Henry Wadsworth Longfellow, William James, and Henry Ward Beecher [11].

Emily Stowe

Emily Stowe (1831–1903) holds a unique place in the history of Canadian medicine (Figs. 3.3 and 3.4). She was born Emily Jennings in 1831 in Ontario, trained professionally as a teacher, and, in 1854, became the first woman principal of a public school on Upper Canada. She married in 1856 and produced three children. The Stowes' third child developed tuberculosis when young, an experience which led Emily to explore homeopathy and herbal medicines. This in turn inspired Emily to become a physician. Her application to enter the Toronto School of Medicine in 1865 was rejected, the university's vice-president telling Emily that "The doors of the University are not open to women and I trust they never will be" [12]. From this rejection, Stowe resolved to pursue her training elsewhere and to do all she could to ensure that other women have the same opportunities. She entered the New York Medical College for Women and graduated in 1867, returning to her home country where she

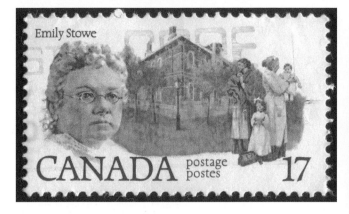

Fig. 3.3 Emily Stowe. Commemorative postage stamp, Canadian Postal Service. Available from: http://www.123rf.com/photo_9585044_canada--circa-1981-stamp-printed-by-canada-shows-emily-stowe-circa-1981.html

Fig. 3.4 Emily Stowe's professional announcement. The Globe, November 11, 1867. In the public domain (*Source*: Famous Canadian Physicians. Library and Archives Canada)

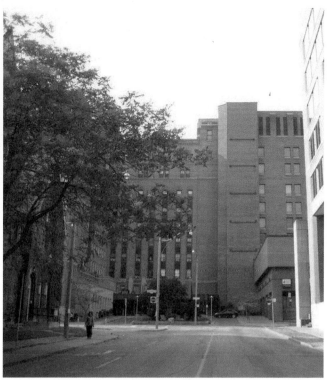

Fig. 3.5 Women's College Hospital, Toronto. July 2006. This hospital was founded in 1898 by Emily Stowe. In the public domain (*Source*: w/ Image:Wch c1219.jpg. Author w:User:Nephron)

became the first woman in Canada to open a medical practice. Complications arose when Ontario changed its licensing procedures, by introducing a requirement for foreign-trained doctors to take further study in Canada as a condition of license eligibility. Again the university denied entry, until after further attempts Stowe was finally accepted in 1871. Stowe encountered more hostility, which caused her either to fail her exams or to refuse to take them, so she dropped out and resumed her practice, still without a license. From all her hardships, Stowe became an ardent fighter for women's rights and was a major force in creating the Toronto Women's Guild, the first suffragette organization in Canada. The activities of this group (later to be named the Canadian Women's Suffrage Association) lead to increased higher education opportunities in Canada.

Stowe continued with her practice but encountered further difficulty in 1879 when she was charged with performing an illegal abortion. After a long and intimidating trial, at which her character was challenged, Stowe won acquittal and in the next year was finally granted her license by the provincial College of Physicians and Surgeons, thereby making her Canada's second licensed female physician.

Stowe maintained constant pressure on the University of Toronto to accept women into their medical program – pressure which ultimately bore fruit in 1906. Stowe was also able to celebrate the fact that her daughter, Augusta Stowe-Gullen, was the first woman to graduate from a Canadian medical school, Victoria College, in 1883. In the same year, as a result of Emily Stowe's efforts, Canada's first Medical College for Women was established in Ontario. This college was recognized by the College of Physicians and Surgeons and continued in existence until the year when Toronto University accepted women into their program. Besides the women's college, Stowe was instrumental in creating a free dispensary for women in 1898: this small facility grew over the years into a hospital, originally called the Women's College Hospital and Dispensary, and then the Women's College Hospital (WCH). In 1961, WCH became an affiliated teaching and research hospital within the University of Toronto system (Fig. 3.5). It thrives today as a significant component of Toronto's healthcare system and in 2003 offered the first outpatient SARS (severe acute respiratory syndrome) clinic in Canada. Other regional or national "firsts" associated with WCH include a cancer detection clinic, the use of diagnostic mammography, discovery of certain breast cancer genes, provision of ambulatory education for people with diabetes, and a perinatal intensive care unit. In 1995, the World Health Organization (WHO) designated WCH as a WHO collaborating center in women's health, the first in the Western Hemisphere. Perhaps the impact of WCH is best summed up in the words on a plaque which was erected outside the hospital in 1995, designating WCH as a National Historic Site of Canada: "Women's College Hospital has earned a distinctive place in Canadian medical history … the institution symbolizes the struggle of women to claim their place in the medical profession …. The hospital has made innovative contributions to the treatment and diagnosis of disease through its vital focus on health issues affecting women and families." Few would disagree that these words apply in a much broader sense to what has been accomplished by women homeopathic physicians over a period of almost 100 years [13]. Paths Canada has paid tribute to the groundbreaking role of Emily Stowe in bringing the WCH to birth [14].

Stowe is remembered for her medical and suffragist achievements. In 1896, she fell off the podium while giving a medical talk at the Chicago World Fair and fractured her hip. Recovery was slow and led to retirement from medical practice, but she continued her work on behalf of women's enfranchisement and became well known for taking part in the 1896 play *Mock Parliament*, where women and men reversed their roles with men coming to parliament begging for the vote. It was argued by women that giving men the vote would be regressive and lead to moral and social decay – a reminder perhaps of a comment by Stowe's daughter that "when women have a voice in national and international affairs, wars will cease forever." The mock parliament brought further awareness about Stowe to a younger generation of Canadians who were not so familiar with her medical pioneering. In 1889, Stowe founded the Dominion Women's Enfranchisement Association, serving as its president until her death in 1903. Unfortunately, she did not live to see women's enfranchisement, which took place in 1917.

Mary Safford Blake

Mary Safford Blake (1831–1891) was born in 1831 (Fig. 3.6). After her secondary school education, she trained firstly to become a teacher and then later a nurse. She earned the name "Angel of Cairo" for her treatment of sick and injured Union troops in the Civil War. Cairo, Illinois, was a strategically important town occupied by Union forces early in the war. It took no time for epidemic disease to break out, and Blake

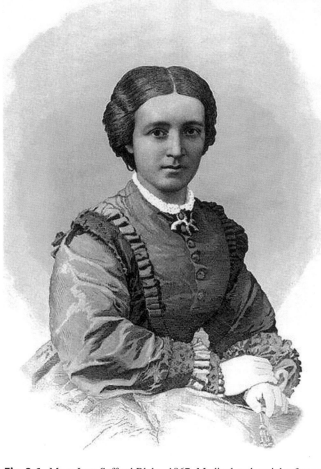

Fig. 3.6 Mary Jane Safford Blake. 1867. Medical and social reformer in Chicago and Boston, Civil War nurse, professor of medicine, Boston University. In the public domain. Author John Sartain

offered her services to visit the sick, to bring them food, and later to act as a nurse. In 1862, she attended the many casualties from the Battle of Shiloh, but exhausted herself to the point of breakdown and took time away to recuperate. Following a long convalescent tour of Europe, this "mite of a woman … with an indomitable soul" [1, p. 44] returned home energized, matriculated as a medical student at the NYMCW, and graduated with a homeopathic degree in 1869. She then returned to Europe for further surgical training and is believed to have been the first woman to perform an ovarian resection on that continent. For some of the time when Blake was in Europe, she studied at the University of Heidelberg with her medical student friend Isabel Chapin Barrows, who became famous as America's first female ophthalmological surgeon; Barrows and Blake shared a commitment to suffrage and women's rights. In 1872, Blake returned to the United States and settled in Boston, joining the Boston University School of Medicine (BUSM) faculty as professor of gynecology, possibly being the first female gynecologist in the United States [15]. At BUSM, Safford Blake gave lectures on menstruation, hysteria, ovarian tumors, and mammary disease. She conducted a busy practice among Boston's poor and, rather unusually for the time, was so well respected by her allopathic peers that she would receive referrals from some of Boston's most prominent male gynecologists.

As with many of the women mentioned here, Safford Blake became deeply involved with the suffrage movement and other initiatives to advance the welfare of women and indigent Bostonians. She was a member of the WEIU, held radical views on sexual relations, and became identified with the cause of free love, which offended at least one of her students [1, p. 70]. Dress reform was another cause dear to her heart, as it was for many other women inside and outside of the homeopathic community. Along with others, Safford Blake saw heavy dresses and tight lacing as a threat to women's health and campaigned for dress reform. In part, this campaign was rooted in health concerns, for there was a belief that such tightly constricting clothes resulted in weak abdominal muscles which did not serve women well when it came to childbearing.

As she grew older, Blake's health again deteriorated, and she retired from the practice of medicine in 1886, to spend much of her later years in Florida, where she passed away in 1891.

Alice Boole Campbell

Alice Boole Campbell (1838–1909) was in the first class to graduate from NYMCHW in 1863 [16]. and she spent her career practicing homeopathy in New York, where she served on the governing board of her medical school. Her clinical appointments included positions at the Woman's Hospital in Philadelphia, and she was a founder of two Brooklyn hospitals for women. Among her numerous activities, Campbell was concerned for the welfare of psychiatric patients, and she presented a paper at the 6th meeting of the Society for Promoting the Welfare of the Insane, advocating paid employment of New York asylum inpatients, regarding it as therapeutic to draw financial reward for their labor [17].

Campbell's activism brought her into confrontation with the male-only King's County Homeopathic Society, when they turned down her membership application. She was unrelenting in her quest to join and eventually took the society to court, where she won her case [1, p. 40]. Campbell also did battle with the General Conference of the Methodist Episcopal Church. The conference, an important legislative body ruling on matters of church doctrine and policy, had refused to allow women as conference representatives. As a result of the church's discrimination against women, Campbell ostentatiously withdrew her membership, rallied national support, and fought successfully to overcome this injustice: in 1906, the church accepted women as conference representatives. Kirschmann characterizes Campbell as one who refused "to compromise on important egalitarian principles," a refusal which "was felt in her chosen profession" [1, p. 40].

Susan Smith McKinney Steward (Also Known as Susan Smith McKinney)

When she graduated from the NYMCW in 1869, Susan Steward (1847–1918) became the third African-American female doctor in the United States (Fig. 3.7). Before entering medical school, Steward had worked for a while as a teacher but, after caring for a sick niece, turned her ambitions towards medicine. She practiced homeopathic medicine in Brooklyn, a part of New York where women's homeopaths dominated in the community. With her prominent social status and African-American heritage, Steward symbolized homeopathy's liberal leanings. She married first William McKinney, who died in 1894, and then later married Reverend Theophilus Steward, a military chaplain to the 25th US

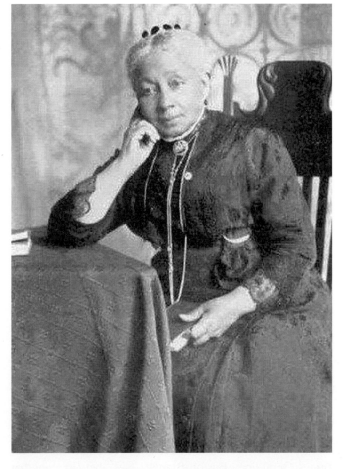

Fig. 3.7 Susan McKinney Steward (1847–1918). Date unknown. The third African–American woman to earn a medical degree. In the public domain

Colored Infantry. Steward's medical career lasted 48 years, and she remained a committed homeopath, active in her local medical society, organizing an alumni society and presenting papers at local homeopathic society meetings. She firmly believed that homeopathy was the treatment of choice for malnourished and starving children [18]. In 1881, Steward helped to found the Brooklyn Woman's Homoeopathic Hospital and Dispensary, where she took a position as surgeon in 1891. Steward did well in practice, ministering to all types: rich and poor, white and black, men and women, and young and old. A local newspaper hailed her as "the most successful practitioner of medicine of her sex and race in the United States" and listed her as one of New York's "famous doctors" in 1891 [18, p. 39]. Steward held a faculty appointment at the New York Medical College between 1892 and 1896 and served on the board of directors of the Brooklyn Home for Aged Colored People. After her second marriage, Steward travelled with her husband to Montana and Wyoming, where she would treat sick and injured soldiers, before returning with him to take up a faculty appointment at Wilberforce University in Ohio, where she taught health and nutrition and served as resident physician to the university. Here she remained until her death in 1918. The causes of women in medicine and African-Americans remained close to her heart. As examples, in 1911 she attended the First Universal Races Congress in London, presenting a talk on women in medicine, and in 1914 gave a paper on "Colored American Women" at a meeting of the National Association of Colored Women's Clubs. At the latter meeting, Steward argued for medical schools to accept men and women, rather than keeping them separate.

Beyond her medical career, Steward founded the Equal Suffrage League of Brooklyn and the Women's Local Union – a leading black women's club – and was president of the Women's Christian Temperance Union [19]. At Steward's funeral, the oration was delivered by W.E.B. Du Bois. Her name lives on today through the Dr. Susan Smith McKinney Steward Junior High School, so named in 1975, and in the Susan Smith McKinney Steward Medical Society for African-American female doctors in the northeastern United States. Steward serves as a role model for what African-American women could achieve in medicine, founding community health clinics, training nurses, creating service agencies for women and the indigent and colored populations and education programs on hygiene. It has been said that once medicine became more scientific and male dominated by the 1920s, many African-American women who might have entered medicine turned to nursing, and their number as physicians was to diminish significantly. Battles won often have to be refought. In a later time, Geraldine Burton-Branch (see below), another homeopathically trained doctor, stepped up once again to this challenge.

Florence Nightingale Ward

Florence Nightingale Ward (1860–1919) described her main causes in life as "heaven, homeopathy and women's rights" (Fig. 3.8). She received her training in New York and then in 1888 returned to San Francisco, where she opened a practice. In 1907, she founded a private clinic named the Florence N. Ward Sanatorium. She obtained an appointment as professor of obstetrics at Hahnemann Medical College and earned a reputation as one of the country's finest female surgeons. Recognition of her abilities came when she was elected as a Fellow of the American College of Surgeons. Although some sources have claimed that she was either the first or second woman to be so elected, in actuality five women had preceded her as Fellows in the first year of the college's existence. Ward was accepted the next year, 1914, so it can reliably be stated that she was one of the earliest woman Fellows [20]. Ward served two terms as president of the

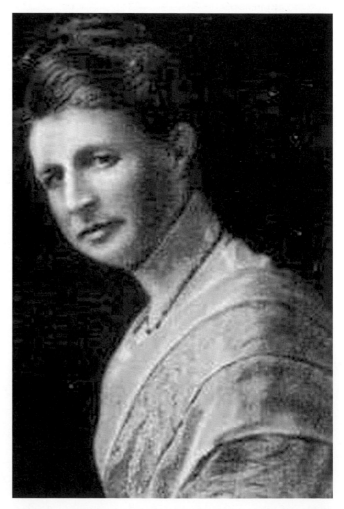

Fig. 3.8 Florence Nightingale Ward (1860–1919), homeopath and surgeon; one of first women to be awarded Fellow of American College of Surgeons. Date unknown (By permission of Sylvain Cazalet, Homeopathe Internationale, Montpellier, France)

American Institute of Homeopathy, as well as of the Institute's Society of Obstetrics. In World War I, she worked on the Medical Board of National Defense and served as head of the base hospital unit of female physicians [21]. Ward was for a time married to James William Ward (1861–1939), dean of the Homeopathic Medical College in San Francisco and a prominent public health physician and homeopathic surgeon in his own right (see below).

Ward "lived her life as though anything was possible" [22]. In her comprehensive review of Ward's life, Mottershead Pfeiffer observed Ward's allegiance to homeopathy in her daily medical practice, as well as devotion to the concept of "individual patient as whole person" that was so integral to homeopathy. Although surgery was her specialty, she would prescribe homeopathic remedies in low potencies, for example, aconite 3× and phosphorus 4× every half hour alternately for laryngitis in one instance, but she was quite willing to mix homeopathy with allopathy, and records exist of orders such as nitroglycerin 1/1,000 g (or 1 mg). True to homeopathic teaching, Ward would strive to individualize her prescribing, for example, adjusting doses of anesthetic based on a person's sensitivity.

In the late nineteenth century, it was fashionable for surgeons to remove healthy reproductive organs from women who had been diagnosed with hysteria, neurasthenia, or other neurotic syndromes. Ward joined the community of female surgeons in a backlash against this practice, and she would reserve hysterectomies and oophorectomies only for situations where, in her judgment, it was necessary for the patient's health.

Maria Augusta Generoso Estrella

Maria Augusta Generoso Estrella (1860–1946) was born and raised in Brazil. As a teenager, she was inspired to study medicine, but there were no such opportunities for women in her country at that time. She prevailed on her father to allow her to study in New York. Although 2 years below the minimum age for admission, the 16-year-old girl was offered a place at the NYMCHW. She passed her exams easily and graduated in 1881. Unfortunately, during this time in New York, her father's business collapsed, and funding was cut off. Fortunately, the Brazilian Emperor, Dom Pedro II, came to her rescue with a scholarship which allowed Estrella to complete her studies. However, another problem arose when, in 1879, Brazilian government legislation made possible the entry of women into medical school, but not until they reached the age of 21. So Estrella remained for two more years in New York, working as a medical intern before officially receiving her MD degree, at the same time being honored as class valedictorian and prizewinner for an essay on skin diseases. Estrella also coedited with a Brazilian friend a

newspaper for Brazilian women: *The Woman – Devoted to the Interests and Rights of Brazilian Women*. Upon her return to Brazil in 1882, the Emperor personally welcomed her home and urged her to dedicate herself to promoting the fortunes of women in Brazil. Her US medical diploma was recognized by the Brazilian Medical board, and Estrella set up practice, serving as an inspirational role model for other women to enroll in higher education. Estrella's husband was a pharmacist, and it was in his pharmacy that she maintained an office from which she prepared and distributed meals to women and children in the community. Estrella continued with medical practice for the remainder of her long life, although at one stage had to reduce her hours after the death of her husband in 1908 left her as a single parent with five children [23].

Geraldine Burton-Branch

Some of Dr. Burton-Branch's (born 1908) achievements are described in Chap. 4, but she could equally well be included in the chapter on public health.

Burton-Branch graduated from New York Homeopathic Medical College towards the end of its existence as a homeopathic institution. She then practiced gynecology and obstetrics, public health, and family planning and was medical examiner and district health officer in the Watts region of Los Angeles. Her adoption of family planning occurred long before it was widely accepted [24]. Her many activities on behalf of African-Americans and the impoverished Watts community are detailed in Chaps. 4 and 7. Without repeating these achievements, it is appropriate to mention that any account of homeopathy's leading women would be incomplete without her name. She exemplifies how homeopathically trained women have created social change and broadened the reach of healthcare to minorities; the same holds true for her work in respect of minority medical education in helping establish the Drew University of Medicine and Science. She was instrumental in convincing the Los Angeles County supervisor to build the Martin Luther King Hospital (now known as the King/Drew Medical Center). One of the guiding principles of her life was: "If you see a need, why sit and complain about it? Do something to straighten it out" [25]. In keeping with this maxim, after she retired as assistant district health officer and seeing the need for a senior center in South Central Los Angeles, she arranged for its construction and the training of firemen to serve as ambulance drivers and paramedics.

Burton-Branch has led an unusually long and productive life. She retired at the age of 98 and, since the age of 103, has given talks to her community, on topics such as "Healthy Sleep," "You Are Never Too Old to Learn," and "Commitment" [26]. In a talk entitled *Attitude and Recovery*, Burton-Branch stated that the body was designed to heal itself and that doctors sometimes gave themselves more credit than they deserve for bringing about recovery from illness [27]. Such a statement comes close to the heart of homeopathy.

Early in life, when Burton-Branch was in fifth grade, she wrote an essay expressing her desire to be a doctor. Her classmates scornfully told her that would never happen because "You're black and you're a woman." She proved them spectacularly wrong.

Boston Graduates and Students

Mercy B. Jackson

Mercy B. Jackson (1802–1877) was one of the many New England women who entered medicine to promote opportunities for their gender. She was ideally connected to pursue these goals through her relatives who introduced her to Ralph Waldo Emerson and other liberal Boston luminaries. Without having any official medical training, Jackson began a small homeopathic practice in 1841 for family and friends. Through the good offices of her family doctor who mentored Jackson, she eventually entered the NEFMC. By this time, she was in her mid-40s and was 48 when she graduated. Eighteen years later, she was nominated as a member of the state homeopathic society, but in keeping with the prejudices of the time, this nomination was rejected. Three years later, in 1871, she applied again and was accepted as the first female member. Jackson was appointed professor of pediatrics at Boston University Medical School [2, pp. 218–219]. As with a number of her homeopathic associates, Jackson waged war on behalf of women, contributing articles to *The Women's Journal*, a magazine edited by the prominent feminist Lucy Stone.

Mary H. Thompson

Mary Harris Thompson (1829–1895) is a distinguished figure in the history of American medicine. She has been referred to as a product of the homeopathic system, but this is questionable, and it would be more accurate to describe her training as eclectic, perhaps with some exposure to homeopathy. Nevertheless, the inclusion of Thompson in this chapter affords an opportunity to discuss the relationship between eclectic and homeopathic schools of medicine, as well as Thompson's important friendship with Lucy Waite, a Chicago homeopath.

Thompson is believed to have been the first female surgeon in the United States [28]. Her name lives on today at the Northwestern University Feinberg School of Medicine through the Mary Thompson Society, one of two Medical Student Societies at the school which were "named in honor of a notable alumnus" and which still represent a critical part of the curriculum structure at that medical school. Thompson became a member of the American Medical Association (AMA), which lists her today as one of the association's pathfinding female doctors. In 1886, she was the first woman to present a scientific paper at the AMA annual meeting. This paper was published a few months later in the association's journal, under the title of *Why diseases of children should be made a special study* [29, 30]. Among her achievements was the founding of the Chicago Women's Medical College, the first of its kind in the Midwest, and later amalgamated with Northwestern University. Thompson recruited to the faculty Sarah Hackett Stevenson, herself a celebrated physician, the first woman to be accepted as member of the AMA. Besides founding the medical school, Thompson established the Chicago Women's and Children's Hospital and the Chicago Nursing School. The hospital was renamed the Mary Thompson Hospital after her death in 1895 and continued in operation until financial circumstances caused it to close in 1988. For most of its 100 years, the hospital was one of only four in the United States to be staffed entirely by women. In the field of clinical practice, Mary Thompson designed a special surgical needle, which became widely used, as well as developed procedures for abdominal and pelvic surgery.

Thompson received her initial medical training at the NEFMC, qualifying in 1863. Although Thompson has been included in one source as belonging to the "pro-homeopathy" group [2, pp. 213, 223–224] , there is no evidence that she embraced its principles. Thompson felt her training at NEFMC was incomplete and that further study was required [10]. This training was obtained at Elizabeth Blackwell's institution in New York, after which Thompson was ready to return to Boston and accept her degree. There is no evidence that she either prescribed homeopathically or taught or wrote about homeopathy. In order to escape the increasingly competitive landscape for female doctors in the northeast, Thompson moved to Chicago where, in 1869, she received a second medical degree from the Chicago Medical College (which is now known as Northwestern University Medical School). The circumstances around her degree are of some interest, since they reflect on the barriers which existed for women to study medicine. The college opened up places for three women in 1869, but of the three who attended, only Mary Thompson was awarded a degree; the other two unfortunate women were dismissed at the end of the session because the male students and faculty complained that the presence of women in the classroom inhibited discussion of "delicate" subjects. The college quickly reverted to its male-only policy, which was upheld until 1926 when it again became coeducational. It is a testimony to Thompson that she was accepted by such a hostile group. Time proved her to be a regional, and then national, force in American medicine.

Thus, while Thompson cannot be regarded as a graduate of the homeopathic system, she did obtain her initial medical training at an eclectic school which was perceived to have homeopathic leanings at the time.

Eclectic Training

The exposure of students like Mary Thompson to homeopathy during their eclectic training warrants consideration, for some other eclectic graduates went on to embrace homeopathy with enthusiasm, such as James Tyler Kent, Jacob Gallinger, Clemence Lozier, and Edward Franklin. Eclectic schools did include homeopathic materia medica in their curriculum and used homeopathic texts, for example, Bartlett's *Textbook of Clinical Medic*ine and Hill's *Textbook of Surgery* (Benjamin Lord Hill was a renowned eclectic and homeopathic surgeon at the time) [2, p. 359, 31]. As Collins stated in 1916, "Eclectics have reaped a valued harvest from the investigations of this [homeopathic] medical school, which they have added to their therapeutic wealth. In return, Homeopathy is indebted to the Eclectic school for the discovery and proving of many new and important remedies, chiefly from the indigenous medical plants of this country" [32]. So it would have been quite possible for eclectic graduates to include the use of homeopathy in their practice. Indeed, a good example can be seen in the paper by Webster on therapeutics of eye, ear, and throat diseases which appeared in the National Eclectic Medical Association (NEMA) Quarterly. In his account, Webster describes his most frequently used remedies, all of which would have been familiar to homeopaths, and some were even recommended at homeopathic doses [33].

Lucy Waite

Thompson established a significant friendship with *Lucy Waite*, who was a prominent homeopathic surgeon in Chicago. Like Mary Thompson, Waite was well respected for her skills in surgery, practicing and teaching gynecology at a homeopathic college in Chicago. (Waite was married to a well-known regular surgeon, Frederick Byron Robinson, professor of gynecology at Chicago Postgraduate Medical School and at Illinois Medical College and one of the "most important surgeon-anatomists of his time" [34]. He was among the first surgeons in America to conduct extensive animal experiments and also other research. Much of his work was the product of collaboration with his wife.)

Thompson had so much respect for her friend that, notwithstanding Waite's homeopathic background, she requested that after Thompson's death, Lucy Waite was to succeed her as director of the Chicago Hospital for Women and Children (CHWC), which Thompson had founded in 1865. After initial opposition by the medical staff, Waite eventually occupied the position on a permanent basis from 1897 until her retirement, and she ran the hospital very successfully. Among her appointees to the staff was Bertha van Hoosen, one of the most famous American female surgeons of the time [35].

Rebecca Lee Crumpler

In 1860, only 300 out of 54,543 doctors in the United States were women with full medical degrees, and none were black. Rebecca Lee Crumpler (1831–1895) is known to posterity as the first to break through this barrier. It is also claimed that she was the product of a homeopathic training [2, p. 223]. but as an 1864 graduate of NEFMC, she would only have been exposed to whatever homeopathy was included in the curriculum (see above in connection with Mary Thompson, who was in the class 1 year ahead of Crumpler at NEFMC). Pertinent to Crumpler's attitude towards homeopathy is her book *Medical Discourses* [36], which offered recommendations for women on how to take care of themselves and their children. Crumpler gave very specific suggestions about treating a range of diseases without anywhere mentioning homeopathy. In recommending medication doses, Crumpler favored small but conventional amounts of standard medicines: she did not advocate the homeopathic approach even though she was mindful of the harm that many medicines could cause. Thus, it is difficult to link Crumpler in any meaningful way with the stream of homeopathy.

Esther Hill Hawks

Esther Hill Hawks (1833–1906) received her medical training at the NEFMC, graduating in 1857. She and her husband, John Milton Hawks, practiced together in Manchester, New Hampshire. John Hawks had misgivings about his wife practicing medicine as he felt her proper place was in the home, but eventually he became more accepting of her career ambitions. As with some other graduates from NEFMC, it is unclear to what extent homeopathy was incorporated into Hawks' practice. It is likely, however, that it was used to a degree since John Hawks sold homeopathic medicines in his pharmacy, and they were known to prescribe from this stock [37]. Of her later career in Lynn (see below), there is no suggestion that homeopathy was part of her practice.

During the Civil War, the Hawks responded to calls by the New York Freedmans' Aid Society for doctors and teachers on the South Carolina coast. Dr. John Hawks offered his medical services, while Esther volunteered to teach, since women could only visit the south at that time in their capacity as teachers. John Hawks was regimental surgeon to the renowned 54th Massachusetts Colored Infantry, known for its valiant attempt to capture Fort Wagner and immortalized in the film *Glory*. Esther Hawks worked mainly as a teacher but did assist her husband in the military hospital for a while. However, she was dismissed from this post when a new medical superintendent determined that Hawks was unfit to practice military medicine because she was a woman and also graduate of a sectarian, or irregular, medical school. Esther Hawks remained in the south for some years. For a short time in 1865, she lived in Charleston SC, where she opened an orphanage and a school and, according to some sources, was later appointed superintendent of the Charleston city schools. Subsequently, the Hawks together moved south to set up a new town in Florida for freed slaves, which they called Port Orange. This latter venture ultimately proved a failure due to local white prejudice and financial hardships [38]. After Hawks' school was deliberately burned down in 1869, she returned to New England and established medical practice with Dr. Lizzie Breed Welch in Lynn, Massachusetts, specializing in gynecology, while her husband remained in Florida [39]. If she practiced homeopathy at this stage, it was probably to a small degree, for she did not belong to any of the local homeopathic medical societies. Esther Hawks was active in her local community on behalf of the Lynn schools, in furthering measures to prevent tuberculosis, in her local medical societies, and on a broader stage through the Women's National Loyal League and women's suffrage. While in Florida, she became vice-president of the state Equal Rights Association and was the first to petition for women's suffrage in the state legislature.

Julia Holmes Smith

Julia Holmes Smith (1838–1929) was born in Savannah, Georgia, in 1838 and grew up in New Orleans. She married Waldo Abbot, who died from yellow fever 4 years later, leaving her with two children. In New Orleans, Smith was drama critic for the *New Orleans Picayune*. In 1872, Holmes Abbot married her second husband, Sabin Smith, and they had a daughter from this union. The Smiths moved to Boston in 1873, where Julia enrolled as a student at Boston University and then transferred to Chicago Homeopathic College, from which she graduated in 1877; she remained in that city practicing homeopathy for the next 40 years. In 1898, Smith became the first woman to be elected dean of a coeducational medical school, the homeopathic National Medical College of Chicago. While not achieving the notoriety of her colleagues, Smith was well respected for her expertise in women's and children's diseases, for her writings, and for her abilities as a teacher. She established a clinic for indigent women at a Chicago church, where she taught her patients better self-management of their health and well-being. For a time, she was personal homeopath to Susan B. Anthony.

Smith retired from practice at the age of 78, but continued to be active in several societies until her death at the age of 91.

Outside of medicine, Smith was energetically involved with other initiatives. In 1886, a group of women met at Smith's home to organize the Illinois Woman's Press Association, whose goal was to provide a means of communication between women writers and to secure the benefits resulting from organized action; the organization still thrives today. Although dedicated to the suffragist movement, Smith invested more of her energies into homeopathic practice than did some of her colleagues. However, she was active outside of medical practice, and she became the first woman to be placed on a political ticket in Illinois and to be appointed by the governor as trustee of the University of Illinois.

Leila Gertrude Bedell

An article appeared in the *New England Medical Gazette* [40] which described the 1878 graduation ceremony at BUSM; it noted that Leila Gertrude Bedell (1838–1914) was honored by being invited to give the salutatory in a departure from normal graduation procedure. Her speech reflected on the positions of medical students and practitioners, the responsibilities of the profession relative to the community, and true worth and loyalty to a particular school. It noted that her thesis was on the topic of "The origin of the two nervous systems, the basis of sex and of man's dual nature," an essay which formed the germ of a larger work for which Bedell is still remembered, entitled *The Abdominal Brain* [41]. Although the phrase from which the book derived its title was introduced much earlier by the French physiologist, Xavier Bichat, it had received relatively little attention until Bedell took up the subject. Bedell's work was among the earliest on this subject, being followed in 1907 and 1920 by publications from other authors such as Byron Robinson (see above) and Théron Dumont. The notion has subsequently been revived in modern psychosomatic medicine, which refers to the enteric nervous system or "little brain," and has been invoked to explain conditions like irritable bowel syndrome [42].

Leila Bedell was an advocate of women's rights in Chicago for many decades. She was president of the Chicago Women's Club and creator of the Chicago Women's League. This league had a short life but did succeed in placing on the table the matter of governmental responsibility to provide directly for Chicago's people [43]. To Bedell goes credit for raising the idea of a national federation of women's societies. In spite of claims to the contrary, it was from Bedell's suggestions in 1880 and 1888 that the General Federation of Women's Clubs (GFWC) came into being [44]. (The GFWC continues to exist and make its presence felt in contemporary life.) It was also due to Bedell that the GWFC designed an identification badge for members to purchase [45]. Other initiatives with which Bedell was involved included the Chicago Protective Agency for Women and Children and Hull House, the well-known settlement where reform-minded, educated women provided social and educational opportunities for working class women in Chicago and, later on, around the nation. Bedell was a member of the American Institute of Homeopathy and served on the Board of Visitors at BUSM. In the last years of her life, Dr. Bedell moved to Tryon, NC, where she became president of the Lanier Library and took an active part in the local writers' community.

Martha George Ripley

Martha George Ripley (1843–1912) came from a family known for its "resolute concern for practical justice" [1, p. 44], working for abolition of slavery by means of an underground railroad station next to their home (Fig. 3.9). Martha inherited progressive views and, in turn, became a fighter for the oppressed. She identified with the cause of women's rights, befriending Julia Ward Howe, Lucy Stone, and others prominent in the movement, including two doctors, Maria Zakrzewska and Mercy Jackson (see above). Ripley impressed her more prominent colleagues and was appointed by them in 1876 to the executive councils of the New England and Massachusetts Women's Suffrage Associations, posts which she held until departing for Minnesota in 1883 [46]. Later she joined the Women's Rescue League, an organization devoted to the rehabilitation of prostitutes, as well as becoming president of the Minnesota State Suffrage

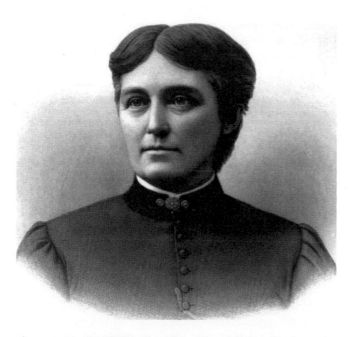

Fig. 3.9 Martha Ripley. Founder of the Minneapolis Maternity Hospital, suffragist. In the public domain

Association. Her home was center to many gatherings for reformers desirous of equal representation for women in suffrage and education.

It is believed that Ripley's decision to enter medical school was shaped by the perspectives obtained from her suffragist and medical friends in Boston, and she enrolled at Boston University in 1880. A sister had also previously graduated as an MD from that institution. Other proximate reasons included a desire to provide care for her family and for the New England mill workers. One story illustrative of Ripley's outspokenness tells how, during a dissection class, she brandished a vertebra in front of the class insisting that this (i.e., "backbone") was what the faculty needed since they persisted in giving male students the best appointments and that the time had come for women to be given equal treatment. After Martha's husband, William, was seriously injured in a mill accident and forced to retire, the burden of wage earner fell entirely on Martha's shoulders. Following graduation in 1883, Ripley left for Minneapolis, where opportunity seemed better and where William had relatives.

Ripley slowly gained acceptance in the community, as her suffragist connections enabled her to become better known. She was outspoken on issues in which she believed strongly saying, according to Solberg, that her conscience imposed "the duty of not keeping silent when … wrong exists." In due course, her practice flourished, and she campaigned on the broader front of public health and community medicine, being an early and vigorous advocate of cremation as a public health issue, at a time when this practice was beginning to be used more widely: the first American crematorium was built in Pennsylvania in 1876.

Ripley's single most enduring monument was the creation in 1887 of the Minneapolis Maternity Hospital, which accepted both married and unmarried mothers. This venture, with which Ripley was to remain closely involved for the rest of her life, embodied her concern for the welfare of women and children and of her compassion in reaching out to the disadvantaged regardless of opprobrium. Interestingly, the articles of incorporation required that the hospital admit all comers, including the destitute, and that care was to be given to destitute children who were born in the hospital. The one non-amendable clause directed that the medical department must be under the care and control of homeopathic female physicians, although any doctor of good standing could treat patients there. In spite of many local obstacles and prejudice against acceptance of "sinful" women who had children out of wedlock, the hospital grew steadily and underwent several moves to larger quarters. In 1916, it took Ripley's name and was thereafter known as the Ripley Memorial Hospital, continuing in existence until financial problems forced its closure in 1957. Subsequently, funds were used to create the Ripley Memorial Foundation, which remains active today as a donor-advised fund of the Women's Foundation of

Minnesota and honors the legacy of Martha Ripley by supporting programs which focus on preventing teenage pregnancy. The Maternity Hospital was remarkably forward looking and claimed three "firsts" in the city: (1) a social service department, (2) parenting and natural childbirth classes, and (3) a maternity facility for the rooming of infants with their mothers. Ripley's name is also perpetuated in the Ripley Gardens, a low-income housing project in Minneapolis. One cannot disagree with Solberg's appraisal of Ripley as one who "committed herself to extending the area of human freedom and equal rights for all."

Anna Howard Shaw

Anna Howard Shaw (1847–1919) was born in England on February 14, 1847 (Fig. 3.10). She came to the United States with her parents when she was 6, first to Massachusetts and then to Michigan, where she grew up in the tough midwestern wilderness. At the age of 16, Shaw took her first paid job

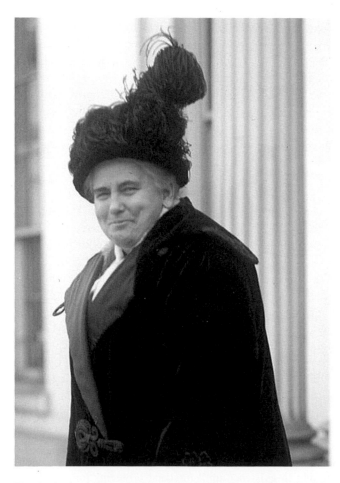

Fig. 3.10 Anna Howard Shaw. 1914. Suffragist and women's rights leader; president National Woman Suffrage Association; first ordained woman in the US Methodist church. In the public domain. Author Harris and Ewing Photographer

as a teacher. She was determined to obtain a college education and moved to Boston where she enrolled at the BU Theology School. She graduated in 1878, but her application to become an ordained Methodist Episcopal minister was rejected. Fortunately, the Methodist Protestant Church accepted her, and she became the first woman to be ordained in the Methodist church in the United States. For 7 years, she was pastor of the church in East Dennis, Massachusetts, and during this time, she studied medicine at BU, graduating in 1885. Upon obtaining her medical degree, Shaw resigned her pastorate and took up medical practice in the poorer areas of Boston, albeit without emphasizing that she was homeopathically trained [1, p. 53], Her main passion, however, lay in women's suffrage, and she devoted the rest of her life to this cause. Shaw has been called a "master orator" for social justice, and in the course of her lifetime she gave over 10,000 lectures worldwide [47]. She was president of the National Woman Suffrage Association between 1904 and 1915, was a close friend of Susan B. Anthony, and gave the eulogy at Anthony's funeral. Her tireless effort was an important factor behind passage of the 19th Amendment to the US Constitution in 1919. Shaw was invited to serve as head of the women's committee of the United States Council of National Defense in World War I and was the first woman to receive the Distinguished Service Medal. For her services to women and soldiers in the war, Shaw received commendation letters from Queen Mary of the United Kingdom, President Woodrow Wilson, General Pershing, and the wife of the French president. In 2000, she was inducted into the National Women's Hall of Fame, and she is now regarded by her church as being an agent of change both for the church and for society: "It was due in great part to Shaw's leadership in the fight for women's suffrage that women were given the right to vote" [48].

Rebecca Lee Dorsey

Rebecca Lee Dorsey (1859–1954) must be one of the more colorful characters to have graduated from BUSM; she was certainly a person who had strong self-belief. After completing her studies there in 1883, she spent 2 years in Europe studying under Louis Pasteur, Robert Koch, and Joseph Lister. Upon her return home, she settled in Los Angeles, where she spent the next 60 years in practice. According to McNamara, she accomplished several noteworthy firsts. Among her achievements were the following: delivering the first baby in a Los Angeles hospital, administering the city's first diphtheria vaccination and the first injection of adrenaline to prevent heart failure, performing the area's first three successful appendectomies and a nephrectomy, founding the first nursing school in the city, and delivering over 4,000 babies, including Earl Warren, who became governor of

California and a Supreme Court Justice [49]. Dorsey boasted that she never lost a baby or mother during delivery because she adhered to the following four principles: perfect understanding of the measurement of the mother's pelvis, advocacy of good prenatal care, strict aseptic technique, and complete delivery of the afterbirth. She experienced no cases of septicemia, which she attributed to her knowledge of sterilization. Among her more exotic accomplishments was the transplant of a lamb's thyroid gland into a Civil War veteran whose thyroid had been destroyed by a bullet at the Battle of Bull Run. This undertaking was done in secret and had a good outcome for the patient. However, angry colleagues found out and demanded her resignation from the hospital staff. It is reported that Dorsey was the country's first female endocrinologist. Her surgical experience was extensive, and she allegedly performed 90 % of the operations conducted at St. Vincent's Hospital, one of the few facilities to admit Latino, Chinese, and black patients. She was always politically minded and "eventually became a thorn in the side of the City Council with her public health campaigns for better drinking water, food inspection, and cleaner streets and playgrounds. When councilmen saw her coming, they literally shut the chamber doors" [50]. Like Geraldine Burton-Branch, Dorsey was one of homeopathy's pioneers in Los Angeles medicine, promoting public health, surgery, and access to treatment for minorities.

After 60 years in practice, Dorsey retired and invested her money in date farming. It is to her that credit has been given for bringing the date industry to California [51].

Clara Barrus

Clara Barrus (1864–1931) is best known as the literary executrix of John Burroughs, the essayist, naturalist, and early American conservationist (Figs. 3.11 and 3.12). Barrus met Burroughs in 1901, when she was 37 and Burroughs 64. Barrus became the love of Burroughs' life and eventually moved into his home upon the death of Mrs. Burroughs. Less well known (today) is Barrus the psychiatrist. Barrus had received her medical training at Boston University School of Medical School, after which she took an appointment as assistant psychiatrist at Middletown State Hospital and as professor of psychiatry at New York Women's Medical College. Ozarin referred to Barrus' paper on gynecological disorder in relation to insanity as one of the earliest scientific publications by women in this field [52]. This paper [53] appeared in the *American Journal of Insanity* in 1895 and was followed 1 year later by a report in the *Journal of Nervous and Mental Disease* on the subject of insanity in young women [54].

The first of these papers described 100 patients who had been examined by Barrus at the Middletown State Hospital

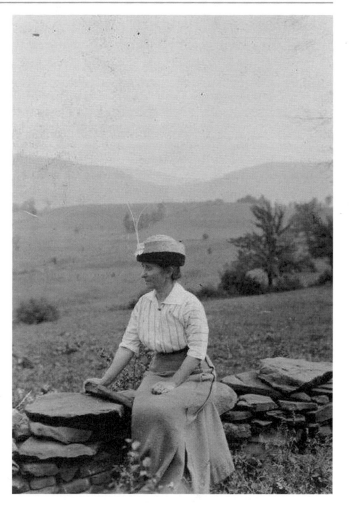

Fig. 3.11 Clara Barrus (1864–1931). Psychiatrist, writer on mental health issues in women, companion, and executrix of John Burroughs. Date unknown. In the public domain

and reflects her careful physical and psychological assessments. She pointed out that, while women no doubt differed somewhat from men in causative factors for mental illness, it was important not to lose sight of their shared risks. "The causes of insanity in women … are as varied and many of them identical with the causes of insanity in men … *with the addition* [her emphasis] of those which come to her as a human being of the female sex." Barrus also recognized that mental illness often had two types of cause. These were (1) the predisposing vulnerability (or the "tyranny of a bad organization" to borrow a phrase from Henry Maudsley, a contemporary British psychiatrist) and (2) life's trials and tribulations which became "the last straw that broke the camel's back." She concluded that gynecological disorders may sometimes be relevant causative factors, while at other times, they can be the consequence of mental illness, and it was her belief that overall doctors made too much of them as a cause of mental illness. Nevertheless, she argued that when an abnormality was found, it should be treated whenever

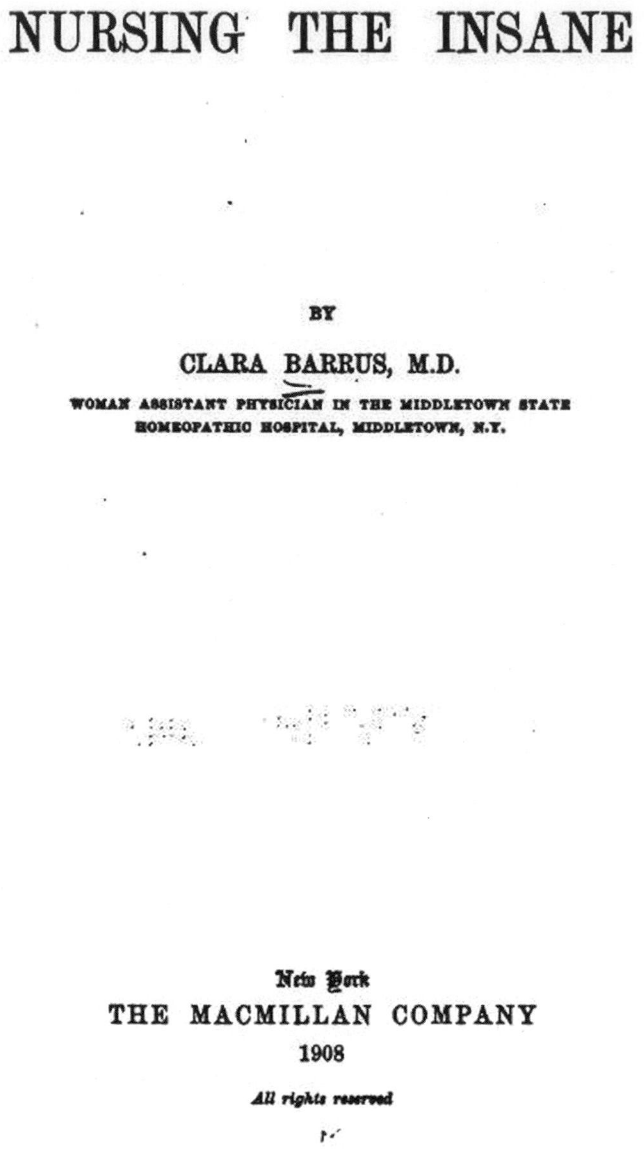

NURSING THE INSANE

BY

CLARA BARRUS, M.D.

WOMAN ASSISTANT PHYSICIAN IN THE MIDDLETOWN STATE
HOMEOPATHIC HOSPITAL, MIDDLETOWN, N.Y.

New York

THE MACMILLAN COMPANY

1908

All rights reserved

Fig. 3.12 Title page: Nursing the Insane. In the public domain

possible, so that one of the stumbling blocks to recovery might be removed.

In Barrus' second paper, she presented an analysis of 121 girls and young women with psychosis. Of interest was the frequency with which rapid switches between mania (the "highs") and depression (the "lows") were seen. In this respect, the symptoms of bipolar disorder differed from the classical picture of marked cycling between the two poles, or *folie circulaire*, as it was called. Gynecological abnormalities were found in three-quarters of those examined, but the relationship to insanity of these abnormalities, as well as menstruation, was unclear. Interestingly, subtle physical alterations like asymmetries and mild deformities were quite common and thought by the author to be of some relevance. These observations foreshadow by about a century the more

recent interest in psychiatry of so-called "soft" neurological signs which characterize a number of psychiatric disorders. Another fascinating aspect of Barrus' paper is her suggestion that, by paying closer attention to innate vulnerability and to external stressors, it may be possible to prevent the onset of psychosis, which has become another promising area of investigation in recent times [55].

These two publications have been described as significant from a sociological standpoint. Hirshbein observed, for example, that power structures in society created sharp demarcations on the basis of sex, ensuring that women were kept subordinate and denied the opportunities given to men. To support this state of affairs, rationalizations were often made that women were more delicate and prey to the vicissitudes of hormonal fluctuations and other gender-specific influences. Hirshbein noted that in her 1895 paper, Barrus agreed with this view only up to a point, holding that sex-specific influences were less of a determinant in causing mental illness than experiences which were shared by men and women [56] In Barrus' 1896 paper on insanity in young women, she expressed her belief that women could be empowered to make decisions in respect of their health. It was her opinion that adolescent girls could cure themselves "with the help of a doctor who encouraged self-control, meaningful work and exercise" [57].

It is perhaps for her textbook on nursing in psychiatry that Barrus the psychiatrist was best known in her day [58]. This book was published in 1908, after Barrus had been on the Middletown staff for 15 years. Although not the first book on the topic, *Nursing the Insane* was acclaimed in the *American Journal of Psychiatry* [59] as "probably the best that has appeared," while the *California State Journal of Medicine* "unhesitatingly recommend[ed] the perusal of it to all classes of nurses, as well as physicians in touch with insane patients" [60]. Even the *Journal of the American Medical Association* reviewed Barrus' book and found its perusal "will do no harm and may serve to sharpen the observing faculties" [61], a recommendation as positive as one might expect from an AMA publication. Unlike most homeopathic textbooks, which were published by homeopathic publishing companies, *Nursing the Insane* was published by Macmillan, a stalwart of the publishing industry.

Two years after her book was published, Barrus left Middletown, travelled to the southwest with John Burroughs and their friend John Muir, and then returned to New York where she commenced private practice at a sanitarium in Pelham. After resigning from this position in 1914, Barrus gave up psychiatry and devoted the remaining 17 years of her life to literary and conservation activities with Burroughs and, after his death in 1921, edited his works and published *Life and Letters of John Burroughs* in 1928 and *Whitman and Burroughs* in 1931.

Eliza Taylor Ransom

Eliza Ransom (1867–1955) is best known as a women's suffrage advocate and champion of twilight sleep in childbirth. Ransom was born in Ontario, Canada, in 1867, educated in New York, and worked as a teacher before entering medical school at BUSM, where she qualified in 1900. She commenced practice shortly after, specializing in psychiatry, neurology, and obstetrics. Ransom was active in her local homeopathic society, serving as vice-president of the Boston and Massachusetts Homeopathic Medical Societies. In 1901, she was appointed professor of histology at BUSM, where she remained for many years. At one stage, she took significant administrative responsibility on an interim basis, while the dean, John Sutherland, was temporarily indisposed. However, the greater part of Ransom's career was devoted to furthering the cause of painless childbirth, and she was the first person in America to establish a maternity hospital devoted entirely to this practice, which was known as twilight sleep [1, pp. 49–50, 62]. She founded the New England Twilight Sleep Association and was one of the leaders in the National Twilight Sleep Association, which had come about largely in response to public anger at the medical profession's reluctance to pursue pain-free childbirth [63]. The association staged rallies, presentations, and published pamphlets and campaigned for the construction of a teaching hospital.

Twilight sleep had been developed in Germany at the end of the nineteenth century and later promoted by two physicians in that country, Drs. Gauss and Krönig. To lessen the experience of pain and obliterate memory of labor, Gauss and Krönig administered scopolamine and morphine at the onset of labor and then throughout. While this produced the desired effects, it was not without danger and many doctors refused to use it. But countervailing arguments were made as to its safety when properly administered, which in effect meant by trained physicians in the hospital setting, and the practice spread, reaching a peak around 1915. Thereafter, it began a decline, spurred on by the unfortunate death in childbirth of one of its strongest advocates, Frances X. Carmody. Although Mrs. Carmody's doctors and her husband denied that scopolamine had any part in her death, the movement was dealt a heavy blow. Nevertheless, twilight sleep continued to be quite popular in the parts of the United States until the 1930s.

Not surprisingly, many twilight sleep advocates were the same people who worked hard on behalf of women's suffrage, of whom Eliza Ransom was one and Florence Ward another. Ransom was Ward Eleven's representative to the Massachusetts Woman Suffrage Association, and she also spoke out for coeducational medical schools. The twilight sleep movement in the United States began as a means to empower women, and one may ask whether it achieved this goal. The movement left an impact in the following ways [64]: (1) by turning childbirth from a home-based procedure into one requiring hospitalization, it hastened the growth of obstetrics as a specialty; (2) it forced physicians to search for ways to reduce pain in childbirth; and (3) it became harder to ignore women's challenge to the American Medical Association, thereby paving the way to reforms in women's medical care, including prenatal care, aseptic techniques, and reduced maternal mortality. Ironically, progress in obstetric anesthesia was slower to arrive, and scopolamine remained in use until the 1960s, when regional anesthesia took over. At the same time, while twilight sleep was seen as a form of empowering women in managing childbirth, it left them in some ways even more dependent on doctors who kept control and used heavy doses of medicine. This imbalance was later partly corrected by the natural childbirth movement which allowed for fully conscious participation and choice.

Cleveland Graduates

Caroline Brown Winslow

Caroline Brown Winslow (1822–1896) was born in England and came to Utica, New York, with her parents when she was quite young. She trained at the Cincinnati Eclectic Medical College and then later in homeopathy at the Western College of Homeopathy in Cleveland. For some years afterwards, she practiced homeopathy in Utica, specializing in surgery. Following the death of her parents, she moved to Washington, DC, where she continued in practice. This was during the Civil War, and because the government excluded homeopaths from providing medical services to soldiers, Winslow and her colleague Susan Edson made furtive visits to the city's military hospitals to provide care for sick and injured soldiers. In the years which followed, Winslow was active in opening a free homeopathic dispensary, the National Homeopathic hospital and the local chapter of the American Institute of Homeopathy [65]. She played a crucial mentoring role in the life of Grace Roberts, who was to become the first African-American woman to graduate from the University of Michigan School of Medicine and later became a visible presence in the Washington DC medical scene. As a young girl, Roberts had been cured from a serious disease by Winslow, and, when Roberts had already obtained a regular medical degree, she then decided to enroll in the homeopathic school in Michigan, where she lived with members of the Winslow family [66]. Roberts worked together with Winslow on many of the projects in DC with which Winslow was associated.

Outside of medical practice, Winslow was an active participant in women's rights, suffrage, and moral reform. In

1873, she served as vice-president of the National Women's Suffrage Association and then as editor of Alpha, the newspaper for the Moral Education Society, an organization with a broad agenda which focused on sex education, voluntary parenthood, dress reform, divorce, providing financial aid to striking women, the welfare of prostitutes, temperance, and general social and political reform. During her involvement with this society, Winslow became closely associated with Helen Pitts, who assisted Winslow in writing articles for the magazine and who eventually became Frederick Douglass' second wife [67].

Susan Edson

Susan Edson (1823–1897) is best known as the female doctor who provided medical care to President James Garfield and for being the first woman or homeopath to provide medical care to a US president [1, p. 41, 68, 69]. Edson had been a family doctor to the Garfield family for many years, and they held her in high esteem; one of Garfield's sons referred to her as "Dr. Edson, full of med'cin." When Garfield was shot, Edson was called upon to provide further care by Mrs. Garfield, with the president's full agreement. However, this produced considerable friction within the president's medical team, because Edson was both a woman and a homeopath. The superintending doctor, D.W. Bliss, was strongly opposed to collaboration of any sort with a homeopath, having previously been censured by the American Medical Association for consulting with a doctor who in turn had once consulted with a homeopath, in violation of the AMA's code of ethics. Since the Garfields wished for Edson to provide care, Bliss could hardly dismiss her, although he would surely have liked to do so. By way of compromise, he insisted that Edson and another homeopath with connections to the family, Silas Boynton, serve in the capacity of nurses. Although this was clear demotion for two fully qualified doctors, Edson and Boynton agreed since it enabled them to stay involved in the president's care. As Garfield deteriorated, they rightly became quite critical of the poor care which Bliss gave, complaining that some abdominal symptoms came about from the side effects of large doses of quinine. They also objected to the incessant probing of the wound, as Bliss searched in vain for the bullet. It turned out that Edson was right in her concerns, for Garfield's death was due to the complications of care, including massive infection and malnutrition, rather than to the effects of the bullet, which in all probability could have safely remained in its place.

Susan Edson received her medical training at the Cleveland Homeopathic Hospital College, qualifying in 1854. She later moved to the capital city, where she became Washington's first practicing female doctor. During the Civil War, she served the Union troops, along with her colleague Mary Jane Safford Blake. However, this had to be in a nursing capacity, owing to government restrictions against medical practice by homeopaths. She continued to live in Washington after the war and cofounded the Homeopathic Free Dispensary, which provided care, mainly to blacks and to women, seeing over 2,000 patients per year. In the 1880s, along with Caroline Brown Winslow, Edson organized the District Women's Suffrage Association, which became the national headquarters for the National Women's Suffrage Association. Around the same time, Edson set up a regional center of the WEIU, the organization which had been established in Boston by her colleague Harriet Clisby.

Others

Laura Matilda Towne

Laura Matilda Towne (1825–1901) received her training at the sectarian Penn Medical University, a short-lived (1853–1881) medical school in Philadelphia. It is unclear whether or not she graduated [70], but Towne supplemented her training with personal supervision in homeopathy by Constantine Hering, one of the nation's foremost homeopaths. Among her patients was the abolitionist and author Thomas Higginson, who recuperated from a wartime illness on Towne's South Carolina plantation. He wrote: "… Miss Laura Towne, the homeopathic physician of the department, chief teacher and probably the most energetic person this side of civilization … I think she has done more for me than anyone else by prescribing homeopathic arsenic as a tonic, one powder every day on rising, and it has already, I think (3 doses) affected me" [71].

In 1861, Federal forces occupied St. Helena Island in South Carolina, and many of the established white planters abandoned their estates, leaving behind thousands of freed slaves. In response to this, the Federal government called for teachers and doctors to volunteer their services. Laura Towne was one of the first to provide medical and teaching services, arriving at Port Royal early in 1862. A few months later, she was joined by her friend and future life partner Ellen Murray. Towne and Murray founded a secondary school, which they named the Penn School, after William Penn. It was for a time the only school to teach the black population and some years later expanded its reach by offering courses in teacher training. In addition to teaching, Towne continued to practice medicine and spread the gospel of temperance. She found it hard to obtain basic supplies, including homeopathic remedies [72], so she was obliged to become adept in the use of native and folk remedies. Eventually, however, Towne abandoned medicine in order to devote her time to the school [73]. She became fully acquainted with local Gullah culture and music, was accepted into the Gullah culture, and rarely left the Sea Islands in the remaining 40 years of her life. The Penn Center lives on today as one the nation's most historically significant African-American educational and cultural institutions and is remembered for being Martin Luther King's retreat, where he would find privacy and time for reflection and where he held the annual conferences of his Southern Christian Leadership Conference on the Penn campus [74]. To gauge the full impact of Towne's work, we can turn to Cross, who pointed out that Towne did more than help a few small Gullah communities on the South Carolina coast. "She was laying the groundwork for programs that over the next century would help to save an entire culture from slow extinction … the Gullah culture" [72, p. 42].

Conclusions

From the mid-nineteenth century into the first part of the twentieth century, most homeopathic medical schools welcomed women into their ranks. Several graduates went on to shape society by promoting women's enfranchisement; creating welfare services; establishing women's medical schools, hospitals, and free clinics; and elevating the standards of medical education. They played a key role in the empowerment of women. Some of these gains were rolled back in the twentieth century as medicine again became a male-dominated profession for several decades, but others were more enduring. The influence of these homeopathic women was felt not only in the United States but also in other countries such as Canada and Brazil.

Even today, in technologically advanced countries, the battle for equal opportunity for women in medicine continues to be waged [75]. Many of the women in this chapter are reminders of homeopathy's contributions on a broad social front to progress in medicine. Much came from their determination, vision, boldness, and civic responsibility.

References

1. Kirschmann A. A vital force. Women in American homeopathy. New Brunswick: Rutgers University Press; 2004.
2. Ullman D. The homeopathic revolution. Berkeley: North Atlantic Books; 2007.
3. Slawson RG. Medical training in the United States prior to the Civil War. J Evid Based Complement Altern Med. 2012;17:11–27.
4. Young S. Israel Tisdale Talbot 1829–1899 [Internet]. Sue Young Histories; 2007 [Cited 2012 Aug 18]. Available from: www.sueyounghistories.com/archives/2007/12/09/israel-tisdale-talbot-and-homeopathy.htm.
5. Cazalet S. New England Female Medical College & New England Hospital for Women and Children [Internet] 2001 [Cited 2012 Aug 18]. Available from: www.homeoint.org/cazalet/histo/newengland.htm.
6. Waite FC. History of the New England Female Medical College 1848–1874. Boston: Boston University School of Medicine; 1950.
7. Yacorzynski GK. Book review: history of the New England Female Medical College, 1848–1874. J Am Med Assoc. 1951;146:686–7.
8. Morantz-Sanchez RM. Women physicians in American medicine. New York: Oxford University Press; 1985.
9. Godlee F. A modern approach to mental health. BMJ. 2012;344:e1322.
10. Frist WH. Public policy and the practicing physician. Ann Thorac Surg. 2001;71:1410–4.
11. Thompson K. 'Clisby, Harriet Jemima Winifred (1830–1931)' [Internet]. Clisby. Australian Dictionary of Biography, National Centre of Biography, Australian National University [Cited 2012 Feb 22]. Available from: http://adb.anu.edu.au/biography/clisby-harriet-jemima-winifred-3235/text4879.
12. Famous Canadian Physicians [Internet] Library and Archives Canada 2007 [Cited 2012 Feb 28]. https://www.collectionscanada.gc.ca/physicians/030002–2500-e.html.
13. Women's College Hospital [Internet]. 2012 [Cited 2012 Feb 29]. Available from: http://en.wikipedia.org/wiki/Women's_College_Hospital.
14. Canada's historic places [Internet]. 1999 [Cited 29 Feb 2012]. Available from: http://www.historicplaces.ca/en/rep-reg/place-lieu.aspx?id=7738&pid=0.
15. Sammarco A. The Dorchester Community News. 4 Nov 1994 [Internet] [Cited 2012 Mar 1]. Available from: www.dorchesteratheneum.org/page.php?id=919.
16. Young S. Alice Boole Campbell 1836–1909 [Internet]. Sue Young Histories 2008 [Cited 2012 Mar 9]. Available from: http://sueyounghistories.com/archives/2008/01/28/alice-boole-campbell-and-homeopathy.
17. Employment for the insane: Dr. Alice B. Campbell's suggestions on the value of some kind of work [Internet]. The New York Times. 10 Oct 1883 [Cited 2012 Mar 9]. Available from: http://query.nytimes.com/gst/abstract.html?res=F60815FE3B5F15738DDDA90994D8415B8384F0D3.
18. Seraile W. Susan McKinney Steward: "New York State's First African-American Woman Physician". Afro-Americans New York Life History. 1985;9(2):34.
19. Women in history. Susan McKinney Steward biography [Internet]. Last updated: 11/7/2012. Lakewood Public Library [Cited 2012 Nov 7]. Available from: www.lkwdpl.org/wihohio/stew-sus.htm.
20. Susan Rishworth, Archivist, American College of Surgeons. Personal communication to author. 6 Mar 2012.
21. Florence Ward [Internet] San Francisco History, SF Genealogy. The San Francisco Examiner. 16 Dec 1919 [Cited 2012 Mar 6]. Available from: www.sfgenealogy.com/sf/history/hgoe16.htm.
22. Mottershead E. Florence Nightingale Ward, M.D. Medical sectarian or medical scientist? [Internet]. 2004. p. 22 [Cited 2012 Mar 6]. Available from: http://www.berkeleyhomeopathy.com/articles-and-research/.
23. Maria Estrella [Internet] [Cited 2012 Mar 5]. Available from: http://www.dec.ufcg.edu.br/biografias/MariAGEs.html.
24. Under the microscope: Geraldine Burton Branch, MD, MPH Receives Honorary Membership [Internet]. Charles R. Drew Medical Society Newsletter. 1 Nov 2010. p. 3 [Cited 2012 Aug 19]. Available from: http://charlesdrewmedicalsociety.org.
25. Ponder J. Loma Linda University TODAY. Wednesday, 9 Dec 2009;22(18):5 [Cited 2012 Aug 19]. Available from: http://www.llu.edu/assets/news/today/documents/2009/2009December9.pdf.
26. News/Press Releases. Hollenbeck Palms Newsletter [Internet]. Hollenbeck Headlines. Spring 2013 [Cited 2013 Apr 24]. Available from: http://www.hollenbeckhome.com/news.aspx.
27. Dr. Geraldine Branch [Internet]. Hollenbeck Headlines. Fall 2011. 5 [Cited 2012 Aug 19]. Available from: http://www.hollenbeckhome.com/news.aspx.
28. Ward Rounds, Northwestern University, Feinberg School of Medicine [Internet] History Making Personified, Mary Harris

Thompson 2009 [Cited 2012 Feb 18]. Available from: http://archives.wardrounds.northwestern.edu/archive/2009/spring/Features/Feature4.html.

29. Available from: http://www.ama-assn.org/ama/pub/about-ama/our-history/timelines-ama-history/1941-1960.page? Women Physicians and the AMA. [Internet] [Cited 2012 Feb 18].

30. Thompson MH. Why diseases of children should be made a special study. J Am Med Assoc. 1886;13:399–402.

31. Eighth Annual Announcement, Bennett Medical College for the Session 1875–76. [Internet] Chicago: Metropolitan Printing Company; 1875. p. 3–6 [Cited 2012 Dec 31]. Available from: www.archives.org/details/annualannounceme00benn.

32. Collins AH. Principles, practice and progress of the eclectic school of medicine. National Eclectic Medical Association Quarterly. 1916;7:29–46 [Internet] [Cited 2013 Jan 18]. Available from: www.henriettasherbal.com/eclectic/journals/nemaq1915/03-eclectics.html.

33. Webster HT. Therapeutics of eye, ear and throat diseases. National Eclectic Medical Association Quarterly. 1916;7:19–28.

34. Rutkow IM. American surgery: an illustrated history. Philadelphia: Lippincott-Raven; 1998. p. 283.

35. Fine E. Pathways to practice: women physicians in Chicago, 1850–1902. Dissertation. Madison: University of Wisconsin; 2007.

36. Young S. Rebecca Lee Crumpler 1831–1895 [Internet]. Sue Young Histories 2007 [Cited 2012 Jan 26]. Available from: http://sueyounghistories.com/archives/2007/09/06/rebecca-lee-crumpler-and-homeopathy/.

37. Schwartz G, editor. A Woman Doctor's Civil War: Esther Hill Hawks' Diary (Women's Diaries and Letters of the Nineteenth Century South). Columbia: University of South Carolina Press; 1984. p. 25.

38. Anonymous. Esther Hill Hawks Civil War Women Blog [Internet] 2006 [Cited 2012 Mar 19]. Available from: http://www.civilwarwomenblog.com/2006/12/dr-esther-hill-hawks.html.

39. Schultz JE. Women at the front: hospital workers in Civil War America. Chapel Hill: University of North Carolina Press; 2007. p. 174.

40. Commencement exercises. N Engl Med Gazette. 1878;13:169.

41. Bedell LG. The abdominal brain. Chicago: Grass and Delbridge; 1885.

42. Lydiard RB. Irritable bowel syndrome, anxiety, and depression: what are the links? J Clin Psychiatry. 2001;62 Suppl 8:38–45.

43. Flanagan MA. Serving with their hearts: Chicago women and the vision of the good city 1871–1923. Princeton: Princeton University Press; 2002. p. 35–7.

44. Frank HG, Jerome AJ. Annals of the Chicago Women's Club for the first forty years of its organization, 1876–1916 [Internet]. The University of Illinois Library [Cited 2012 Dec 17]. Available from: http://archive.org/stream/annalsofchicagow00chic/annalsofchicagow00chic_djvu.txt.

45. 2010–2012 Club Manual. Know Your Organization. V4. 6 June 2011 [Internet]. General Federation of Women's Clubs [Cited 2012 Dec 17]. Available from: www.GFWC.org.

46. Solberg WU, Martha G. Ripley: pioneer doctor and social reformer. Minnesota History. 1964;39:1–17.

47. Young S. Anna Howard Shaw [Internet]. Sue Young Histories 2007 [Cited 2012 Feb 25]. Available from: www.sueyounghistories.com/archives/2007/11/26/anna howard-shaw-and-homeopathy.html.

48. Thompson P (adapted text). Through the front doors: methodist women's journey toward ordination – Anna Snowden Oliver and Anna Howard Shaw [Internet]. Emory University, Candler School of Theology [Cited 2012 Mar 9]. Available from: www.pitts.emory.edu/community/exhibits/womensord/page3.cfm.

49. McNamara O. Generations. A history of Boston University School of Medicine 1848–1998. Boston: Trustees of Boston University; 1998. p. 35.

50. Rasmussen C. A medical pioneer's many firsts. The Los Angeles Times. 1997 Feb 3.

51. Bakken GM, Farrington B. Encyclopedia of women in the American West. Thousand Oaks: Sage Publications; 2003. p. 99.

52. Ozarin LD. Women in psychiatry: 19th century obstacles [Internet]. Psychiatric News. 18 Apr 1997 [Cited 2012 Feb 17]. Available from: www.psychnews.org/pnews/07–04–18/hx.html.

53. Barrus C. Gynaecological disorders and their relation to insanity. Am J Insanity. 1895;51:475–91.

54. Barrus C. Insanity in young women. J Nerv Ment Dis. 1896;21:377–87.

55. Bond CH. Part III, – psychological retrospect: American. Br J Psychiatry. 1897;43:174–85.

56. Hirshbein L. Sex and gender in psychiatry: a view from history. J Med Human. 2010;31:155–70. doi:10.1007/s10912-010-9105-5.

57. Thierot NM. Negotiating illness: doctors, patients, and families in the nineteenth century. J Hist Behav Sci. 2001;37(Fall):349–68.

58. Barrus C. Nursing the Insane. New York: The Macmillan Company; 1908.

59. Book reviews. Am J Psychiatry. 1908;65:550.

60. Book review. Nursing the Insane. Cal State J Med. 1908;6:399.

61. The public service. Nursing the Insane. J Am Med Assoc 1908;51:239.

62. Bacon EM. The book of Boston. Boston: The Book of Boston Company; 1916. p. 307.

63. Leavitt JW. Birthing and anesthesia: the debate over twilight sleep. J Women Cult Soc. 1980;6(1):147–64.

64. Hairston AH. The debate over twilight sleep: women influencing their medicine. J Womens Health. 1995;5(5):489–99.

65. Young S. Caroline Brown Winslow, 1822–1896 [Internet] Sue Young Histories 2007 [Cited 2012 Aug 18]. Available from: http://sueyounghistories.com/archives/2007/11/18/caroline-brown-winslow-and-homeopathy/.

66. Calkins LM. "Roberts, Grace" [Internet]. African American National Biography, edited by Ed. H.L. Gates, Jr., edited by Evelyn Brooks Higginbotham. Oxford African American Studies Center [Cited 2012 Feb 24]. Available from: http://oxford.aasc.com/article/opr/t0001/e3610.

67. Czerkas J. Helen Pitts Douglass 1838–1903[Internet] [Cited 2012 Mar 2]. Available from: http://www.fomh.org/Data/Documents/HelenPittsDouglass.pdf. Accessed 7 Mar 2012.

68. Millard CB. Destiny of the republic. New York: Doubleday; 2011. p. 155–6, 217–9.

69. Deppisch LM. The white house physician. Jefferson: McFarland & Company; 2007. p. 52–4.

70. James ET, James JW, Boyer PS. Notable American women. A biographical dictionary. Boston: Harvard University Press; 1971. p. 472.

71. Looby C. The Complete Civil War Journal and Selected Letters of Thomas Wentworth Higginson [Internet]. Chicago: University of Chicago Press: 2000. p 316 [Cited 2012 Mar 15]. Available from: http://books.google.com/books?id=w_ak6M_fza8C%pg=RA1-PA316&1pg=RA1-PA316&dq=Thomas+Wentworth+Higginson+homeopath.

72. Cross W. Gullah culture in America. Westport: Praeger Publishers; 2008. p. 124–6.

73. Richards MS. Towne, Laura Matilda (1825–1901) [Internet]. In: Edgar W. The South Carolina Encyclopedia. Columbia: University of South Carolina Press; 2006 [Cited 2012 Mar 19]. Available from: http://sc150civilwar.palmettohistory.org/edu/people/Towne-LauraM.htm.

74. Penn Center, St. Helena Island, Beaufort Co, SC [Internet]. 2004 [Cited 2012 Mar 19]. Available from: http://www.beaufort-sc.com/penn/.

75. Editorial. Bringing women to the forefront of science and medicine. Lancet. 2012;379:867. doi:10.1016/50140-6796(12)60286-4.

The Homeopathic Scalpel: Contributions to Surgery from the World of Homeopathy

4

In the 1830s and 1840s, American homeopaths and allopaths displayed a respect for one another that was short-lived. During these early years, it was possible for physicians of both schools to consult with one another and cross-refer patients. By the late 1840s, however, professional rivalry had intensified, and newly created institutions such as the American Institute of Homeopathy (AIH) and American Medical Association (AMA) defended and promoted the respective interests of each school. As homeopathy became increasingly marginalized from mainstream American medicine, dialog between the schools ceased, no doubt stimulated by the AMA's code of ethics prohibiting its members from consulting with a homeopath. Thus, whereas a homeopath at first experienced little difficulty in referring a patient to a surgeon, this had become practically impossible by the 1850s. William Tod Helmuth remarked, "In those days the opposition of Allopathists to everything Homoeopathic handicapped those of our own school who attempted surgical performances. If an error should chance to be committed, or an operation prove a failure, or the patient succumb, such results were given as additional grounds to prove the incompetency of the Homeopathists" [1]. During the Civil War (1861–1865), homeopaths were excluded from all military medical appointments in the Union army, unless they confined their practice to conventional medicine, although there were some exceptions, such as George Beebe. Thus marginalized, homeopaths took the only course open to them: they trained their own surgeons and included lectures on surgery and practical experience in their medical school curricula. In going their own way, they achieved some notable success.

Homeopaths participated in the development of surgery, yet their role has been airbrushed out of the official narrative. As an example, in response to a question about the activity of homeopaths in ophthalmology, the author learned that the American Academy of Ophthalmology has no such record and that the main ophthalmic textbooks were silent on the matter. The director of the Museum of Vision of the American Academy of Ophthalmology, Jenny Benjamin, stated that: "After hours of searching, I have to conclude that homeopathy has been purposely left out of the official ophthalmic literature … because of the backlash against it by the AMA and allopathic physicians." She then noted that, having come up empty, after some "digging around online," she came up with a wealth of information [2]. Much the same applies to other surgical specialties in relation to homeopathy.

In his exhaustive compendium of early surgical history from 1775 to 1900, Rutkow identified a large number of published textbooks and monographs relating to the development of surgery in the United States [3]. Rutkow undertook this survey because, as he put it, his mentors and colleagues either ignored their nineteenth-century ancestors or knew little about them. As he collected source material, he was struck by the originality and "crude eloquence" of many nineteenth-century surgical tomes and the "ingenuity and boldness with which early American surgeons approached seemingly unsolvable surgical problems" [3, p. xviii]. If, as Rutkow states, the legacy of regular surgeons has been neglected, then it could be said that the very existence of homeopathic surgeons has sunk without trace. Indeed, the term "homeopathic surgeon" may strike some as the description of an extraterrestrial being. Yet, in counting the surgeons mentioned in Rutkow's textbook, around 40 were trained as homeopaths. As with their regular counterparts, there was variability in scholarship, productivity, and influence, but some homeopaths clearly stand out. Unfortunately for the entire field of medicine, the apartheid-like status of homeopathy has resulted in the two cultures running on separate tracks, and whatever mingling took place on a personal level has not been well recorded. Homeopaths certainly acknowledged and respected orthodox surgery and incorporated its advances into their practice. It was not infrequent for homeopaths to train under regular surgeons or attend clinics for postgraduate education, and there was clearly a level of direct professional contact. However, allopathic surgeons generally failed to acknowledge the innovations made by surgeons of the homeopathic school until homeopathy was a dying force, and even then such surgeons were not remembered for their homeopathic heritage. Nevertheless, in some

J. Davidson, *A Century of Homeopaths*,
DOI 10.1007/978-1-4939-0527-0_4, © Springer Science+Business Media New York 2014

cases, the contributions of homeopathic surgeons, such as with William Tod Helmuth (1833–1902) and Edward C. Franklin (1822–1885), were recognized by regular surgeons. Moreover, a number of twentieth-century homeopathic surgeons were accepted as fellows of the American College of Surgeons.

It is clear from Rutkow's accounts that homeopaths shared in the "originality and eloquence" of which he spoke. They were quite creative in inventing new procedures and devices and in describing clinical signs. The gynecologist Henry Guernsey developed a "uterine elevator" for retroversion of the uterus [4]. E.A. Munger designed a new splint for compound fractures of the femur [5, pp. 501–502], Ralph Lloyd developed a stereocampimeter for assessing visual fields, Butler was an innovator in the surgical application of electricity [5, pp. 949–959], Copeland achieved fame for corneal transplantation, and Munson's name has been perpetuated by Munson's sign, as found in keratoconus. George Beebe of Chicago reportedly performed the first successful intestinal anastomosis on record and pioneered the use of carbolic acid to treat sarcoma; Alonzo Boothby of Boston is believed to have been the first to perform a nephrectomy (as well as being father to one the twentieth century's most famous anesthesiologists, Walter Boothby, who is discussed in Chap. 5). Dr. N. Schneider was yet another early homeopathic surgeon who commanded respect from his allopathic competitors and performed one of the first successful excisions of an intracranial glioma (tumor) from within the cranial cavity [1, 6–8]. Many decades later, Emmons Briggs earned fame as a gallbladder and intestinal surgeon [9–11], codeveloped a new method for aseptic anastomosis of the intestine, and published in leading medical journals – he also contributed to the homeopathic materia medica of the remedy stramonium, providing indications for its use [12, 13]. (Briggs also played a critical role in the transformation of the Boston University School of Medicine from a homeopathic to an allopathic institution, when, as college registrar, he chaired the committee to recommend on future directions of the medical school. It was the committee's recommendation to abandon homeopathy and make major changes to the curriculum.)

In the manner they practiced surgery, homeopaths were indistinguishable from conventional surgeons, apart from their readiness to incorporate homeopathic remedies, either (1) in preparation for surgery, (2) to aid postoperative recovery, (3) as an alternative to surgery, or (4) to treat problems that the operation might have not helped.

Joseph Fobes, a faculty member at New York Medical Center () and one-time president of its alumni association, asked rhetorically how it was possible to be a homeopathic surgeon. He went on to elaborate that such a person differed from the regular surgeon by knowing the homeopathic materia medica, which put them in the position of understanding the person with the disease, as well as understanding the disease itself. In consequence, the homeopathic surgeon "has all the advantages of any other surgeon, and added to that he has a working knowledge of the individual action of homeopathic drugs on individuals. He must be a student of symptoms" [14].

Not surprisingly, to the homeopath, any surgical practice that made use of homeopathic remedies was superior to practice that did not make such recourse. W.A. Guild boldly asserted that "This superiority, particularly distinct in preoperative and post-operative care of cases not considered the best of surgical risks, is not established by isolated cases, but by large numbers of varied ones." Not only was homeopathy useful, according to Guild, but it showed itself to good advantage in the higher-risk cases. Guild then provided the interesting example of August Bier, who used pre-etherization with a homeopathic 3X dose 1 day prior to surgery as a prophylactic against postanesthetic respiratory complications; Guild said that his experience in over 300 cases bore out Bier's practice and that few if any patients experienced postoperative nausea and other problems. In addition, ether pretreatment reduced the degree of fear that occurred during induction of anesthesia at surgery [15].

Proceeding from this general overview, the detailed story of individual homeopathic surgeons will be chronicled by specialty. Those singled out here are the more distinguished homeopathic surgeons, but it is worth remembering that surgery was a lucrative profession for many homeopaths, which gave rise to much lament among the leaders of organized homeopathy who saw their discipline sliding into decline in the 1920s. As part of the blame, they attributed diminished commitment to homeopathic principles and practice – an arduous pursuit with poorer recompense – in favor of the greater lure of surgery.

Dental Surgery

Josiah Foster Flagg

The Flagg family occupies a prominent place in the history of American dentistry, surgery, and anesthesia. Josiah Foster Flagg (1788/1789–1852/1853) belonged to a famous family of American dentists, some of whose names are so similar that they can easily be confused. Some effort will therefore be made to clear up the matter of identification. Lt Col Josiah Flagg served in the Revolutionary War and married Hannah Collins, who produced a son also named Josiah Flagg Jr. (1763–1816). The younger Josiah is known as the father of American dentistry, having designed what is believed to have been the first dental chair. After the death of his first wife, the older Josiah married Eliza Brewster, who gave birth to a son named John Foster Brewster Flagg (1802–1872), who in turn had a son called Josiah Foster Flagg (1828–1903). All the Flaggs were dentists, and because of their similar names, professions, and, to some extent, achievements (e.g., their work with ether), it is no surprise that at times they have been confused, especially the half brother contemporaries Josiah Foster Flagg and John Foster Brewster Flagg [16, 17].

Josiah Flagg graduated from Harvard Medical School in 1815 and pursued further study with John Warren, one of the country's foremost surgeons. Warren must have thought well of the young Flagg, for he asked Flagg to provide many of the illustrations in Warren's book on the mammalian nervous system [3, p. 26]. Flagg was a man of many talents, being known for his anatomical art, wood engraving, and possibly also his silversmith work [18]. He specialized in dentistry but never abandoned the practice of medicine. Among his contributions were the development of forceps for extracting different types of teeth and the invention of porcelain ("mineral") teeth to replace the ivory, hippopotamus, and human teeth which were then in use. His 1822 book *The Family Dentist* is believed to have been the first dental book written for the general consumer and had three goals: (1) to provide a clear and concise description of the structure and formation of human teeth, (2) to describe the most common dental diseases and how the reader might better prevent or treat them, and (3) to guard against "the injurious practice of ignorant operators" [19]. It has been said that the book revolutionized American dentistry through its first analysis of the human teeth [20]. As the earliest consumer guide to promote better dental hygiene, it is a significant work.

Flagg was a well-regarded member of the Boston medical and dental communities. At a time when ether anesthesia had just been introduced by Morton, a Boston dentist, on October 16, 1846, Flagg created controversy by a series of letters to the *Boston Medical and Surgical Journal* challenging Morton's patent, as well as his intention to keep the ingredients secret and retain exclusive marketing rights. Morton found an initial ally in the surgeon Henry Bigelow, who agreed with the need for patents, although he offered different justifications at different times, ranging from secrecy, the assurance of competent use, and protection of intellectual property, before finally rejecting the basis for any patent of ether for scientific reasons [21]. In reaction to Morton and Bigelow, Flagg wrote to the journal on December 2, 1846, attacking their motives and claiming that Morton misrepresented the ingredient as "letheon" when in fact it was simply sulfuric ether. Flagg predicted that local doctors would obtain ether without purchasing it from Morton and stated that he himself had already used it hundreds of times on his patients. He doubted that ether gas was patentable, saying "It would seem to me like patent sun-light or patent moonshine" [22]. Flagg was annoyed by Bigelow's insinuations that dentists were more secretive in their work than physicians and that dentistry was a trade rather than a higher skill. Bigelow

not unexpectedly replied at length, followed again by a second letter from Flagg. Although neither man changed his position as a result of this exchange, other correspondence suggested that Flagg's views were representative of the larger community of doctors and dentists in Boston [23]. Flagg later began to use chloroform in his practice and reported his experience in the *Boston Medical and Surgical Journal* in 1848. Having found it safe, rapid in onset and offset, he preferred it for simple dental operations, while he used ether for more complicated procedures [24]. On the matter of ether, Flagg's half brother John Foster Brewster Flagg wrote a book entitled *Ether and Chloroform*, which he dedicated to Josiah Foster Flagg, "with my sincere thanks for the independent course manifested by yourself at the commencement of Ether inhalation in your city" [25]. As with his half brother, John Foster Brewster Flagg wished to give as impartial an account of ether as he possibly could and recognized the various conflicts of interest that surrounded its introduction and its many claimants to original ownership.

Phrenology was emerging as a popular movement in medicine. Flagg adopted it with gusto, as did many prominent doctors in Boston, including Flagg's mentor John Collins Warren. Flagg served on the publication committee of the Boston Phrenology Society's (BPS) journal, the *Annals of Phrenology*, and was engaged in the pursuit of phrenology as a legitimate scientific topic. Two volumes appeared, each of about 500 pages in length. Interestingly, the BPS disbanded after they reached the conclusion that phrenology's fundamental tenets had been demonstrated to their satisfaction [26]. Phrenology has long been discounted as a pseudoscience, but in the early nineteenth century, many respected scientists considered that the shape of the skull revealed important information about the size of brain regions, each of which had its own function. In Boston, as in other cities of Europe and North America, groups of medical doctors would meet to discuss this topic, and many of the inner cadre who established the *Boston Medical and Surgical Journal* (now the *New England Journal of Medicine*) subscribed to the creed. Flagg was part of this esteemed circle, attesting to his stature in the Boston medical community.

Flagg played a seminal role in the professional organization of homeopathy [27, 28], being joined by Samuel Gregg and the Wesselhoeft brothers in this effort. On Christmas Eve in 1840, Flagg met with two homeopathic members of the Massachusetts Medical Society to discuss Hahnemann's approach to prescribing; other similar meetings followed over the next weeks, and on February 2, 1841, the group resolved to form an association to investigate the teachings and practice of homeopathy. A constitution and set of bylaws were established, including the requirement that members should also be members of the Massachusetts Medical Society. They referred to this new organization as the Homeopathic Fraternity and presided over its growth to

50 members by 1852, at which time it changed its name to the Massachusetts Homeopathic Medical Society, an organization which continued to exist into the mid-twentieth century. In 1843, the New York Homeopathic Physicians' Society invited homeopaths across the country to attend a meeting with the express purpose of forming a national association. A planning committee was formed, and on April 10, 1844, the American Institute of Homeopathy (AIH) held its first meeting. The AIH set forth two major objectives: (1) to reform and augment the materia medica and (2) to restrain physicians from claiming to be competent homeopaths without proper study and training. The elected president and vice-president at the first meeting were, respectively, Constantine Hering and Josiah Flagg, who also was called on to chair the meeting. Six boards of censors were appointed to examine the credentials of applicants for AIH membership, and Flagg served on one of these. Flagg was a man of great creativity and open to the unprejudiced examination of new ideas. He played an important role in organizing homeopathy as a force in the nineteenth-century American healthcare.

Gynecology and Obstetrics

George Taylor

George Herbert Taylor (1821–1896) was a well-known author who wrote *Diseases of Women: Their Causes, Prevention, and Radical Cure* and at least seven other books. Besides being proficient in gynecology, he was famous for introducing the Swedish mechano-movement cure into the United States. As the specialty of orthopedics was taking shape in the United States, massage, Swedish mechano-movement, was the subject of considerable interest, and Taylor was an early leader in this field.

Rebecca Lee Dorsey

Rebecca Dorsey (1859–1954) was a respected and experienced obstetrician for 60 years in Los Angeles, where she delivered over 4,000 babies without loss of baby or mother or even one case of puerperal infection. She has been referred to in greater detail in Chap. 3.

George Southwick

George Southwick (1859–1930) taught on the faculty at Boston University Medical School and authored two books on obstetrics and gynecology, one for students and the other for consumers. He was elected fellow of the American College of Surgeons.

James Wood

James Wood (1858–1948) authored *A Textbook of Gynecology*, which was unique for including a large collection of illustrations from the English Royal College of Surgeons' medical museum.

James Ward and Florence Nightingale Ward

James and Florence Nightingale Ward were (for a time) a husband-and-wife team in the San Francisco area, and both were distinguished homeopathic surgeons.

Florence Nightingale Ward (1860–1919) has been described in the chapter on women in homeopathy. She received additional training in Europe and befriended many eminent surgeons and homeopaths in the United States, including the Mayo brothers, William Tod Helmuth, the Lilienthals, and E. Beecher Hooker. She was known as one of the country's finest female surgeons and was elected fellow of the American College of Surgeons. Although some sources, including the *San Francisco Examiner*, have claimed that she was the first woman to be so elected, five women had preceded her as fellows in the first year of the college's existence. Ward was accepted the next year, 1914, making her one of the earliest women fellows [29]. Ward served two terms as president of the American Institute of Homeopathy, as well as of the Institute's Society of Obstetrics. In World War I, she worked on the Medical Board of National Defense and served as head of the base hospital unit of female physicians [30].

At a time in medicine when surgeons treated women with neurosis by removing healthy reproductive organs, Ward lent her voice to those female surgeons opposed to this practice.

James Ward (1861–1939) trained at the New York Homeopathic College and spent two periods in Europe to further his experience. He was hired as professor of physiology at the Hahnemann Medical College of the Pacific in 1883 and in 1893 became one of the country's first professors of gynecology [31]. In 1901, he was appointed health commissioner of the city of San Francisco, a position he retained until 1907. In 1903, he was elected president of the commission, although not without some struggle due to opponents of homeopathy who at first succeeded in electing Michael Casey, a nonphysician who was a popular Teamsters Union official. During Ward's term as commissioner, the San Francisco earthquake struck on April 20, 1906, and he had to deal with the enormous public health challenge of preventing typhoid and cholera epidemics. He provided effective leadership in working with civilian and military authorities to inspect food, test drinking water, repair plumbing and latrines, and teach those living in temporary accommodation about sanitation and prevention of disease [31]. Perhaps by virtue of his power in local politics and friendship with the mayor, Ward was able to advance the cause of homeopathy in San Francisco by acquiring two wards in the city and county hospital for use by local homeopaths. Other accomplishments include service as president of the California State Homeopathic Medical Society. In 1923, Ward announced the formation of the Homeopathic Foundation of California, which some years later played an important role in bringing Otto Guttentag (see Chap. 15) to the United States from Germany. In 1920, Ward had a hand in procuring a historically important document when he co-purchased the long unpublished 6th edition of Hahnemann's *Organon*, which he obtained for the Hahnemann Library in San Francisco and where, at the University of California San Francisco (UCSF), it can still be found.

Among his publications was a comprehensive review of ovarian surgery [32], in which he described the progress made in this form of surgery throughout the nineteenth century, as well as his own experience and recommendations on practical management. All in all, the tone of the article is such that it could have been written by an allopathic surgeon and all the references, except for two of Helmuth's papers, are to conventional surgeons. Ward was moved to write this review because of the varied rates of mortality associated with ovarian surgery, "which overshadows in importance and interest any other chapter in the study of the subject." Of interest is the fact that he makes no mention of homeopathy in the immediate aftermath of surgery, although he did teach homeopathy at the University of California San Francisco until the time of his death in 1939. Ward wrote a series of papers on the fundamentals of homeopathy, which were based on lectures he gave to homeopathic nurses [33–38].

Lucy Waite

Lucy Waite (1860–1943) rose to fame as one of Chicago's most eminent surgeons. However, the path to success did not come easily. After qualifying with a homeopathic degree in 1883, Waite was not accepted by her allopathic peers until she obtained an orthodox medical degree. Until that occurred, Waite was denied her rightful place as director of the Mary Thompson Hospital for Women and Children. It had been Thompson's wish that Waite succeed her as director of the hospital, but the all-male allopathic hospital staff blocked her approval. Only after Thompson's replacement resigned a few years later, and Waite had in the interim obtained her regular degree, did she receive the votes to take over as director, a post which she held for many years and which she filled with distinction. Waite not only obtained two medical degrees but also spent some years in Europe developing her

surgical skills and returned to Chicago to transition from general practice to the practice of gynecology and abdominal surgery. She married the famous allopathic surgeon Byron Robinson – a marriage which resulted in much productive academic work together. Waite published a number of papers and book chapters, including a critique of current surgical practices for retrodeviations of the uterus, which was published in the *Journal of American Medical Association* [39]. This paper is notable for the clarity with which it frames and answers three key questions as to the necessity, safety, and success of the procedures, which the author determined to be unnecessary, unsafe, and unsuccessful.

Although Waite became increasingly detached from homeopathy in her practice, she remained active in homeopathic affairs, presenting at homeopathic congresses and serving on committees of homeopathic societies well into her career. She also joined the American Medical Association, founded a nursing school at the Mary Thompson Hospital, cofounded the Chicago Women's Club, and was president of the Medical Women's Club of Chicago in 1904–1905. Waite received accolades from some of Chicago's finest male surgeons, such as Nicholas Senn and Christian Fenger, both of whom were well known nationally. Senn, for example, described Waite as "one of the ablest and most successful surgeons in this city" and said that "under her supervision [the Mary Thompson Hospital] has prospered wonderfully." Fenger observed that "Dr. Lucy Waite has attained high rank in the profession by hard work of a superior kind and this in spite of the difficulties which attend the pioneer … As an operator and an abdominal surgeon, she has an enviable reputation" [40].

Walter Crump

Walter Crump (1869–1945), poet, physician, and champion of civil rights, trained at the New York Homeopathic College (NYHMC), where he later held an adjunct faculty position in obstetrics and gynecology; in 1936, he was made emeritus professor (Fig. 4.1). He belonged to the county, state, and national homeopathic societies and is best known for his creation of medical training opportunities for African-Americans. It is more than likely that Crump's liberal attitude was shaped by his father, who was an ardent Civil War abolitionist and friend of John Brown. In 1928, Crump established at NYHMC the first scholarship program in the United States to support minority medical students. A 1944 tribute in the *Journal of the National Medical Association* stated, "We wish Dr. Crump to know how greatly appreciated is his service to this Clinic, and in more ways than one, to the Negro race. We regard him as a stalwart champion for the civil, professional, and economic rights of minorities, the Negro race in particular" [41].

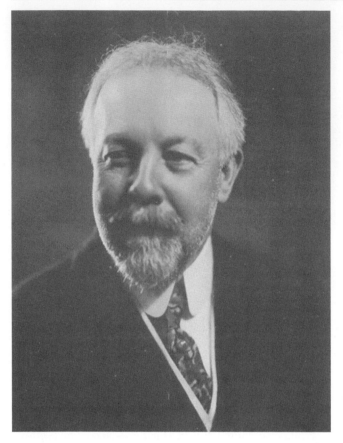

Fig. 4.1 Walter Crump. New York surgeon and advocate for training of African-Americans (Courtesy of Journal National Medical Association)

He was a trustee of the Tuskegee Institute and of Howard University. In recognition of his dedication and visionary contributions to the college, he was appointed emeritus professor at NYHMC. Although Crump is not remembered today for being a homeopath, in the early stages of his career, he was substantially involved in homeopathic research as director of the proving committee that tested the effects of different homeopathic remedies in healthy volunteers [42]. As Anschutz noted in 1902, "For the past few years the Alpha Chapter through the special efforts of Dr. Walter Crump and others has appointed committees to consider and map out plans for the proving of remedies according to the most approved methods." This amounted to quite an ambitious project, and it was interesting to note that because of the onerous nature of the proving protocols, which required numerous visits and exceedingly detailed physical examinations and scrutiny of symptoms, the drop-out rate of subjects was often high; at times, even the assessors, as in Crump's case, were unavailable for the assessments because of clinical obligations. Crump was part of the team that tested homeopathic doses of radium in the 2X to 6X potencies [43].

Geraldine Burton-Branch

Geraldine Burton-Branch (born 1908) was one of the first recipients of the Crump fellowship, which enabled her to enroll at NYHMC in 1932. She graduated MD in 1936 and, 30 years later, supplemented her qualifications with a Master's in Public Health (MPH) degree from the University of California at Los Angeles (UCLA) in 1962. The story behind her acceptance into medical school is a curious one. While working as a high school teacher in New York City, she was about to undergo orthopedic surgery, and the doctor asked her to take a sleeping pill the night beforehand. Resisting his request, the doctor told Geraldine that, as it was his last day on the service, she would be doing him a great favor. When she asked what favor he would repay her with, he asked her what she wanted. Her reply was, "I want to go to medical school," whereupon he remarked, "Oh, I know who can send you to medical school! Walter Crump" [44]. Dr. Burton-Branch went on to practice gynecology and obstetrics, as well as public health and family planning, and serve as a medical examiner and district health officer. Early in her career, she moved to California, spending the rest of her professional life in the Watts area of Los Angeles, working up to 2001. Progressive in her outlook, she set up a pre-paid health plan in Watts many years before health maintenance organizations (HMOs) came into existence. She was instrumental in creating a new middle school to relieve overcrowding in the Watts school system, and as district health officer she gained praise for her handling of the health department merger between county and city, a crucial move that enabled the area to receive federal and state health funding. In 1965, the infamous Watts riots occurred, taking the lives of over 34 and injuring over 1,000; Burton-Branch was one of several community leaders who committed themselves to repair the damage. She played a key role in dismantling the enormous and unwieldy Los Angeles County, which was then the nation's most populous, into five smaller and more manageable districts. She was named senior health official for the southern parts of the county, paving the way for the Watts Health Center and Health Foundation and the Golden Age Adult Day Health Center. She played a lead role in establishing the Charles Drew University of Medicine and Science in 1966, an institution which has proved to be a vital resource for African-American medicine in the Los Angeles area and on the national stage. Burton-Branch was awarded an honorary degree by Drew in 2010 [45], which established the Geraldine Burton-Branch Scholarship, awarded to a graduate who best exemplifies potential to build, shape, and improve the overall health of underserved communities. Also, in 2010, Burton-Branch followed the example of her mentor Walter Crump in setting up an Adopt-a-Scholar program at her alma mater in New York. Both Crump and

Burton-Branch are outstanding examples of homeopathy's social conscience. Their labors have kept alive into the twentieth and twenty-first centuries the tradition set by those nineteenth-century homeopaths who opened the doors into medicine for American minorities, as well as provided access to healthcare for minorities and the impoverished.

Urology

Bukk Carleton

Bukk Carleton (1856–1914) was trained at the New York Homeopathic College and practiced urology. He served as chair of genitourinary and kidney diseases at the Metropolitan Postgraduate School of Medicine and, between 1902 and 1913, as chair of urology at NYMC. Carleton's *Manual of Genito-Urinary and Venereal Diseases* was the first homeopathic text on the subject and became a best seller. Among his other books were *Medical and Surgical Diseases of the Kidneys and Ureters*, *Uropoietic Disease*, *Disorders of the Sexual Organs of Men*, and *A Practical Treatise on Urological and Venereal Disease*. He was one of America's most prolific authors on urological surgery, yet remains an obscure figure in surgical history today [3, p. 360].

Sprague Carleton

Bukk Carleton's son, Sprague, followed in his father's footsteps and succeeded him as chair of the department at New York Medical College, a position he held until 1948. It was under his leadership that a urology training program was established and the department recognized as an independent program. He participated in homeopathic activities, for example, serving as discussant on the topic of bladder tumors at the AIH meeting in 1921 [46]. He served as chairman of the institute's committee on amendments to the constitution and bylaws, as well as a term as trustee. He wrote a paper entitled *Moral Prophylaxis*: *A Criticism with Suggestions*, published by the Homeopathic Society of Pennsylvania [47]. Carleton was elected as fellow of the American College of Surgeons. In 1956, he received the NYMC Medal of Honor. His name is perpetuated through the establishment of the Sprague Carleton, MD, Award at NYMC, given for proficiency in urology.

George Nagamatsu

George Nagamatsu (1903–2000) graduated from NYHMC in 1934, at a time when the school was still homeopathic.

He was the first Nisei Japanese American to be named chairman of an academic urology department [48]. Nagamatsu is considered to have been an outstanding urologist. He developed a surgical approach for removing kidney and adrenal tumors, known as the Nagamatsu dorsolumbar incision, which is still used to remove large retroperitoneal masses. Before entering medical school, Nagamatsu earned a doctoral degree in electrical engineering and was employed by the Otis Elevator Company, an experience that positioned him favorably to develop new instruments for urological surgery. Among many honors that he was accorded are the following: president of the American Urology Association (AUA), New York Section; chairman of the AUA biomedical device group; consultant to the armed forces on biomedical devices; American Japanese Medical Ambassador; Golden Cane Award of the AUA; Order of the Treasure from the Emperor of Japan; and NYMC Medal of Honor. Nagamatsu has been accorded much of the credit for Japanese prominence in urology over the last 50 years [49].

Leonard P. Wershub

Leonard Wershub (1902–1969) was a well-regarded urologist who graduated from NYHMC in 1927. He joined the faculty, where he rose to the rank of professor in urology. He was well known as a surgeon and medical historian. Wershub published in the peer-reviewed literature, including a large series on renal tuberculosis in the *Journal of the American Medical Association*, and authored books including *The Human Testis*: *A Clinical Treatise*, *Urology and Industry*; *Urology from Antiquity to the twentieth Century*; *Sexual Impotence in the Male*, and *One Hundred Years of Medical Progress*: *A History of the New York Medical College, Flower and Fifth Avenue Hospitals*. Wershub was president of the NYMC Alumni Association between 1947 and 1950, and his name is remembered there through the Leonard P. Wershub Medal of Honor. At the time of his death, he was president of the medical board of Flower and Fifth Avenue Hospitals. Internationally, he was recognized by the Spanish Academy of Surgeons, who made him an honorary fellow.

General Surgery

Edward C. Franklin

Rutkow and Rutkow [50] have written about Franklin as follows: "Not only was Franklin important to homeopathic surgeons, but his influence extended well into the ranks of the allopaths. He is among the most active and prolific of all mid-nineteenth century American surgeons, both regular and

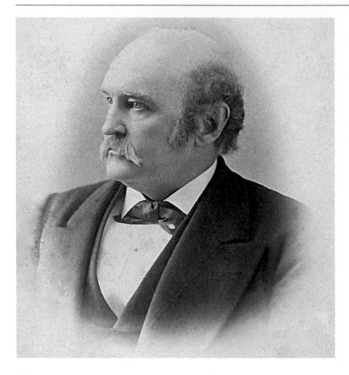

Fig. 4.2 Edward Franklin. Leading homeopathic general surgeon, author of textbooks (Image reproduced by permission, Bentley Historical Library, Box 2, University of Michigan Faculty Portrait Collection)

sectarian." Nonetheless, Franklin is a forgotten figure in the history of American surgery [3, p. 346]. Franklin (1822–1885) was a grandnephew of Benjamin Franklin and trained in New York under one of the country's leading surgeons, Valentine Mott (Fig. 4.2). He began his career as an allopathic practitioner and was appointed deputy health officer for California and then as physician to the Panama Railroad Hospital. While in Panama, he acquired malaria and failed to respond to regular treatment but did respond to homeopathy, an experience that convinced Franklin about the value of this form of medicine. He returned to the United States in the mid-1850s, initially to private practice and later to an academic position at the Homeopathic Medical College of Missouri. In 1861, and by now a well-regarded physician, he volunteered his services in the Union army and was accepted as Brigade Surgeon of Volunteers; he was also put in charge of the US army general hospital at Mound City, Ill. Apparently, he neither volunteered nor was asked about his record as a homeopath, but after it was discovered that he was treating soldiers homeopathically, he was ushered out of the military in 1863. However, he left his mark by being mentioned positively for the management of over 30 cases in an authoritative government publication on medicine in the Civil War. The same document included his extensive report on management of the medical corps and military hospital where he served.

Franklin returned to the world of academia, clinical practice, and medical politics. He was appointed professor of surgery at the Missouri College and distilled his wartime experiences into an 800-page textbook, *Science and Art of Surgery*, which became standard at all homeopathic medical schools. The book also contained a detailed section on surgical history. The role of homeopathic medicines received attention, with *Calendula* being recommended for suppurating wounds, *Lachesis* for traumatic gangrene, *Corydalis formosa* for syphilis, and *Hypericum perforatum* for painful wounds and nerve injury [51]. In 1873, Franklin published the second edition of his book. A review from that year describes Franklin as "first in the field, and the ripe experience which as Surgeon of Volunteers he gathered during our late unpleasantness, he spreads now before his students (and every reader is his student) in this volume" [52]. As with most homeopathic texts on surgery, what was written about the technical aspects of operating differed little from what was found in orthodox texts, but more attention was given to conservative management with (homeopathic) remedies or on their use pre- and postoperatively. In 1877, Franklin completed a monograph on *The Homeopathic Treatment of Spinal Curvatures According to the New Principle*, followed shortly afterwards by *A Monograph on Mammary Tumors*. Three more books followed: *A Complete Minor Surgery*, *The Practitioner's and Student's Manual of the Science of Surgery*, and *A Manual of Venereal Disease*. Within the homeopathic community, Franklin served as president of the Western Institute of Homeopathy and the American Institute of Homeopathy, as well as dean of the Homeopathic Medical College of Missouri.

Franklin did not escape conflict and was embroiled in one particular scandal when he was professor of surgery at the Homeopathic College of the University of Michigan [53]. He had challenged the professional and moral character of one Professor Maclean, which came to the attention of the University Regents who, on May 3, 1882, investigated Franklin's charges and found them to be baseless. In return, Maclean accused Franklin of deceiving and misleading the public with an untruthful treatment outcome report and falsification of university statistics. Allegations were also made that Franklin incorrectly claimed the famous orthopedic surgeon, Professor Lewis Sayre, adopted some of Franklin's techniques in applying plaster of Paris casts, and referred patients to Dr. Franklin in St. Louis. When Dr. Maclean asked Sayre about these claims, Sayre replied that they were absolutely untrue. When the Board of Regents gave Franklin the opportunity to defend himself, he failed to do so beyond issuing a general denial. He then left Michigan and returned to St. Louis, where he lived for another two years, suffering from angina pectoris before dying of a myocardial infarction in 1885. Exactly where truth lay in the matter of the Michigan allegations may be difficult to determine as turbulent relations between the university's regulars and homeopaths led to constant infighting at the time.

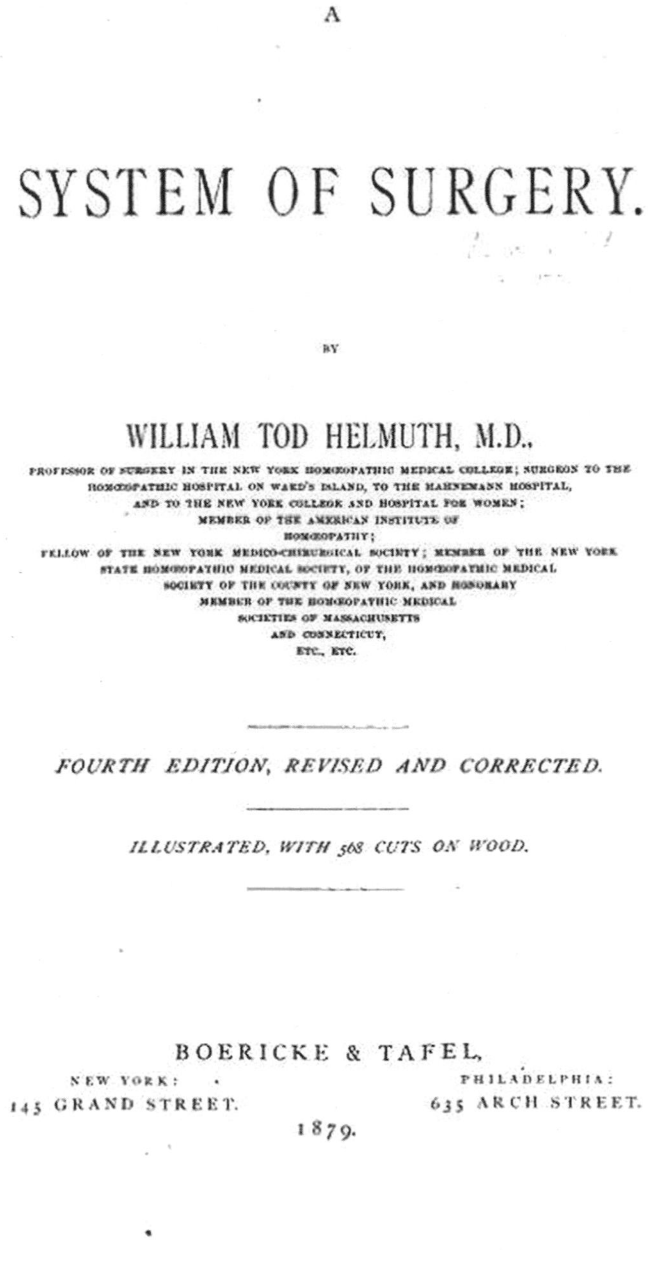

A

SYSTEM OF SURGERY.

BY

WILLIAM TOD HELMUTH, M.D.,

PROFESSOR OF SURGERY IN THE NEW YORK HOMŒOPATHIC MEDICAL COLLEGE; SURGEON TO THE
HOMŒOPATHIC HOSPITAL ON WARD'S ISLAND, TO THE HAHNEMANN HOSPITAL,
AND TO THE NEW YORK COLLEGE AND HOSPITAL FOR WOMEN;
MEMBER OF THE AMERICAN INSTITUTE OF
HOMŒOPATHY;
FELLOW OF THE NEW YORK MEDICO-CHIRURGICAL SOCIETY; MEMBER OF THE NEW YORK
STATE HOMŒOPATHIC MEDICAL SOCIETY, OF THE HOMŒOPATHIC MEDICAL
SOCIETY OF THE COUNTY OF NEW YORK, AND HONORARY
MEMBER OF THE HOMŒOPATHIC MEDICAL
SOCIETIES OF MASSACHUSETTS
AND CONNECTICUT,
ETC., ETC.

FOURTH EDITION, REVISED AND CORRECTED.

ILLUSTRATED, WITH 568 CUTS ON WOOD.

BOERICKE & TAFEL,
NEW YORK: PHILADELPHIA:
145 GRAND STREET.   635 ARCH STREET.
1879.

Fig. 4.3 Title page, Helmuth's System of Surgery, 1879 (In the public domain)

William Tod Helmuth (1833–1902)

Rutkow observed that Helmuth's talent brought homeopathic surgery to its highest level. Within a year of graduation from the Homoeopathic Medical College of Pennsylvania, the remarkably precocious Helmuth had published his first edition of *Surgery and Its Adaptation to Homoeopathic Practice*, a comprehensive and influential book that compared well with conventional texts of the time [54] (Fig. 4.3). The book was hailed by homeopaths as groundbreaking in that, for the first time, a bridge was forged between homeopathy and surgery: or more accurately, one might say that homeopathy

began to embrace surgery as one of its own specialties. As noted, the two disciplines had become disconnected, and, by 1853, scarcely any homeopaths possessed adequate surgical skills. Helmuth's book was to change all that.

Helmuth attained prominence in the homeopathic community, cofounding the Homeopathic Medical College of Missouri and later becoming chair of surgery at the New York Homeopathic Medical College and Flower Hospital and then dean of that institution in 1893. According to Rutkow, he enjoyed outstanding success and was regarded as the doyen of homeopaths. Wershub notes that he was a "gentle, magnetic, humorous, eloquent and brilliant surgeon" [55]. He was one of the first surgeons in the United States to operate under antiseptic conditions when, in 1876, he performed an ovarian resection. It is believed that he was teaching his students the importance of antisepsis in surgery at a time when many US surgeons had not accepted it as a necessary part of their art [56]. Helmuth was a firm advocate of mutual respect between homeopaths and allopaths, arguing that the levels of bigotry, intolerance, and jealousy exceeded the actual differences between the two systems.

Israel Tisdale Talbot

Israel Talbot (1829–1899) was a nineteenth-century homeopathic colossus (Fig. 4.4). He graduated from the Pennsylvania Homeopathic Medical College in 1853 and then from Harvard Medical School in 1854. He was of "mechanical talent" and thus attracted to surgery and is credited with being the first US surgeon to perform a successful tracheotomy on June 5, 1855 [57]. That said, other attempts had already been made with varying success, and even in the eighteenth century, it was a procedure known to American doctors, one of whom had recommended its use in George Washington. Talbot's more modest claim was to have performed the "first successful operation … by Trousseau's method in this country." (Trousseau had previously introduced in France a safer method of tracheotomy.) In Talbot's report, he referred to having conducted 15 operations, 5 of which were associated with a successful outcome [58]. Talbot is known to have perfected tracheotomy techniques long before the procedure was routinely used for acute respiratory distress. As distinguished as he was as a surgeon, Boston University remembers him even more as one whose "principal concern was medical education" and for having had a "lasting effect on the School of Medicine's curriculum" [59, pp. 31–32].

Talbot was the founding dean of Boston University Medical School, holding office from 1873 until 1896, and his name is perpetuated on campus today in the form of the Talbot building (Fig. 4.5). Talbot was one of several well-qualified doctors who were expelled from the state medical

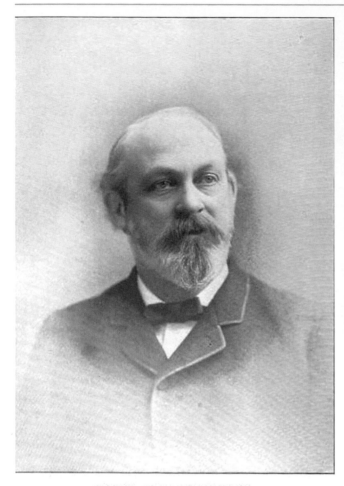

ISRAEL TISDALE TALBOT
Late Dean of Boston University School of Medicine

Fig. 4.4 Israel Tisdale Talbot. Founding dean of Boston University School of Medicine, surgeon and leader in American homeopathy (Image courtesy of Boston University Alumni Library Archives)

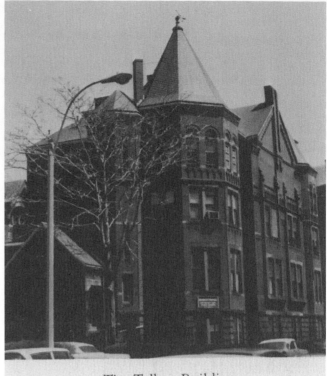

The Talbot Building

Fig. 4.5 Talbot Building (Courtesy of Boston University Alumni Library Archives)

society because of their homeopathic leanings, and he was also forbidden to participate in established hospitals and medical schools. As a result, he threw his energies into creating a parallel system that included a homeopathic society, hospital, and medical school. He was a leader in homeopathic education throughout the nation, serving 15 years as chair of the intercollegiate committee of the AIH and ultimately as its president. He founded and edited the *New England Medical Gazette*. Talbot was a dynamic and attractive personality, although at times he could be something of a martinet. Because he so often emphasized idiopathic and traumatic diseases, he was known to students as "Idiopathic Traumatic Talbot," playing on his initials ITT [59, p. 31].

Other general surgeons have left their mark. *Homer Ostrom* (1852–?) wrote himself into American surgical history with *A Treatise on the Breast and Its Surgical Diseases*, which was the first textbook devoted solely to breast disease.

John Butler (1844–1885) authored two books, *Electricity in Surgery* and *A Text-book of Electro-therapeutics and*

Electro-surgery, as well as edited the *American Journal of Electrology* (Fig. 4.6). At a time when electrosurgery and electrocautery were coming into vogue, his books were in the vanguard, with *Electricity in Surgery* perhaps being the first monograph on the topic [3, p. 191]. It received a positive review in the journal *The Electrician* [60] and was used as a textbook. Rutkow noted that a chapter on cautery as a hemostatic (bloodless surgery) was "an interesting forerunner to Harvey Cushing … and W.T. Bovie's classic paper on electrocoagulation in neurosurgery" [3, p. 84]. which appeared in 1928. While Butler was far from being the first to use electricity in surgery, as he acknowledged in his book, it appears that his use of diathermy as a hemostatic preceded by many years the work of d'Arsonoval and Thompson, who have been credited as the earliest pioneers in this field [61]. In the preface to his book [62]. Butler stressed the need to acquire precision in using electrosurgical techniques, the lack of which he believed was a problem among surgeons who increasingly used electrotherapy. Butler believed that casual use of the technique led to unnecessary failure of surgery. The contents of his book represented a distillation of various papers he had published previously. Butler asserted that "although the knowledge of the use of electricity to medicine and surgery has advanced rapidly, it has not kept pace with the progress of electricity in other branches of science." He went on to

ELECTRICITY

IN

SURGERY.

BY

JOHN BUTLER, M.D.

BOERICKE & TAFEL:

NEW YORK: PHILADELPHIA:

145 GRAND STREET.   1011 ARCH STREET.

1882.

Fig. 4.6 Title page, Electricity in Surgery, by John Butler. 1882 (In the public domain)

UNITED STATES PATENT OFFICE.

JOHN BUTLER, OF NEW YORK, N. Y.

IMPROVEMENT IN ELECTRICAL RHEOSTATS.

Specification forming part of Letters Patent No. **217,331**, dated July 8, 1879; application filed November 8, 1878.

To all whom it may concern:

Be it known that I, JOHN BUTLER, of the city, county, and State of New York, have invented a new and Improved Rheostat, of which the following is a specification.

The object of this invention is to provide a rheostat for electric circuits in which the desired amount of resistance can be quickly obtained and accurately determined and measured.

It consists of a plate of non-conducting material, on which is placed, either on the surface or in a groove, a film of plumbago or a plating of nickel or other suitable resisting material. One end of this resistant is connected with the battery, and the circuit is completed through a movable key, one end whereof is on the resistant, so that by changing the distance of the key from the extremity of the resistant joined to the wire from the battery the amount of resistance is determined at pleasure.

In the accompanying drawings, Figure 1 is a plan of my improved rheostat. Fig. 2 is a section of the same on line *x x*, and Fig. 3 shows a modified form of the improvement. Similar letters of reference indicate corresponding parts.

Referring to the drawings, A represents the bed-plate, supported on legs B. It is made of hard rubber, glass, or any other suitable non-conducting material. In the upper surface of this table is a segmental groove, *a*, having at one end a slotted screw or stud, *b*, passed through the plate and joined underneath to a metal strip, *c*, the other end whereof is connected with the under end of the binding-post *d*, to which the wire *d'* is joined above. In this groove is placed a film of plumbago, (indicated by *a'*,) or other suitable resisting material, as will be hereinafter referred to.

The key C, for regulating the resistance, is composed of the horizontal arm *e*, one end pivoted to the stud *f*, (the center whereof coincides with the center from which the groove *a* is struck.) The opposite end of the arm is joined to the right-angular stud *g*, in the free end of which is pivoted a friction-wheel, *h*, resting in groove *a* on the resistant *a'*.

The lower end of stud *f* projects through plate A, and is connected with one end of metal strip *i* under the plate, the opposite end of said strip being joined to the binding-post *j*, to which wire *k* is connected.

Across the groove *a*, in radial lines, are placed strips of tin-foil *l*, at regular or irregular intervals. These strips graduate the groove and are intended to indicate the point to which the key must be moved in order to obtain a certain required resistance.

The operation of my improvement is as follows: When the key is turned so that the friction-wheel is in the slot in screw *b*, the current flows from metal connection *c*, through key C, thence through metal strip *i* to wire *k*. When resistance is required the key is moved over the groove until it reaches the point marked by the tin-foil strip indicating the number of ohms of resistance desired. Now, the current has to flow through the resistant in the groove *a* before reaching the key, and thus the resistance desired is obtained.

In Fig. 3 a modification of the invention is shown. Here the groove is straight, lined with a film of plumbago, or a metal resistant where low resistance will answer, and graduated like the above.

The arm of the key is slotted and passed upon the straight metal bar *m*, so as to slide freely back and forth, and is provided with a set-screw to fix it in any required position on the bar.

The roller or wheel *a'* on the key runs on the side off the resistant *o*, but parallel to it. Narrow strips *p*, of tin-foil, with right-angular end pieces, are placed across the resistant at right angles, so as to be crossed by the friction-wheel when moved back and forth. In this way the resistant is brought into the circuit. The tin-foil strips serve to graduate the resistance, as before described.

The advantage of this arrangement is, that the plumbago, being free from the friction of the wheel, is not worn away, and thus its conductivity is not lessened, and greater accuracy is obtained. This arrangement may be applied to the segmental groove first described, as well as to the modification shown in Fig. 3.

As a resisting medium I employ the film of plumbago, or else, where a low resistance is sufficient, there may be a plating of nickel or other metal instead of the plumbago.

To plate the hard-rubber plate it is first

Fig. 4.7 Patent to John Butler for improvement in electrical rheostats, 1879, page 1 (In the public domain)

---

2   **217,331**

dipped in silver-strike, and then a deposit of nickel or other plating metal is made upon the plate at the proper place, either in the groove or on the surface in the path of the key.

Another way is to plate the plumbago with a deposit of copper when a very low resistance will answer. The plumbago film can be placed on the plate by rubbing the point of a lead-pencil in the groove, if employed, but if not, on the roughened surface of the plate in the line of the movement of the key.

While a groove is shown and described it is not essential that the resistant should be placed therein under all circumstances. In cases where a groove could not conveniently be made in the plate, (where the latter is of glass, for example,) a segmental or straight band of the plumbago or metal plating can be placed upon the plate, forming a track upon which the key moves; or, in case the tin-foil graduating-strips are employed, the key

can be moved in a parallel line to the resistant, so as to cross these strips, as before described.

Having thus described my invention, I claim as new and desire to secure by Letters Patent—

As an improvement in rheostats, the plate A, with a resistant of plumbago or metal plate, (placed on the surface or in a groove in said plate, so as to form a connection with a movable key,) one end of said resistant being joined to one of the wires of the battery, in combination with the movable key C, joined to the other wire of the battery, whereby the full force of the current or a diminished force accurately measured and determined can be utilized at pleasure, substantially as described.

                JOHN BUTLER.

Witnesses:
   C. SEDGWICK,
   WILTON C. DONN.

Fig. 4.8 Patent to John Butler for improvement in electrical rheostats, 1879, page 2 (In the public domain)

---

state that there were a looseness of practice, inattention to detail, and neglect of the laws governing electricity, all of which "has led to much blind and ignorant experimenting, which is to be deplored" [62, p. 8]. His book was intended to make up for the deficiencies of the literature and encourage more exact use of electrotherapy. In order to enhance accurate delivery of electricity, Butler devised and patented (US patent number 217331, issued July 1879) a new and less costly rheostat to replace the expensive Wheatstone bridge which was considered gold standard at the time [63] (Figs. 4.7 and 4.8). Butler said that his equipment had stood the test of time and "answers almost all purposes" [63, p. 99]. It was made from graphite, based on a suggestion he obtained from Thomas Edison. The rheostat became well known, was used in allopathic medicine, and gave rise to two modifications about 10 years later when Massey and Goelat both further refined Butler's rheostat. Massey claimed that his invention was less prone to malfunction, while Goelat's rheostat was smaller and portable and could be self-administered at home [64].

Butler was born in Ireland, trained in Edinburgh and Dublin, divided his career between New York and Wales, and died at a young age from septicemia secondary to otitis media. Among his various interests outside of surgery were microscopy, music, photography, and mesmerism [65].

John Mallory Lee

Lee is best known for his early leadership in radiology (Chap. 8), but he later became a well-established surgeon. Midway into his career, he undertook 4 years of postgraduate training in general surgery and obstetrics and subsequently built up a successful surgical practice. He authored a chapter in the *Homoeopathic Textbook of Surgery*, edited the journal *Physicians' and Surgeons' Investigator*, was a state examiner in surgery for the homeopathic school, and wrote or presented many papers and addresses on the topic of surgery. He was chief surgeon at the Rochester Homeopathic Hospital.

Ophthalmology and Otolaryngology

It could be argued that the surgical influence of homeopaths was at its greatest in ophthalmology. In 1894, *Joseph Buffum* (1849–?), professor of ophthalmology and otology at the Chicago Homeopathic Medical School, wrote *Diseases of the Eye and Ear in Children*, one of the earliest books devoted entirely to pediatric diseases. When the New York Homeopathic Medical College (NYHMC) affiliated with the New York Ophthalmic Hospital (NYOH) in 1867, the latter became a homeopathic facility and remained so for the next 60 years. The appointment that year of *Carl Theodore Liebold* as professor and chair of ophthalmic surgery was one of the earliest such appointments in the United States [66]. Even before its amalgamation with NYHMC, the ophthalmic hospital was a well-established institution. In 1879, the NYOH began to confer a unique postgraduate degree "*oculi et auris*," which was abbreviated as "*O. et A. Chir.*"

Edwin Sterling Munson

Edwin Munson (1870–1958) was trained at the NYHMC and remained on the faculty as professor of histology and assistant surgeon at the NYOH. He was actively involved with homeopathy, being treasurer of the Homoeopathic Medical Society of New York County and member of several homeopathic societies. He published in the homeopathic literature, including papers on ophthalmoscopy [67]. the etiology of comitant convergent strabismus [68] and the use of homeopathic medicines in eye conditions [69]. The last of these publications is interesting insofar as it reflects the experience of a surgeon who enjoyed a good reputation in the field of ophthalmology as a whole and not merely within homeopathy. He begins his paper by acknowledging the laborious nature of learning about homeopathic materia medica and the attendant difficulty in finding time to master the specialty. He writes about the four main medicines for cellulitis, noting that *Rhus toxicodendron* is indicated when there is restlessness, burning, itching, tingling, and abscess and when warmth produces

some improvement in symptoms. On the other hand, remedies like *Euphrasia*, *Mercurius*, and *Pulsatilla* have different indications, such as in the case of *Pulsatilla*, which would be recommended when coldness and fresh air improve the symptoms. He writes in similar vein about corneal ulcer, keratoconjunctivitis, iritis, and cataract. Munson believed that early senile-type cataract could be helped by homeopathic remedies, especially *phosphorus*, *causticum*, and *sulfur*. For *phosphorus*, the general tendency to avoid mental or physical effort was a telling clue. Today, most surgeons would find Sterling's recommendations bewildering, yet they were given in all seriousness by a well-trained, sober, and experienced eye surgeon who said that, while he was of the habit to discard from his bookshelves all books over 10 years old, the exceptions were books on ophthalmology and homeopathic materia medica. It might be valuable to test the efficacy of Munson's remedies in modern-day ophthalmology: it is not inconceivable that such remedies still have a place in surgery. There is limited evidence, for example, that homeopathic arnica is more effective than a placebo for bruising after face-lift surgery [70], for pain and swelling after cruciate ligament reconstruction [71], and for post-tonsillectomy pain [72].

According to Wershub, Munson had an international reputation, and his name lives on in Munson's sign, a V-shaped indentation of the lower eyelid when the gaze is directed downwards – a sign that is characteristic of advanced keratoconus [55, p. 171].

The life and political impact of *Royal S. Copeland* (1878–1938) have been described elsewhere (Chaps. 7 and 14), but as large as his impact was in the US Senate, his reputation as a surgeon was not far behind. He is mentioned by Rutkow [3, p. 518] as a leading specialist, and Robins wrote about Copeland's daring pioneer work [73]. He received his training in Michigan and later in Germany and earned recognition for his surgical expertise both in the popular press and by his peers when he was accepted as a fellow of the American College of Surgeons. One surgical operation for which Copeland became nationally famous occurred in Flower Hospital on June 7, 1910, and was widely covered in the press (Figs. 4.9, 4.10, and 4.11). A detailed article in the New York Herald of June 8 described how Copeland performed what was believed to be the first human-to-human corneal

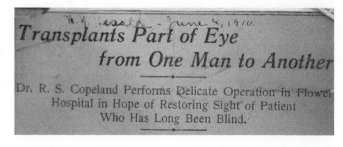

Fig. 4.9 Corneal transplant by Royal Copeland. Headline from NY Herald June 8, 1910 (Image permission PARS International Group)

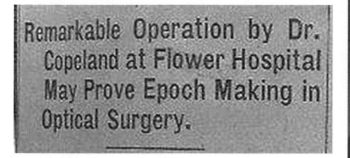

Remarkable Operation by Dr. Copeland at Flower Hospital May Prove Epoch Making in Optical Surgery.

Fig. 4.11 From article in NY City World. June 1910 (In the public domain)

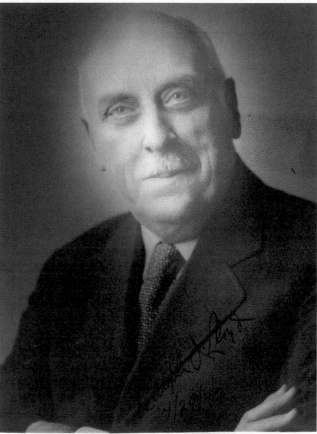

Ralph J. Lloyd
1942

transplant in the United States [74]. There had been a report of such an operation in Austria, as mentioned by Copeland, but with less than ideal outcome [75]. Throughout the nineteenth century, the results of keratoplasty had been poor, and it was not until 1905 that a successful human-to-human corneal transplant took place in Slovakia [76, 77]. Perhaps because of innate conservatism, surgeons in the United States had been slow to adopt the new European approaches, so Copeland's daring step was followed with keen interest, although his contributions do not seem to have left any enduring impact in the annals of American surgery. Copeland was drawn more to the popular press than to the scientific literature, and as far as is known, he did not publish any of his corneal transplant work in the academic literature.

Ralph Lloyd (1875–1963) achieved great distinction in his field (Fig. 4.12). Having graduated as an MD in 1896, he served as house physician at the Brooklyn Homeopathic Hospital and then at the Pittsburgh Homeopathic Hospital. He returned to New York for further training at NYOH and in 1899 obtained the degree of *O. et A. Chir.* Between 1900 and 1929, he held faculty appointments at his alma mater and then later at New York University Medical School, an allopathic facility. Early in his career, Lloyd was involved in the homeopathic community and published a paper in the *North American Journal of Homoeopathy* in 1903 on the importance of urinalysis to diagnose infections and renal problems [78]. He took part in several homeopathic drug provings and

continued to publish in the homeopathic literature as late as 1933, when he wrote on the topic of chronic uveal disease [79]. He also held clinical or consulting appointments at numerous hospitals in New York. In 1925, he obtained certification by the American Board of Ophthalmology, later being elected as fellow of the American Academy of Ophthalmology and Otolaryngology (AAOO). In 1942, he became president of AAOO. Lloyd published 40 articles in the ophthalmology literature on topics related to congenital abnormalities, perimetry, and macular degeneration. He also authored the book *Visual Field Studies* in 1926, wherein he described his stereocampimeter [80] to assist in diagnosing eye diseases by facilitating eye fixation during the measurement of visual fields (Fig. 4.13). This instrument was well known and widely used. Lloyd was a popular teacher and for many years conducted a course on corneal diseases at the annual meeting of AAOO [81]. In 1966, on the occasion of his 90th birthday, the Brooklyn Ophthalmological Society, which Lloyd had founded, honored him by establishing an

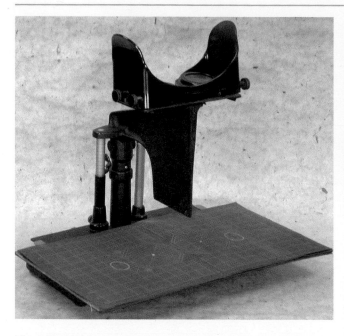

Fig. 4.13 Lloyd stereocampimeter. Manufactured by Bausch & Lomb 1918. Gift of Roger Atkins, MD (Printed with permission of the American Academy of Ophthalmology, all rights reserved)

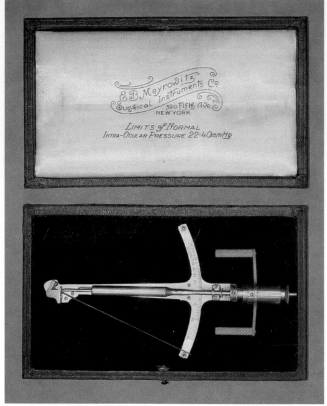

Fig. 4.14 McLean tonometer. Manufactured by EB Meyrowitz, c.1925. Gift of G. Peter Halberg, MD (Reproduced with permission of the American Academy of Ophthalmology, all rights reserved)

annual Ralph I. Lloyd Lecture, citing his "untiring devotion and significant contributions to ophthalmology" [82].

William McLean was another graduate of NYHMC/NYOH. As a homeopath, he took part in institutional activities, being president of the American Institute of Homeopathy's O.O. & L. Society in 1919–1920. McLean is known for the McLean tonometer, an instrument he designed to enhance the reliability of measuring intraocular pressure (Fig. 4.14). Prior to that time, the Schiotz and Gradle tonometers were widely used. McLean hoped that his tonometer would improve on its predecessors by (1) avoiding the need to change weights, (2) eliminating the chart to determine pressure in millimeters of mercury, (3) making it easier for the observer to apply the instrument and take a reading, and (4) preventing capillary attraction between the tonometer plunger and its barrel from fluid in the eye's conjunctival sac [83]. McLean published a preliminary report in the homeopathic *Journal of Ophthalmology, Otology and Laryngology* in 1914 [84] and presented further findings at a congress in Oxford in 1919, which were later published in full in the *British Journal of Ophthalmology* [85]. Freiman noted that McLean was one of first surgeons to perform experiments on living human eyes by connecting the interior of the eye to a manometer [86]. For many years, the McLean tonometer was considered standard in the United States, although even with its purported advantages over the Schiotz tonometer, the latter has continued in use. McLean's son, John, followed in his father's footsteps and became one of America's leading eye surgeons in the late twentieth century, setting up the first eye bank among many other

achievements. However, he did not travel along the path of homeopathy which, at the time of his training, was no longer a presence in the US medicine.

Joseph Ivimey Dowling (1872–?) entered the Philadelphia Medico-Chirurgical College, completing his first year and earning the freshman prize. He then transferred to the NYHMC, from which he graduated in 1895. He worked in New York, becoming medical supervisor of schools in the city and practicing eye, ear, nose, and throat surgery. After some years, he moved to Albany. Between 1902 and 1908, he was president of the Albany County Homeopathic Society and later secretary of the American Homeopathic O.O. & L. Society [87]. During 1906, he took a sabbatical in Europe and shortly thereafter began development of the Argyrol tampon to treat sinus infection. This treatment was used for other conditions, such as allergic rhinitis and sinus headache, and could be widely applied in general practice [88]. During the 1919 influenza epidemic, Dowling's method was also found useful by army surgeons [89]. Argyrol tampons were of value in detecting hidden infections by means of a color change in the packs and therefore could be a valuable diagnostic tool in situations where the x-ray was normal. Dowling administered the Argyrol tampon in ethmoid sinus infections, noting that in some circumstances it could be used to cure the condition and in others to prepare the patient before surgery to obtain a better outcome [90]. The use of Dowling's method extended beyond the confines of homeopathy, and it became quite popular in regular practice worldwide [91].

L. Grant Selfridge

L. Grant Selfridge is described more fully in the chapter on allergy (Chap. 10), being best known for his work in this area. However, he was in his day a well-respected ENT surgeon and champion of the role of vitamins for treating deafness and sinusitis. Selfridge acquired substantial experience as a plastic surgeon and wrote papers in which he reviewed the topic of cosmetic surgery for the nose and ears and presented his personal experiences [92, 93].

Cardiac Surgery

Homeopathy established an early presence in cardiology, as described in Chap. 9, including the innovative contributions of those at the Hahnemann Cardiovascular Institute (CVI). Prominent at the CVI was the surgeon Charles Bailey.

Charles Bailey

Charles Bailey (1910–1993) was arguably the most famous, controversial, and volatile of the CVI group [94] (Fig. 4.15). Rutkow described him as follows: "Long considered a maverick personality…. His professional career was somewhat uneven because of his aggressive and volatile nature … an intrepid pioneer in cardiac surgery and [he] performed the first successful operation for mitral stenosis" [95] an operation which was a "significant landmark in modern heart surgery" because "it demonstrated that the human heart could withstand manipulations previously considered impossible." Bailey graduated from Hahnemann in 1932 and joined the faculty in 1940, becoming professor of surgery and head of the new Department of Thoracic Surgery in 1950. This intrepid surgeon found Hahnemann to be a welcome place to explore new possibilities in heart surgery. In a time that antedated open heart surgery, he was the first to perform a closed-heart repair of mitral valve stenosis (narrowing) and gained international recognition for this achievement. Bailey was a founder of the American Board of Thoracic Surgery and author of an authoritative textbook, *Surgery of the Heart*. In 1957, *TIME* magazine saluted his achievements with a front cover portrait. No greater praise for Bailey can be given than the words of Hahnemann's dean, Joseph DiPalma: "There is little doubt that Bailey by his daring and brilliant exploits put

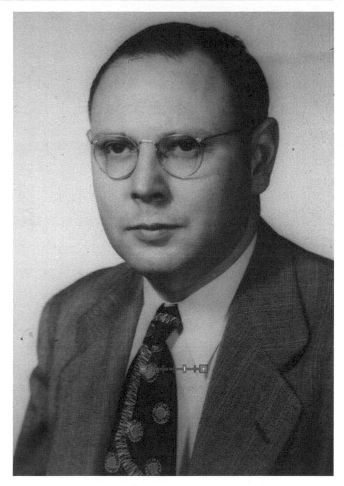

Fig. 4.15 Charles Bailey. Thoracic surgeon and pioneer (Image courtesy of National Library of Medicine)

an obscure homeopathic medical school on the map" [96]. Bailey's enthusiasm as a teacher and researcher inspired all those who came into contact with him, and it was a grievous loss to Hahnemann when he left in 1959, due to conflicts with the new administration. Bailey's willingness to explore new realms again manifested itself when he entered Fordham Law School in his late 50s, obtained qualification, and became an expert in medical malpractice both as lawyer and as medical educator – activities he kept up until the end of his long life.

To better understand what Bailey achieved, a brief detour will set in context the state of heart surgery in the 1940s, a time when there had been some spectacular surgical advances with the stubborn exception being the treatment for heart disease. Responsible for 27 % of all deaths, heart disease had become America's leading cause of death by 1940, and the rate climbed to 39 % in the 1950s. Two formidable challenges stood in the way of further progress in this field of surgery: (i) the large quantities of blood flowing through the operative area and (ii) the incessant movement of a living heart [97, p. 224]. By tying off the blood vessels, it was possible to purchase 3–4 min to complete the operation, and further time could be obtained by cooling the patient to a body temperature of around 85°, a procedure that also lowered the risk of stroke. The Hahnemann group was among the first to develop and apply cooling for cardiac surgery. Even with this, surgeons still had to "blindly grope around the inside of the heart, trusting in their experience and knowledge of anatomy, pathology and physiology" [97, p. 225]. Bailey put it thus: "one must have … eyes on the tips of the fingers" [98]. He likened such operations to surgery which a blind man might perform with great skill and that it was essential to acquire during training "palpatory or tactile vision." Until the development of cardiopulmonary bypass ("heart-lung") machines, which supported circulation and oxygenation of the blood outside of the body, this was the best that could be achieved. Using this approach with skill and daring, Bailey was able to successfully correct many cases of mitral and aortic valve disease, as well as defects in the wall separating the two main chambers of the heart (atrioseptal defects) – all this even while the heart continued to beat. It has been said that Bailey "opened up the field of valvular heart surgery" [99]. A lesson can be drawn from this man who "refused to be hampered by … the prediction of imminent failure by some of [his] colleagues or be stopped by serious obstacles that might hinder [his] professional life." He was a giant upon whose shoulders others have since stood as mitral valve surgery has progressed [100].

During a seminal time for cardiology, when new ideas were being developed and new techniques and drugs introduced, a team of homeopathically trained doctors contributed to major advances in closed-heart surgery, the use of hypothermia, coronary bypass operations, developments in cardiac anesthesia, and establishment of a cardiac nurses' training program. A supposedly second-rate homeopathic medical school was pioneering some first-rate research that captured the world's attention.

Others

While not a practicing surgeon, *Rufus Weaver* (1841–1936) belongs in this story. Weaver was a lecturer on surgical anatomy at Hahnemann half a century before the emergence of the CVI team, and he is famous for two quite unrelated achievements.

Weaver lived for 95 years and held a faculty appointment at Hahnemann from 1869 to 1925, when he retired at the grand old age of 84. He was a native of Gettysburg, PA, and trained as a homeopath at the Penn Medical College. During the post-Civil War years, Weaver did as much as anyone to help the former Confederacy honor its dead and work through its collective grief. Taking up a cause dear to his recently deceased father, Samuel Weaver, Rufus listened to entreaties of various southern women's organizations and

took upon himself the onerous task of identifying the Confederate dead at Gettysburg. The bodies of these dead had lain neglected and become prey to desecration by still-hostile northerners. Starting in 1871, which was already 8 years after the Battle of Gettysburg, and working until 1873, Weaver disinterred the remains of 3,247 Confederate dead and shipped them back for proper burial and honor. In Richmond, senior Confederate military led the procession down Main Street for formal burial of the Virginia dead. For his amazing dedication, Weaver never received payment of the more than $6,000 he was owed by the sponsor, which was unable to raise sufficient funds. Weaver revealed the depth of feeling to this mission with the following words: "If all could see what I have seen, and know what I know, I am sure there would be no rest until every Southern father, brother and son would be removed from the North" [101].

Weaver was also renowned in his day for being the first (and as far as is known, only) person to complete a dissection of the entire human central nervous system, a task which his colleagues had said was impossible. Weaver undertook this labor for 10 h each day over a period of 5 months in 1888 on the body of a former Hahnemann College janitor who had bequeathed her body for medical science. The janitor, named Harriet, has been immortalized by Weaver's work, which stands on display in the Drexel University Medical College. The dissection involved removing all traces of bone and flesh, lifting out every minute filament of the nervous system, wrapping it in alcohol-soaked gauze, and coating it with lead to harden and preserve the tissue. The exposed nervous system was then mounted and pinned to a board. Harriet was an indispensable teaching tool for generations of Hahnemann students and earned a gold medal and blue ribbon Premium Scientific Award at the 1893 Columbian Exposition in Chicago. Even today, colleges and schools request photographs of Harriet and Weaver's work that still appears as reference material in peer-reviewed literature [102–104]. Weaver was the first honorary fellow elected by the Philadelphia Academy of Medicine [105].

References

1. Helmuth WT. Surgery in the homeopathic school. Med Century. 1893;1:192–7.
2. Benjamin J. (Director, Museum of Vision & Stanley M. Truhsen, MD, Director of Ophthalmic Heritage). Personal communication to author. 6 Feb 2012.
3. Rutkow IM. The history of surgery in the United States 1775–1900, vol. 1. San Francisco: Norman Publishing; 1998.
4. Guernsey HN. The application of the principles and practice of homoeopathy to obstetrics and the disorders peculiar to women and young children. Philadelphia: Boericke & Tafel; 1867. p. 116–7.
5. Helmuth WT. A system of surgery. Philadelphia: Boericke & Tafel; 1879.
6. Death of Dr. Schneider. Medical Century. 1895;III:116.
7. Halsey FW. Presidential address. N Engl Med Gazette. 1905;XL: 49–58.

8. Reports of societies and institutions. N Am J Homeopath. 1891;VI:465.

9. Briggs JE. Surgery of the biliary tract. Boston Med Surg J. 1918;178:116–20.

10. Whitaker, Dr. Lester Ray, Surgeon. Prominent whitakers in history [Internet] [Cited 2012 Dec 27]. Available from: www.reocities.com.

11. Briggs JE. Non-perforating ulcers of the stomach and duodenum. Boston Med Surg J. 1924;191:1102–5.

12. Clarke JH. A dictionary of practical materia medica [Internet]. Presented by Médi-T™ [Cited 2012 December 27]. Available from: www.homeoint.org/clarke/s/stram.htm.

13. Bartlett C, Pritchard FH, Lawrence FM. Monthly retrospect: on homoeopathic materia medica and therapeutics. Hahnemannian Mon. 1895;30:558.

14. Fobes JH. The homeopathic surgeon. J Am Inst Homeopath. 1935;28:281–3.

15. Guild WA. The homeopathic side of surgery. J Am Inst Homeopath. 1931;21:1148–9.

16. Haddad FS. Dentist, John Foster Brewster Flagg of Philadelphia, vs. Dentist, J.F.Flagg of Boston. Letter to the editor. Anesthesia History Association Newsletter. 1990;8:4.

17. Secher O. Did you know…? Letter to the editor. Anesthesia History Association Newsletter. 1990;8:3.

18. Voss W. American Silversmiths. Josiah Foster Flagg [Internet]. William Erik Voss 2005 [Cited 2012 June 27]. Available from: http://freepages.genealogy.rootsweb.ancestry.com/~silversmiths/makers/silversmiths/45927.htm.

19. Flagg JF. The family dentist. Boston: J.W. Ingraham; 1822.

20. Historical Notes from OHSU: Josiah Flagg's The Family Dentist [Internet]. Posted by Maija 3 Oct 2011 [Cited 2012 June 27]. Available from: http://ohsu-hca.blogspot.com/2011/10/josiah-p-flaggs-family-dentist.html.

21. Browner S. Ideologies of the anesthetic: professionalism, egalitarianism and the ether controversy. Am Q. 1999;51:101–43.

22. Flagg JF. The inhalation of an ethereal vapor to prevent sensibility to pain during surgical operations. Boston Med Surg J. 1846;35:356–9.

23. Mansfield JD. The inhalation of ethereal vapor &c. Boston Med Surg J. 1846;35:424–5.

24. Flagg JE. Sulphuric ether and chloroform. Boston Med Surg J. 1848;37:521–3.

25. Flagg JFB. Ether and chloroform: their employment in surgery, dentistry, midwifery, therapeutics, Etc. Philadelphia: Lindsay & Blakiston; 1851.

26. Walsh AA. Phrenology and the Boston medical community in the 1830s. Bull Hist Med. 1976;50:261–73.

27. Haller Jr JS. The history of American homeopathy: the academic years, 1820–1935. New York: Pharmaceutical Products Press; 2005. p. 46. 47, 175–6.

28. Bradford TL. Homeopathic societies [Internet]. In: King WH, editor. History of homoeopathy and its institutions in America. New York: Lewis Publishing Company; 1905. p. 254–6, [Cited 27 June 2012]. Available from: http://books.google.com/books?id=bSkJAAAAIAAJ&pg=PA261&lpg=PA261&dq=josiah+foster+flagg+homeopathy&source=bl&ots=xW6RdVpYKJ&sig=e2rJECMLO9DUzBI5HvoPMJkebaE&hl=en&sa=X&ei=ZK7rT5ueHoKo8gSojJX1BQ&ved=0CEEQ6AEwAA#v=onepage&q=josiah%20foster%20flagg%20homeopathy&f=false.

29. Personal communication from Susan Rishworth, Archivist, American College of Surgeons. 6 Mar 2012.

30. Florence Ward [Internet]. The San Francisco Examiner. 16 Dec 1919 [Cited 2012 Feb 3]. Available from: www.sfgenealogy.com/sf/history/hgoe16.htm.

31. Mottershead E. Florence Nightingale Ward, M.D. Medical Scientist or Medical Sectarian? [Internet]. 9 May 2004. p. 17 [Cited 2012 Mar 6]. Available from: http://www.berkeleyhomeopathy.com/articles-and-research/.

32. Ward JW. The present status of ovarian surgery. N Am J Homeopath. 1897;45:20–41.

33. Ward JW. Life, health and disease. J Am Inst Homeopath. 1926;19:591–9.

34. Ward JW. Recovery and cure. J Am Inst Homeopath. 1926;19:695–702.

35. Ward JW. Homeopathic posology (dosage). J Am Inst Homeopath. 1926;19:783–94.

36. Ward JW. Foreward: the principles and scope of homeopathy delivered at the University of California. J Am Inst Homeopath. 1926;19:291–301.

37. Ward JW. The philosophy of homeopathy. J Am Inst Homeopath. 1926;19:387–99.

38. Ward JW. The scope of homeopathy. J Am Inst Homeopath. 1926;19:483–93.

39. Waite L. The present status of surgical interventions in retrodeviations of the uterus. JAMA. 1905;XLIV:468–71.

40. Sperry FM. A group of distinguished physicians and surgeons of Chicago. Chicago: JH Beers and Company; 1904. p. 62–4.

41. Jones RF, Dickerson SC, Dibble EH, Kenney JA. Tribute to Dr Walter Gray Crump. J Natl Med Assoc. 1944;36:100–1.

42. Anschutz EP. New, old and forgotten remedies. New Delhi: B. Jain, Publishers; 2002. p. 276.

43. Clarke JH. A dictionary of practical materia medica. Radium Bromatum [Internet]. Presented by Médi-T 2000 [Cited 2012 June 30]. Available from: www.homeoint.org/clarke/r/rad_b.htm.

44. Alumni & Development. Geraldine Burton-Branch, M.D.'36 [Internet]. New York Medical College undated [Cited 2012 June 2]. Available from: http://www.nymc.edu/AlumniAndDevelopment/AlumniRelations/AlumniProfiles/GeraldineBBranch.html.

45. Honorary Degree [Internet]. Charles Drew University of Medical Sciences. Undated [Cited 2012 June 27]. Available from: http://www.cdrewu.edu/assets/pdfs/drewfinal6Page.pdf.

46. Annual Meeting, American Institute of Homeopathy, Washington, DC. June 19–24. Tumors of the Urinary Bladder. Discussant, Sprague Carleton J Am Inst Homeopath. 1921;12:1170.

47. Carleton S. Moral prophylaxis: a critique with suggestions. Homeopathic Soc Pennsylvania. 1907;1–9.

48. Department of Urology History, New York Medical College [Internet]. [Cited 2012 Oct 11]. Available from: www.nymc.edu/urology/history.html.

49. Dr. George R. Nagamatsu. Engineering & Urology Society [Internet]. 2012 [Cited 2012 Oct 21]. Available from: http://engineering-urology.org/memoriam.html.

50. Rutkow LW, Rutkow IM. Homeopaths, surgery, and the Civil War. Edward C. Franklin and the struggle to achieve medical pluralism in the Union army. Arch Surg. 2004;139:785–91.

51. Reviews. The Science and Art of Surgery, Adapted to Homoeopathic Therapeutics. Br J Homeopath. 1869;27:321–6.

52. Review. The Science and Art of Surgery. By E.C. Franklin, M.D., of St. Louis. 1872. N Am J Homeopath. 1873;21:429.

53. Book Reviews. A statement in brief, by Donald Maclean. Physician Surg: Prof Med J. 1882;4:265–6.

54. Rutkow IM. William Tod Helmuth and Andrew Jackson Howe. Surgical sectarianism in 19th-century America. Arch Surg. 1994;129:662–8.

55. Wershub LP. A history of the New York Medical College, flower and fifth avenue hospitals: One hundred years of medical progress. Springfield: Charles C. Thomas Publisher; 1967.

56. Rothstein WG. American physicians in the 19th century. From sects to science. Baltimore: The Johns Hopkins University Press; 1972. p. 259.

57. Obituary. Israel Tisdale Talbot. Bostonia. 1900;3:14.

58. Talbot IT. Tracheotomy in croup. A paper read before the Massachusetts Homoeopathic Medical Society. October 8, 1862. Pamphlets: Homoeopathic Surgery. Boston: John Wilson and Son; 1866;2:12–25.

59. McNamara O. Generations. A history of Boston University School of Medicine 1848–1998. Boston: Trustees of Boston University; 1998.

60. Anonymous. Book review, "Electricity in Surgery". The Electrician. 1882;1:168.

61. Mitchell JP, Lumb GN. The principles of surgical diathermy and its limitations. Br J Surg. 1962;50:314–20.

62. Butler J. Electricity in surgery. Philadelphia: Boericke & Tafel; 1882.

63. Butler J. A new rheostat. Am J Electrol Neurol. 1879;1:150–4.

64. New York Obstetrical Society. A new rheostat. Am J Obstet Dis Women Child. 1890;23:1385.

65. Obituary. Trans Am Inst Hom. 1885;38th Session:100–101.

66. Rutkow IM. Ophthalmologic surgery. Arch Surg. 2000;135: 1371.

67. Munson ES. A clinical lecture on ophthalmoscopy. J Am Inst Homeopath. 1933;26:29–33.

68. Munson ES. Etiology of comitant convergent strabismus. J Am Inst Homeopath. 1931;24:139–46.

69. Munson ES. The use of homeopathic remedies in eye conditions. J Am Inst Homeopath. 1927;20:323–32.

70. Seeley BM, Denton AB, Ahn MS, Maas CS. Effect of homeopathic *Arnica montana* on bruising in face-lifts: results of a randomized, double-blind, placebo-controlled clinical trial. Arch Facial Plast Surg. 2006;8:54–9.

71. Brinkhaus B, Wilkens JM, Ludtke R, Hunger J, Witt CM, Willich SN. Homeopathic arnica therapy in patients receiving knee surgery: results of three randomized double-blind trials. Complement Ther Med. 2006;14:237–46.

72. Robertson A, Suryanarayanan R, Banerjee A. Homeopathic *Arnica montana* for post-tonsillectomy analgesia: a randomized placebo control trial. Homeopathy. 2007;96:17–21.

73. Robins N. Copeland's cure. Homeopathy and the war between conventional and alternative medicine. New York: Alfred A. Knopf; 2005. p. 115–6.

74. Transplants part of eye from one man to another. The New York Herald. 8 June 1910. University of Michigan, Bentley Historical Library, Copeland Collection, Box 35.

75. Copeland RS. Transplantation of the cornea: The preliminary report of a single case. Unpublished manuscript. University of Michigan, Bentley Historical Library, Copeland Collection, Box 21.

76. Laibson PR. History of corneal transplantation. In: Brightbill FS, McDonnell PJ, McGhee CNJ, Farjo AA, editors. Brightbill's Corneal surgery: theory, technique, tissue. 4th ed. Maryland Heights: C.V. Mosby; 2008. p. 1.

77. Zirm E. Eine erfolgreiche totale keratoplastic. Graefes Arch Clin Exp Ophthalmol. 1906;64:580–93.

78. Lloyd RI. Urinalysis. N Am J Homoeopath. 1903;51:495–7.

79. Lloyd RI. Glaucoma and cataract as the result of chronic uveal disease. J Am Inst Homeopath. 1933;26:177–8.

80. Lloyd RI. Visual field studies. New York: The Technical Press; 1926. p. 126.

81. Perera CA. Ralph irving lloyd. Trans Am Ophthalmol Soc. 1970;68:12–4.

82. Straatsma BR. News and comment. Arch Ophthalmol. 1966;76:311.

83. Keeler R, Singh AD, Dua HS. Pressure to measure pressure: the McLean Tonometer. Br J Ophthalmol. 2009;93:9.

84. McLean W. Preliminary report of a new tonometer. J Ophthalmol Otol Laryngol. 1914;20:432–40.

85. McLean W. Further experimental studies in intraocular pressure and tonometry. Br J Ophthalmol. 1919;3:385–99.

86. Freiman G. Clinical study and review of tonometry. Arch Ophthalmol. 1943;30:526–46.

87. Schenectady digital history archive. Hudson-Mohawk genealogical and family memoirs: dowling. Cuyler Reynolds 30 July 2009 [Cited 2012 Sept 29]. Available from: http://www.schenectadyhistory.org/families/hmgfm/dowling.html.

88. Green CR. The Dowling method of nasal tamponade in general practice. N Engl Med Gazette. 1916;LI:444–9.

89. Heseltine B. Results of the Dowling Tampon in nasal work in army hospitals. N Am J Homeopath. 1920;68;8:766–70.

90. Dowling JI. Non-surgical treatment of ethmoiditis. Laryngoscope. 1930;40:633–9.

91. The union of the New York Ophthalmic Hospital and the New York Homeopathic Medical College and Flower Hospital. J Am Inst Homeopath. 1933;26:120–30.

92. Selfridge G. Plastic surgery of nose and ears. A further contribution. Cal State J Med. 1918;XVI:416–23.

93. Selfridge G. Intranasal cosmetic surgery, with special reference to rib with cartilage, and cartilage transplants. Cal State J Med. 1917;XV:445–51.

94. Pace E. Obituary: Dr. Charles P. Bailey, 82, pioneer in new methods of heart surgery. The New York Times. 1993 Aug 19.

95. Rutkow IM. American surgery. An illustrated history. New York: Lippincott-Raven Publishers; 1998. p. 452.

96. Rogers N. An alternative path. The making and remaking of Hahnemann Medical College and Hospital of Philadelphia. New Brunswick: Rutgers University Press; 1998. p.187.

97. Rutkow IM. Seeking the cure: a history of medicine in America. New York: Scribner; 2010.

98. Bailey CP, Glover RP, O'Neill TJE. Transcardial palpatory surgery of the heart. Can Med Assoc J. 1952;66:529–35.

99. Dobell ARC. Rival trailblazers: the origins of successful closed valvular surgery. Ann Thorac Surg. 1996;61:750–4.

100. Gonzalez-Lavin L, Charles P. Bailey and Dwight E. Harken – the dawn of the modern era of mitral valve surgery. Ann Thorac Surg. 1992;53:916–9.

101. Faust DG. This republic of suffering. New York: Vintage Books; 2008. p. 246–7.

102. From the collections: Harriet [Internet]. A movable archives. Posted by Lisa Grimm 17 Feb 2010 [Cited 2012 Nov 2]. Available from: http://amovablearchives.blogspot.com/2010/02/from-collections-harriet.html.

103. Dr Rufus Benjamin Weaver [Internet]. Phototheque Homeopathique 2004 [Cited 2012 Nov 2]. Available from: www.homeopint.org/photo/wz/weaverrb.htm.

104. Clark K. Harriet Cole: Drexel's longest-serving employee [Internet]. Drexel Now 2012 June 19 by Katie Clark [Cited 2012 Nov 2]. Available from: http://drexel.edu/now/features/archive/2012/July/Harriet/.

105. Personal and general items. Anon. N Engl Med Gazette. 1909;44:573.

Homeopaths and the Dawning of Anesthesiology

5

Many who helped shape anesthesiology into an independent specialty came from the ranks of homeopathy, while others who achieved distinction in anesthesiology later embraced the cause of homeopathy. A short account of the history of anesthesia will first be given to provide context.

For many centuries, surgery was held in lower esteem than medicine or pharmacy. The risks of pain, sepsis, and mortality were so great that surgery was usually a course of last resort and sometimes a barbaric one at that. Traditional measures to reduce pain included the use of plants containing opium, mandragora, or henbane or the consumption of alcohol, all of which were unsatisfactory. Towards the end of the eighteenth century, the chemist Sir Humphrey Davy experimented with nitrous oxide gas in animals, noting its ability to deaden pain. He then self-administered the gas and gave it to his poet friends William Wordsworth and Samuel Taylor Coleridge, who both noted a similar effect. Davy was led to suggest that nitrous oxide held promise as an anesthetic gas in surgery, but this idea failed to gain traction. Michael Faraday also made the same suggestion for ether, but to no avail. Shortly afterwards, in the 1830s and 1840s, John Esdaile, a doctor employed by the East India Company, found that hypnosis induced sleep during surgery, and he used it in thousands of major and minor operations with great success and a negligible fatality rate. Unfortunately, hypnosis had already gained a poor reputation, being tainted with the charlatanry of mesmerism. Esdaile was the target of many attacks in the Indian medical literature and his ideas failed to spread, leaving an uncontested field for the introduction of anesthetic drugs.

It has been said that the modern anesthetic era began in the United States with the use of ether by Crawford Long in 1842, followed by the use of nitrous oxide as a dental anesthetic by Horace Wells in 1844 and again with ether by WTG Morton in 1846. In the 1850s, the Scottish surgeon Sir James Young Simpson introduced chloroform to relieve the pains of labor, and around the same time in England, John Snow (famous for his work in tracing the spread of cholera) introduced chloroform more widely as a general anesthetic, devising an inhalation apparatus for safer administration.

When in 1853 and again in 1857 Queen Victoria requested and received this new gas for the birth of two of her children, chloroform anesthesia had truly arrived.

Despite these advances, anesthesia continued to be a risky affair. For one thing, in England, for example, anyone could administer an anesthetic, even the hospital porter or the surgeon's coachman! Peripatetic anesthetists travelled about the country equipped with "rag and bottle." In the early twentieth century when Winston Churchill, as British Home Secretary, was asked to enact legislation to make anesthesia an exclusively physician-administered specialty, he declined. The situation was little different in the United States, where anesthesia remained loosely regulated until well into the twentieth century. Many times, when a physician gave anesthesia, it was entrusted to the most junior doctor with minimal experience, and when patients died, it was simply put down to their inability to tolerate the anesthetic.

Other problems included the fact that gases like ether, chloroform, and nitrous oxide variously caused heartbeat irregularities, blood pressure changes, liver damage, or postoperative nausea and vomiting. At the beginning of the twentieth century, there was still need for safer anesthetics and for the development of a cadre of practitioners who had sufficient skill in the administration of anesthesia. In this regard, individual homeopaths made some notable contributions, chiefly in (1) the creation of anesthesia as a fully recognized specialty within medicine and (2) the introduction of new anesthetics. Some important anesthetic devices and procedures were also introduced by doctors who initially started their careers as orthodox practitioners and then adopted homeopathy.

To explain why homeopaths became so connected to anesthesia defies simple answer as there is no inherent philosophical affinity between the two specialties. One speculation is that homeopathy has traditionally been on the margins of medicine and that many of its practitioners may tend to think "out of the box." As a result, perhaps some homeopathic graduates found greater opportunity in branches of medicine which were still in their infancy and where the power structures and "old boy's clubs" were not closed to

J. Davidson, *A Century of Homeopaths*,
DOI 10.1007/978-1-4939-0527-0_5, © Springer Science+Business Media New York 2014

outsiders. Possibly, anesthesiologists were more open-minded than some of the other medical disciplines and less prejudiced against homeopaths. Certainly, morbidity and mortality were common complications from administering "too much" of a single anesthetic drug, thereby appealing to those who favored the small dose.

The creation of anesthesiology as a specialty illustrates how the medical profession has evolved. Professionalism can be seen as a form of contract between society and a profession, as has been elaborated in the Physicians' Charter [1, 2]. Three fundamental principles apply to the medical profession, (1) primacy of patient welfare, (2) patient autonomy, and (3) social justice, and 10 subsidiary principles, among which included professional competence, improving quality of care, professional responsibilities, allocation of limited resources, advancing scientific knowledge, and improving access to care. Until the mid-1920s, the practice of anesthesia was more of an art whereby skilled clinical practitioners learned how to use old and new treatments and passed on their learning to (the few) doctors who wanted to specialize in this branch of medicine. One excellent example is demonstrated by Thomas Drysdale Buchanan (see below), who described his introduction to anesthesia at the Homeopathic College, where it was the practice to take on four senior students to administer anesthetics in the clinic. Lobbying for the chance to obtain such experience, Buchanan approached one of the junior surgeons to let him give an anesthetic. The surgeon replied: "Yes indeed, you may bring me a case for surgery and I will let you give the anesthetic." Buchanan said, "that was about the only instruction I had in anesthesia, more than most interns received at that time" [3].

In order to achieve the goals listed in the Physicians' Charter, it would be essential to establish good teaching and training facilities, to set standards for credentialing, to advance research and practice, and to attract sufficient numbers of doctors into the field. With the Physicians' Charter in mind, how did academic homeopathic physicians contribute to anesthesiology?

A number of the main players came from Hahnemann Medical College in Philadelphia. Despite its low status as a medical school, Hahnemann exerted an influence on anesthesiology far out of proportion to its station. Nine of their graduates will be described, along with Thomas Buchanan, who graduated from the New York Homeopathic College. Following a chronological account of these ten individuals, the careers of other anesthetists, who embraced homeopathy later in their careers, will be described.

Herbert Leo Northrop

Herbert Leo Northrop was born in 1866, studied medicine at Hahnemann Medical College, and graduated in 1889. After a year as resident physician there, Northrop took up the practice

of surgery and anesthesia, becoming professor of anatomy at Hahnemann in 1895 and later dean of that institution. He was among the first to train surgeons to administer anesthetics, and, partly as the result of his efforts, Hahnemann enjoyed a national reputation for anesthesiology among medical schools. Northrop wrote: "To hear of an official American anaesthetic authority … is a rare thing, while the ether-soaking process and the careless, not to say ignorant, method of administering chloroform are daily practices. Much reform is needed … in this direction. Too little attention is given to this subject in our colleges. Special lectures and practical instruction on the proper administration, means of resuscitation and the effects of anaesthetics are demanded and should constitute a prominent part of our curricula. It is gratifying to know that the Hahnemann College in this city is at the front in this respect …. The Hahnemann Hospital of Philadelphia has for a number of years enjoyed a high reputation for the careful administration of anaesthetics. It has recently been stated by one well informed that much more scientific attention is given to the subject in the Hahnemann Hospital than in the majority of hospitals, while its surgeons are looked upon by members of all medical schools as competent, careful administrators of anaesthetics." In the same article, Northrop went on to describe the careful preoperative assessment and preparation that occurred in Hahnemann, as well as the routine (but then unusual) practice of keeping records of important anesthetic events for later discussion and comparison [4]. From this account, it may be concluded that Hahnemann was already in the vanguard of anesthesia practice and teaching, traditions which were already in place when Northrop joined the faculty. However, Northrop strengthened the Hahnemann program even further.

Northrop was a popular anatomy lecturer at Hahnemann. Early in his anesthetic career, he conceived the idea that chloroform and oxygen given together would be an improvement over chloroform alone. In this, Northrop joined the chorus of anesthetists who were beginning to recognize that the addition of oxygen to various anesthetics, including ether, chloroform, and nitrous oxide, might be safer. He was the first to report the combined use of chloroform and oxygen for anesthesia, describing 100 cases thus treated [5]. He subsequently devised and patented apparatus for the delivery of chloroform and oxygen, as a means to increase safety and achieve quicker induction of anesthesia, quicker recovery, and need for less chloroform. Although chloroform was not as popular in the United States as it was in parts of Europe, the "Northrop Method of Anesthesia" was used for a period of time and his new apparatus was hailed in one journal, perhaps with partisan bias, as "second to the discovery of chloroform itself" [6]. It is interesting that an English homeopath, Dr. Theo Nicholson, disputed priority of the invention, claiming that he (Nicholson) first described a similar approach at the Southport Regional Homoeopathic congress in September 1892 and then in the British Medical Journal on December 31, 1892 [7]. He then had obtained a US patent for the principle of giving chloroform with oxygen in May 1893 [8] and devised an apparatus for the delivery of both gases, which he commercialized [9].

Dr. Northrop's talents extended beyond anesthesia. At the time of his deanship, in 1907, he performed brain surgery on a man who had undergone personality change following head injury, which had resulted in the individual becoming psychopathic and unable to regulate his intake of alcohol. After Northrop had cleared the meningeal adhesions which he found at surgery, the patient was followed for 2 years, by which time he was restored to his premorbid condition as a law-abiding, productive member of society, devoted family man, and valued employee who was subsequently twice promoted at work. At the time, this operation was acclaimed as a triumph for surgery in criminology. Northrop himself recognized that while many operations had been performed on the brain, it was rare for the surgeon to care about the correspondence between brain function and mental characteristics [10]. Two years later, he performed surgery on a young woman who had suffered traumatic brain injury as a child, which resulted in aberrant behavior, including kleptomania. Following a similar surgical removal of meningeal adhesions, this patient recovered and was doing well at follow-up [11]. Northrop was an early advocate of surgery to correct clearly localized brain-based psychiatric problems and he was firm in the belief that specific mental and behavioral functions had their own localization within the brain.

With respect to homeopathy, there is an interesting account of Northrop's participation as a subject in a homeopathic proving experiment in 1888, when he was a 23-year-old medical student. The report provides detailed information about his health, vital signs, and medical history of eczema and his "sanguine" temperament and propensity for easy startle in response to toads. He tended to itch after receiving placebo. In the first proving report, Northrop received *zincum metallicum* at a dose of 2X, and on further occasions over the next 11 days. A detailed daily record was kept, typical of the proving methodology, in which Northrop described his condition, noting such things as poor sleep on day 3 and aching eyeballs and stitchlike pain in the left eye on day 8. At 5.50 pm on day 9, he observed perspiration and moist palms, face, and neck and a temperature of 100°F. On day 11, he experienced more thirst than usual. It is notable how much identifying information was revealed in those days, the published report giving the subject's full name and address and other medical information which, under today's regulations, would be a violation of the law [12].

Thomas Drysdale Buchanan

Thomas Drysdale Buchanan (1876–1940) was 1 of 17 graduates of the New York Homeopathic Medical College and Hospital in 1897 (Fig. 5.1). After interning at the Flower

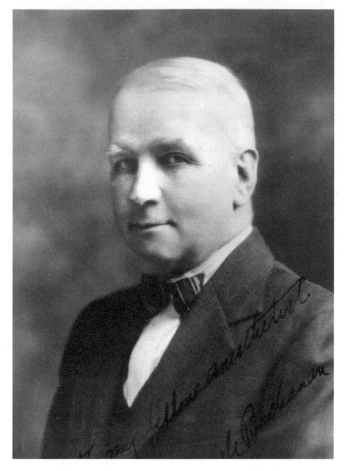

Fig. 5.1 Thomas Buchanan. First board-certified anesthesiologist, first president of American Board of Anesthesiology, and president of American Society of Anesthetists (Image courtesy of the Wood Library-Museum, Park Ridge, Illinois)

Homeopathic Hospital, he took a position as anesthetist at Flower and at Fifth Avenue Hospital in 1902. In 1904, Buchanan established what is claimed to have been the first department of anesthesiology in the United States led by a full-time chairman in the specialty. Thus, it was in a homeopathic medical college that this precedent was set [13]. (Some dispute must be acknowledged on this point, however, as the Department of Anesthesiology at the University of Wisconsin-Madison was founded in 1927 under the guidance of Ralph M. Waters, MD, and claims to have been the first academic program in anesthesiology in the country.)

Buchanan's work did not end there, as he became an energizing force in building the Long Island Society of Anesthetists between 1905 and 1911. After several years of growth, the society was renamed the New York Society in 1911. Due to the urging of Buchanan and his colleague Paul Wood, the American Society of Anesthetists came into being in 1936. Nine years later, in 1945, the society took its final name as the American Society of Anesthesiologists. Wood paid the following tribute to Buchanan in his 1941 memorial address: "Buchanan was a founder and past president of the

American Society of Anesthetists; and at the time of his death (1940) he was President of the American Board of Anesthesiology, both of which organizations his labors so materially helped to establish. The latter was one of the most difficult tasks, as not only was there the usual lack of interest, but in addition much active opposition on the part of the medical profession. His personality, persistence and good judgment finally overcame all opposition" [3].

With reference to the board, Buchanan was not only its first president but also its first examiner and first to obtain board certification – a homeopath as holder of certificate #1.

As part of Buchanan's quest to place anesthesia on firm footing, he accepted a commission as captain in the Army Medical Corps and took charge of the first anesthesia training school in the US army. In 1921, he was appointed Major in the Reserve and advised the surgeon-general over the drafting of plans for a Division of Anesthesia.

Wood provides other insights into Buchanan's legacy. For example, in recognizing Buchanan's clinical vision, he singles out a paper written on shock which, 30 years later, was still considered relevant; as Wood put it, "the reason for his success of many of the suggestions made by Dr. Buchanan in this article has been explained by research during the intervening years."

Emphasis has been placed here on Buchanan's role in creating a sound training program, in achieving academic respectability for anesthesiology, and seeing it grow on the national stage as an accredited specialty. He was also known for developing new anesthetic equipment, including the Buchanan oropharyngeal rebreathing tube and the Buchanan ether drop cup, and for "outstanding" collaboration with Dr. Chevalier Jackson, the father of modern bronchoscopy, in developing the anesthesia portion of part of the Jackson endotracheal and bronchoscopic apparatus [3].

Walter M. Boothby

Walter M. Boothby (1880–1953) grew up in a homeopathic household. His father, Alonzo Boothby, was professor of gynecology at Boston University and became a leading figure in the world of homeopathic surgery. Walter wished to follow in his father's footsteps, to train at the *alma mater* and in turn become a surgeon. He set out to achieve these aims, completing the first 3 years of medical training and passing all the exams at BU, but in Walter's third year there, Alonzo Boothby died suddenly, and for unclear reasons, Walter transferred to Harvard where he completed his final year of medical school. He then trained as a surgeon and established a private practice in Boston, before turning his attention to anesthesia. His career has been described in detail by Vandam, who noted Boothby's many accomplishments [14]. Vandam considers Boothby to have been far ahead of his time and characterizes him as "perhaps the first real investigator in anesthesia." Among many claims to fame are co-invention of the Boothby-Lovelace-Bulbulian ("BLB") oxygen mask, leadership in military and aviation medicine, exceptional skill in administering ether, and work on metabolism. In 1912, Boothby and Cotton designed the Boothby-Cotton apparatus for administering nitrous oxide and oxygen, which was "a milestone for its technical innovations that now form the major ingredients of most modern apparatus." Some of his ideas on respiration, uptake, and distribution of anesthetics and the need for measured dose administration of anesthetics have gone unchallenged. Again, as with most of the anesthesiologists mentioned here, his entry into medicine was through the homeopathic portal – in Boothby's case, at least for three quarters of his initial training. Subsequent contacts with the homeopathic community have not been recorded, although the Boston University sesquicentennial commemorative does claim him as a member of the BU department of anesthesia around 1907 at the time he invented one of his devices to deliver nitrous oxide, oxygen, and ether [15].

Everett A. Tyler

Everett Tyler was born in 1887 and received his medical training at Hahnemann in Philadelphia, graduating in 1913 (Fig. 5.2). He showed an early interest in anesthesiology and spent some time training with Dr. E McKesson in Toledo, Ohio. Tyler returned to Hahnemann and became the first full-time medical anesthetist in Philadelphia. He remained on the faculty there until his retirement in 1950 and taught a number of Hahnemann graduates who made important contributions to the specialty, most notably Henry Ruth. Tyler published in leading medical journals on various aspects of anesthesia and served as president of the American Association of Anaesthetists in 1924. In his presidential address, Tyler made two main points: (1) he urged the necessity to accurately record the outcome of anesthesia during surgery, with particular concern on mortality rates, and (2) he described a series of experiments in which his group looked at alterations of electrical potential as a possible mechanism of action for anesthetics [16]. From 1941, Dr. Tyler was on the governing board of the International Anesthesia Research Society (IARS), an organization which still thrives today. He was also one of the few anesthetists invited to form the fledgling Anesthetists Travel Club, a small coterie of leading academic anesthetists dedicated to promoting academic development of the specialty. Like the IARS, the travel group flourished and eventually grew into the Academy of Anesthesiologists in 1952.

While Tyler advanced his career in anesthetics, he did not let his contacts with homeopathy atrophy. For example, he

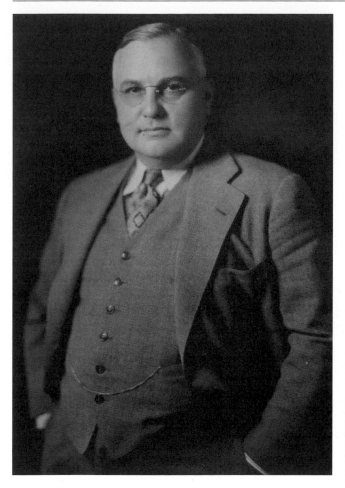

Fig. 5.2 Everett Tyler. Hahnemann anesthetist and president of American Society of Anesthetists (Image courtesy of the Wood Library-Museum, Park Ridge, Illinois)

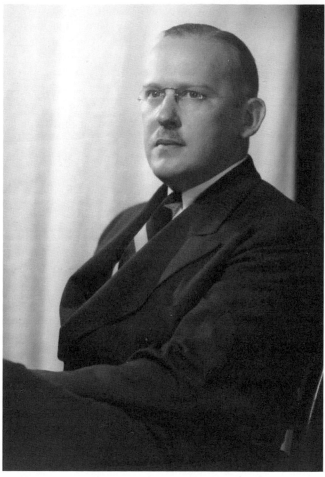

Fig. 5.3 Henry S. Ruth. Hahnemann anesthetist, president of American Society of Anesthetists, and second president of American Board of Anesthesiology (Image courtesy of the Wood Library-Museum, Park Ridge, Illinois)

maintained memberships of the American Institute of Homeopathy, and his local county homeopathic society, and continued to publish scientific papers in the homeopathic literature. He belonged to the Medical Fraternity Alpha Sigma, an organization with active ties to homeopathy.

Henry Ruth

Henry Swartley Ruth was born in 1899, in Lansdale, PA, where his father was the president of a bank (Fig. 5.3). He studied preclinical and clinical medicine at Hahnemann Medical College in Philadelphia, graduating with honors in 1923. Ruth was a classmate of Harold Griffith. Among Ruth's mentors was Everett A. Tyler. Ruth joined the faculty at Hahnemann and remained there for his entire professional life, witnessing its transformation from a homeopathic into an allopathic institution. In addition, he later obtained an appointment at the Philadelphia General Hospital, where he became the chief of anesthesia in 1933; it is thought that he

and Carl Fischer were the first Hahnemann graduates appointed to the staff of that esteemed institution [17]. In the same year, he was promoted to the rank of clinical professor in Anesthesia at Hahnemann [18].

From the beginning, Ruth was a well-regarded teacher and by 1926 was one of the most popular lecturers at Hahnemann, being appreciated for his knowledge of a nascent medical specialty and for championing research into regional anesthesia (the use of local anesthetics to block nerve conduction of pain). The training of physicians in anesthesia was always a high priority for Henry Ruth, who in 1929 instituted one of the first anesthesia residency programs in the United States; he was also a principal force behind creation of the American Board of Anesthesiology Inc. (ABA) in 1938. This important body provides official credentialing that a physician is competent to practice and teach anesthesiology. Ruth was elected vice-president of the board in 1938 and then president in 1942, immediately following the death in office of Thomas Buchanan. Ruth had formerly served as president of the American Society of Anesthesiologists Inc. in 1938. He was instrumental in establishing a Section on Anesthesiology in the American Medical Association (AMA) and served as its representative in the AMA House of Delegates between 1941 and 1955. By his tireless efforts, Ruth takes much credit for eventual acceptance by the AMA House of Delegates that anesthesiologists could practice as a designated specialty and thus submit a professional fee for service. Among other homeopathic colleagues who fought on his side were Rolland Whitacre and BB Sankey (see below). The consequence of their achievement was far-reaching, for as Ruth said in 1944, "if anesthesiologists cannot expect a financial return comparable to other specialties, the desirable type of young physician will little desire to enter or remain in the field" [19].

During World War II, Ruth designed and taught a course at Hahnemann for armed services medical personnel. As testimony to Ruth's activities, it may be noted that, at one time, Hahnemann produced more board-certified diplomates in anesthesia than any other US medical school. To quote Kenneth Keown: "Ruth was unquestionably the role model so many of us followed. Perhaps it was because of his unfailing labors and his concern for the specialty that his death came at such an early age" [20].

Ruth's signal achievements include his roles in creating the Academy of Anesthesiology, the ABA, the American Society of Anesthetists Inc. (ASA), and the journal *Anesthesiology*, of which he was the first and longest-serving editor. For his part in founding the organizations that led to the development of modern anesthesia, Ruth has few rivals. In tribute to his many achievements, the ASA awarded Ruth their Distinguished Service Award in 1952.

With regard to homeopathy, there is no evidence that Ruth practiced or publicly advocated this form of therapeutics, in contrast to his colleague and classmate Harold Griffith. However, he published in homeopathic journals for many years and may perhaps be one of few authors who published in the *Journal of the American Institute of Homeopathy*, *the Hahnemannian Monthly*, *the New England Journal of Medicine*, and *the Journal of the American Medical Association*. His list of published papers and books exceeds 100.

Henry Ruth did not enjoy the best of health, having four heart attacks before he was 42. In addition, he had a stomach ulcer. He died of a brain hemorrhage after falling in his home, at the age of 56.

Harold Randall Griffith

Harold Griffith is one of anesthesia's high priests, being acclaimed for his work with curare and his leadership in establishing this specialty. He was born in 1894 to a devoutly

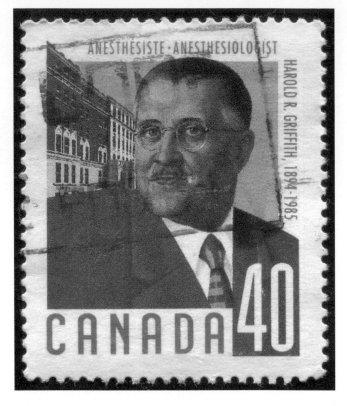

Fig. 5.4 Harold Griffith. Commemorative postage stamp, Canadian Postal Service. Available from: http://www.123rf.com/photo_9381276_canada--circa-1991-stamp-printed-by-canada-shows-harold-griffith-1894-1985--anesthesiologist-circa-1.html

Baptist Canadian family which prized the values of hard work, integrity, and service to others, yet found time for family activities and recreation. Griffith's father, Alexander R. Griffith ("AR"), was a general practitioner of homeopathy, having been trained at the University of Michigan and the New York Homeopathic Medical College. AR's quiet and unworldly manner [21, p. 83] might seem an unlikely mix upon which to build an impressive family dynasty lasting 70 years at the Montreal Homeopathic Hospital (later the Queen Elizabeth Hospital). But build it he did, and one of its shining achievements was the pioneer work of his son, Harold.

In June 1892, after completing his training, AR and his wife left New York and settled in Montreal. Two years later, in 1894, the Montreal Homeopathic Hospital was formed, complete with surgical facilities and a nurses' training school (Fig. 5.4). The hospital became an important part of AR's professional life, and in 1898, he was appointed medical superintendent, a post which he held until his death in 1936 [22, p. 35]. Under the consecutive leadership of AR and Harold Griffith between 1898 and 1966, the Montreal Homeopathic became one of Montreal's most respected training centers, a reputation which it held until its final day. Sadly and suddenly, and despite great protest in the community, the hospital was closed in 1996 – purely and simply a

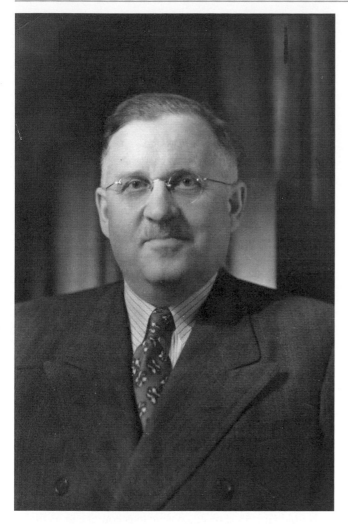

Fig. 5.5 Harold R. Griffith. Hahnemann-trained. Introduced tubocurare, a short-acting neuromuscular blocker, into anesthesia (Image courtesy of the Wood Library-Museum, Park Ridge, Illinois)

THE USE OF CURARE IN GENERAL ANESTHESIA

HAROLD R. GRIFFITH, M.D., AND G. ENID JOHNSON, M.D.*

Montreal, Canada

EVERY anesthetist has wished at times that he might be able to produce rapid and complete muscular relaxation in resistant patients under general anesthesia. This is a preliminary report on the clinical use of a drug which will give this kind of relaxation, temporarily and apparently quite harmlessly.

The physiological action of curare as an interrupter of the neuromuscular mechanism has long been recognized, and its best known practical applications have been by South American Indians as an arrow poison and in the physiological laboratory. The crude curare of the

Fig. 5.6 Title page, Griffith and Johnson 1942 report on first use of curare in anesthesia (Image by permission Wolters Kluwer Health)

*From the Department of Anesthesia, Homoepathic Hospital of Montreal.

Fig. 5.7 Footnote, Griffith and Johnson hospital affiliation (Image by permission Wolters Kluwer Health)

result of politics – thus, ended the 101-year life of the hospital which for almost 70 years of its existence had been capably led by the father and son Griffith team.

AR and his wife Mary produced four sons, Harold, Hugh, James, and Arthur. Harold and James qualified as doctors. Harold received training in orthodox medicine at McGill University and then continued his training in homeopathy at the Hahnemann Medical College in Philadelphia, returning to join his father's practice. His brother Jim was also a surgeon on the hospital staff, serving as chief of service.

The Homeopathic Hospital had played an important role in Harold's early years, as he recalled following his father on hospital rounds and learning some essentials of homeopathic prescribing [21, p. 102]. Later, as a medical student, he lived in the hospital while serving as an intern; in 1923, he was appointed to the hospital staff, where for many years he conducted general practice (Fig. 5.5). An ever-growing interest in anesthetics eventually leads him to full-time specialization,

and by 1933, he had given up general practice in favor of anesthesia and hospital administration. Throughout his professional life, Griffith believed in the "leavening wisdom" of homeopathy, a discipline which he considered to be "rich, unexploited and almost unexplored" [23]. While in clinical practice, he made use of homeopathic remedies and even into the late 1960s continued to remain involved with homeopathy as registrar of the College of Homeopathic Physicians and Surgeons of Montreal [22, p. 38].

Sometimes, the greatest medical breakthroughs are communicated without fanfare in the form of brief communications, like Alexander Fleming's discovery of penicillin. Such was the case with Harold Griffith who, in 1942, published a short 3-page paper [24] which made an immediate impact and cemented his reputation as a great anesthesiologist. The paper, which was written jointly with his trainee coauthor, Enid Johnson, described the successful use of curare in 25 patients undergoing anesthesia (Figs. 5.6 and 5.7). The reasons for this paper's influence will be described.

Until Griffith and Johnson's report, it had at times proved hard to achieve the deep level of muscle relaxation required for safe abdominal, chest, or throat surgery. Deep relaxation could only be obtained at high degrees of anesthesia, mainly with ether or chloroform, but at considerable risk of complications. The great merit of curare was its ability to achieve the desired relaxation with a short-acting drug largely devoid of side effects as long as the anesthesiologist was able to sustain respiration since, as a paralyzing drug, curare blocked the nerve impulses which caused muscle contraction, including the muscles of respiration. Curare had a somewhat formidable reputation as the active ingredient in arrow poisons used by natives of the Amazon to paralyze their victims who would die from inability to breathe. The fascinating story of how curare was introduced to Western medicine has been told in numerous places [25, 26] and involved collaborations between personnel in ethnobotany, psychiatry, industry, homeopathy, and anesthesiology. A comprehensive review has been given elsewhere by Bennett (a psychiatrist). Griffith's contribution is notable because few other anesthetists had the courage to use the drug until Griffith demonstrated that it could be used safely in surgery. Some anesthesiologists had experimented with curare in dogs, often seeing fatal outcomes; in his laboratory at the University of Iowa, Dr. Stuart Cullen had given Introcostrin (the brand name for curare) to over 100 dogs and they all died. The drug had gained a reputation as being too dangerous to use and even some of Griffith's closest professional colleagues kept their distance from the drug for years [21, p. 177]. There had also been some serious complications from the drug in human surgery.

About 30 years earlier, curare had been used in a small number of cases by Läwen, a German physiologist and surgeon, but he pursued it no further since supplies were scarce. Although he published his results, his paper received little attention, and it is not known whether Griffith was aware of the earlier work or if it influenced him in any way.

With its reputation as a dangerous poison, the question arises as to how Griffith could have figured out how to use curare. Dr. Franco Carli, who holds the Harold Griffith Chair of Anesthesiology at McGill University, has gone on record as saying that only a homeopath like Griffith could have understood how to use curare, since the quantity of drug used to produce relaxation is "infinitesimal … ridiculously small" and that no classically trained doctor would have considered such trace doses could be therapeutically useful. Carli stated that "we owe this breakthrough to the way Griffith had been trained – to always use *less* of a chemical instead of more" [21, pp. 117–118]. Tribute to Griffith continues to be paid, as in a recent editorial which stated that "the introduction of neuromuscular blocking drugs (muscle relaxants) into anaesthetic practice 70 years ago revolutionized acute clinical care" and went on to explain that it led to advances in major cardiac, pediatric, and neurosurgery [27]. Others have hailed Griffith's introduction of curare into anesthesia as one of the ten most crucial developments of medicine in the last 100 years [28, 29].

While Griffith is perhaps best known for introducing curare, he achieved much more. Among other things, he established the McGill anesthesia residency training program, the first postoperative recovery room in a Canadian hospital in 1943, and the first intensive care unit in 1961. He served as a vice-president of the American Society of Anesthesiologists in 1945–1946. Between 1951 and 1955, he became involved in what some consider his greatest achievement in anesthesia, the creation of World Federation of Societies of Anesthesiologists, of which he was the first president.

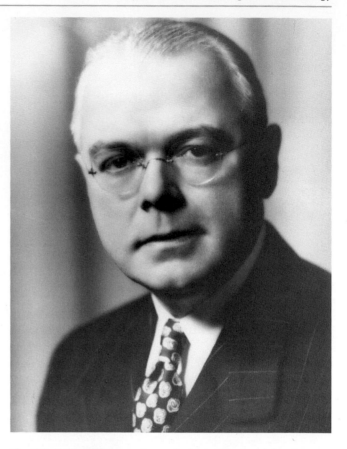

Fig. 5.8 Rolland Whitacre. Innovator in anesthesia training. Inventor of Whitacre needle (Image by courtesy of the Wood Library-Museum, Park Ridge, Illinois)

Harold Griffith showed conspicuous courage in medicine and outside of it: in World War I, he earned the Military Medal for bravery at Vimy Ridge, and it was this same quality that propelled him into unknown territory with his use of curare, confident that any risks would be outweighed by benefit. By introducing curare, he revolutionized the practice of anesthesia.

Rolland Whitacre

Rolland Whitacre was born in Vandergrift, PA, in 1909 (Fig. 5.8). He graduated from Hahnemann Medical College in 1933, having trained under Henry Ruth. At the age of 26, he became the director of anesthesia at the Huron Road Hospital ("Huron Road") in Cleveland. The history of Huron Road is of interest to the student of homeopathy since it was founded by Dr. Samuel Beckwith in 1856 as a homeopathic facility closely linked with the Western College of Homeopathy, which had been formed in Cleveland in 1850. When Whitacre took up his appointment in 1935, Huron Road moved into a new and expanded facility and was about to transition from a largely homeopathic institution to a predominantly allopathic hospital. Even as this was happening, the hospital remained bound by a 1924 injunction which barred allopathic doctors from having staff privileges and it was not until 1959 that this clause was legally dissolved, when there were very few homeopaths left. Therefore, Huron Road for some time continued to attract homeopathically trained physicians, including the Hahnemann-trained anesthetists Rolland Whitacre and BB Sankey, as well as Kenneth Keown whose contributions to cardiac anesthesia are described below.

Under Whitacre's leadership, the Huron Road anesthesia department became one of the largest and best-known teaching departments in the United States. Besides Whitacre's stellar reputation for teaching and practice, he is remembered for inventing the Whitacre needle, a device for delivering spinal anesthesia which is still in use. He was the author of 28 publications on anesthesia.

Whitacre is remembered for being "perhaps the most active individual representative of his specialty in its own societies and in other professional groups striving for the advancement of medical practice in all its phases" [30]. He is also credited as "one of the first to recognize that the welfare of the patient was closely linked to the relationship between the anesthesiologist and the hospital." In this, we may perhaps wonder if some of the Hahnemann College philosophy was reflected in his attitudes: similar words have been used to describe Everett Tyler and Harold Griffith, both of whom placed highest importance on the patient as an individual. Among many offices Whitacre held were the following: president of the American Board of Anesthesiology, vice-president of the board 1950–1954, executive secretary and member of the board of trustees of the International Anesthesia Research Society, and president of the Academy of Anesthesiology. He was the chairman of the Section on Anesthesiology of the American Medical Association in 1953 and was the delegate of that Section to the AMA. He was the chair of the Section on Anesthesiology of the Ohio State Medical Association on more than one occasion. He served on the Joint Commission for Accreditation of Hospitals and was an associate editor of the journal *Anesthesiology* from 1946 until his death. Whitacre served many other organizations in his state and hospital, including a term as president of the hospital medical staff in 1951–1952. His death at 46 brought to a premature end a life of astonishing productivity. His obituary remembered him as "a world leader in the … medical specialty of anesthesia. He long will be remembered for his major role in the evolution of medical practice."

William Neff

William ("Bill") Neff was born in Philadelphia in 1905 and attended Hahnemann Medical College, graduating in 1930 (Fig. 5.9). Initially undecided as to his career path, he took

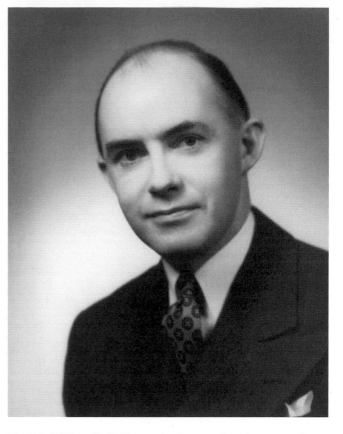

Fig. 5.9 William Neff. Pioneer in the use of cyclopropane (Image courtesy of the Wood Library-Museum, Park Ridge, Illinois)

the suggestion of some friends at Hahnemann to join Harold Griffith's anesthesia training program at the Montreal Homeopathic Hospital, where his academic career quickly took off with a published report on the use of Avertin, which was gradually being introduced, albeit cautiously, by American anesthesiologists. In his publication, Neff described how the use of this drug could be made safer [31]. Following his time in Montreal, Neff obtained further training at the University of Wisconsin and then eventually found his way to the west coast, where he became the chairman of anesthesia at Stanford University, remaining in that position from 1937 to 1950.

Neff wrote the first paper on cyclopropane anesthesia, introduced the concept of "balanced" anesthesia, and established the Arthur Guedel Memorial Center in San Francisco [32]. An interesting but perhaps overlooked contribution was his communication on the use of low-dose sublingual curare for the relief of chronic pain. It is notable that he found very low doses (6–12 mg) of the drug when given sublingually once daily to produce a sometimes long-lasting benefit over several months for chronic pain [33]. He also was recipient of the Distinguished Service Award from the California Society of Anesthesiologists in 1978 and Fellowship of the Faculty of Anaesthetists of the Royal College of Surgeons (United Kingdom) in 1954.

As far as cyclopropane is concerned, the manner in which Neff's report was prepared and published was an interesting process. The first two authors of this initial publication were junior trainees, working under the direction of Dr. Ralph Waters. Dr. Waters requested that each author independently write up the results of the study. These reports were then reviewed and any differences resolved and then the junior collaborators were given "undue prominence to their contributions at the time of publication" by a generous boss [34]. This being said, Neff in fact can be credited with some very important contributions regarding cyclopropane. One major concern about the drug was its explosive nature and the necessity to administer it in a closed system. While the commonly used closed system probably did improve safety, surgeons often blamed it for the many postoperative pulmonary infections which occurred. In 1947, Neff introduced an answer to this difficulty by developing balanced anesthesia, in which nitrous oxide, oxygen, intermittent curare, and meperidine were used together. By use of this procedure, it was possible to achieve the same depth of anesthesia as with cyclopropane, but without the aforementioned concerns about its use [35]. Balanced anesthesia, which is the basis of modern anesthesia, may be seen as a partial implementation of the philosophy of homeopathy: to give as little of each drug where the net effect is good by not having the negative effect of too much of any one drug [36].

Brant Burdell ("BB") Sankey

BB Sankey was born in 1908 and died in 2007 (Fig. 5.10). At the time of his death, he was the oldest surviving past president of the American Society of Anesthesiologists (ASA). Dr. Sankey had received his medical training at Hahnemann Medical College in Philadelphia, where he was a classmate and friend of Rolland Whitacre. BB graduated in 1933 and completed a surgical internship at Huron Road, followed by a 2-year anesthesia residency there under Dr. Whitacre. He stayed on for 6 years at Huron Road before moving to St. Luke's Hospital in Cleveland, where he founded their anesthesia program and spent the next 37 years. Sankey published extensively and achieved high distinction.

BB cofounded the Ohio Society of Anesthesiologists (OSA) and in due course became the president of the ASA in 1955 and the OSA in 1956. He was a founding trustee and treasurer of the Anesthesia Memorial Society and editor of Current Researches in Anesthesia and Analgesia. Between 1961 and 1965, he was the vice-chairman and then the chairman of the IARS and served on its board for 18 years as executive secretary and business manager of the society's journal. Sankey gave 50 years of service to IARS as a trustee and then emeritus trustee. Upon his retirement, the IARS recognized Sankey in the form of its annual BB Sankey Anesthesia Advancement Awards.

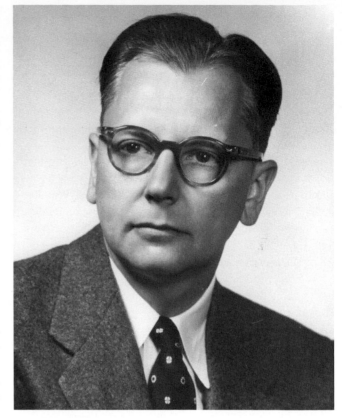

Fig. 5.10 Brant Burdell ("BB") Sankey. Editor of Anesthesia and Analgesia and chairman of International Anesthesia Research Society (Image by courtesy of the Wood Library-Museum, Park Ridge, Illinois)

Dr. Sankey was renowned as one who "loved his profession, going off each morning with a smile and boundless energy." He was a pioneer in the development of anesthesiology, a man with shrewd business skill, and many other talents [37].

Kenneth K. Keown

Dr. Kenneth Keown was another Hahnemann graduate (1941) who belongs in the anesthesia hall of fame (Fig. 5.11). He derived an interest in anesthesia from his father, a general practitioner who had a special interest in pain relief during delivery [38]. Dr. Keown senior was interested in the effectiveness and safety of alcohol, chloroform, and ether (ACE), even trying it on his young son! Keown's father died tragically at the age of 52 following septicemia transmitted from a cut sustained during a surgical procedure. Keown Jr. claimed that he wanted to honor his father and had originally intended to become a general surgeon. He did indeed enter surgical training at the homeopathic hospital in Cleveland. While studying at Hahnemann, however, he had encountered Henry Ruth and was impressed by what Ruth was achieving. Thus, after completing his surgery internship in 1941, he

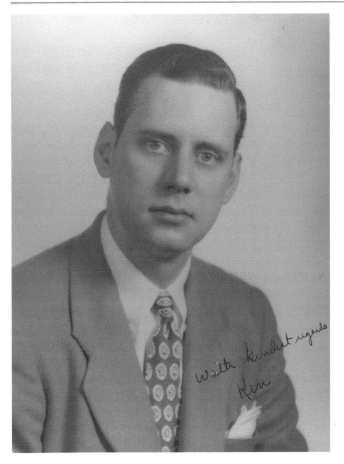

Fig. 5.11 Kenneth Keown. Leader in cardiac anesthesia (Image courtesy of the Wood Library-Museum, Park Ridge, Illinois)

entered Whitacre's training program at Huron Road. World War II interrupted these plans and Keown served for 5 years as a medical officer on the front lines in Europe. He attained the rank of Major in the US Army Medical Corps and earned the Silver Star with cluster and Bronze Star with two clusters. It was during this time that Dr. Keown became acutely aware of the need to train more physicians in anesthetics. Upon his military discharge, Keown entered Dr. Ruth's residency program at Hahnemann.

At Hahnemann, Keown was invited by the cardiovascular surgeon, Charles Bailey, to join his team at the Cardiovascular Institute (CVI), which was rapidly making a name for its groundbreaking work in heart surgery. He became an indispensable member of the CVI group: Bailey acknowledged that "without Ken I could not have gone far … he was a veritable genius in evaluating patients … with respect to getting them through surgery upon the heart" [18]. In 1948, Keown managed the anesthesia in the first US mitral valve commissurotomy operation, which was performed by Bailey. In 1953, Time magazine hailed the 36-year-old Keown as "the grand old man of anesthesia for inside-the-heart surgery" [39].

Keown introduced a method for hypothermic cooling of patients; he published the first paper on anesthesia for mitral commissurotomy, the first textbook on cardiac anesthesia; and he pioneered the use of lidocaine to suppress arrhythmias in surgery. Outside of clinical practice, he is remembered for service as chairman of the board of trustees of the International Anesthesia Research Society, vice-president of the ASA, and chair of the Section of Anesthesiology of the AMA.

Keown died at the age of 68, in 1985.

The physicians who have been described above all entered medicine by way of a homeopathic training and then, in their "post-homeopathic" lives, became distinguished anesthesiologists. In the three who follow next, however, this trajectory is reversed – all were trained as regular doctors, earned their anesthetic spurs, and then embraced homeopathy. The ways in which they have impacted medicine vary considerably.

Caleb Matthews

Caleb Matthews was born in 1801 and graduated from the University of Pennsylvania as MD in 1822. He set up medical practice in Philadelphia, where he spent most of his working life, apart from a spell as ship's surgeon in India. Matthews was well respected in the community and served for a time as editor of the *Medical Recorder*. In 1836, to the surprise of many colleagues, he began to take a serious interest in homeopathy, which had recently been introduced into the United States by German immigrants. He took leadership in forming the homeopathic medical college, was professor of *materia medica* until his untimely death in 1851, and also served as vice-president of the Philadelphia Hahnemann Hospital.

Matthews played a little-known part in the story of ether's introduction to medicine. Initially, the drug was used for non-anesthetic purposes; there are reports of ether being used in England for stomach disorders and cough in the eighteenth century, as well as quite extensive use for tuberculosis during the time of pneumatic medicine [40]. In 1805, Dr. Warren gave ether to a tuberculous patient at the Massachusetts General Hospital and later to patients with asthma. In 1818, Michael Faraday suggested that ether was a promising anesthetic, but conducted no experiments to support his contention [41]. Crawford Long has been mentioned above as the first to use ether during surgery, in 1842. Out of caution, he delayed the publication of his finding and as a result was beaten to the punch by Morton, the Boston dentist who reported on its successful use in 1846. However, it appears likely that neither Long nor Morton was the first; the *National Intelligencer* of June 1836 advertised ether for painless tooth extraction, and a Dr. Samuel Woolsten from

New Jersey recalled using ether with morphine for operative pain as far back as 1836 [42]. Between the reports of Faraday in 1818 and Morton in 1846, there was widespread interest in the use and study of ether in medicine. It is interesting to note that a careful assessment of ether's effects was carried out by Caleb Matthews in 1824, long before Woolsten, Long, and Warren. At the time, Matthews was a medical student at the University of Pennsylvania. Although this account was not published until 1855, the report was completed as part of his graduation thesis and its existence was known to Dr. Callisen in volume 12 of his lexicon, which was published before 1835 [43]. Helmuth credits Matthews being one of the earliest doctors to test the effects of ether inhalation and recognize that it could produce "profound slumber." At all events, his experiments took place over a decade before Morton's work. Matthews admitted that as a student he was quite constrained in how far he could take his work. Among the various obstacles was the fact that ether produced such alarming symptoms that Matthews' friends dissuaded him from further work. Secondly, ether "frolics" were quite a popular pastime and gave ether a bad reputation as an abusable drug. And lastly, perhaps, Matthews was more concerned at that point in his career to develop his medical practice and establish a good reputation. Had he pursued his experiments, however, it is conceivable that the anesthetic benefits of ether would have been better understood many years earlier.

Thomas Skinner

Thomas Skinner was born in Edinburgh, August 11, 1825. He received his medical training there and graduated in 1853 as Licentiate of the Royal College of Surgeons in Edinburgh (LRCS Ed.) and as Doctor of Medicine (MD) from St. Andrews in 1857; as a student, he won the prestigious Simpson Gold Medal of the University of Edinburgh. Following a brief period in private practice, he was appointed as chief assistant to Sir James Young Simpson, the famous obstetrician who introduced chloroform anesthesia into medicine and whose influence on Skinner was twofold.

1. Four years with the master afforded Skinner the opportunity to develop into a competent obstetrician as well as gaining unique experience with chloroform anesthesia in the practice of midwifery. In 1859, Skinner moved to Liverpool, where he established a flourishing practice and served as obstetric physician at the Liverpool Dispensaries. Administration of chloroform was risky, including the occurrence of chemical burn on the face due to spillage, difficulty regulating the dose, and, with the traditional method of administration, inability of the physician to see where he was dropping the chloroform. Skinner therefore devised a dropper bottle and wire mask which overcame these deficiencies and, as a further advantage, required

only one-third the amount of chloroform per hour [44]. Skinner was concerned to preserve chloroform's availability in the face of opposition by colleagues who believed the drug to be unacceptably toxic. Skinner was convinced that chloroform mortality was largely due to unskilled application by the anesthetist and that, as far as he was concerned, chloroform is "as safe as milk." The Skinner mask raised the safety and effectiveness of chloroform anesthesia and was in widespread use for decades. Even as late as 1938, the mask was still available in medical equipment catalogues, at a price of 7/6 (i.e., about $2) at that time [45]. The Skinner mask also served as prototype for other derivatives. Ever conscious of convenience and portability, Skinner's mask was designed to be folded up and carried inside one's top hat! While one might cavil at the unhygienic practice of keeping it in such a place, Skinner was at pains to stress how his device differed from the inhalers in common use by offering the patient a mask which was clean. Unbelievably from today's perspective, inhalers and mouthpieces were neither cleaned nor replaced, but passed along from one patient to the next, "loaded with grease, and filthy enough to upset any one's digestion and sleep for a considerable time to come" [43]. As Westhorpe noted, Skinner was ahead of his time in drawing attention to the health hazards associated through transmission during anesthesia [46]. In addition to his chloroform mask, Skinner devised and marketed equipment for the safer delivery of ether [47].

2. Simpson's influence over Skinner extended to his attitude towards homeopathy. Simpson was a well-known opponent of homeopathy and homeopaths, as in the case of William Henderson, an esteemed Scottish physician. At first, Skinner followed in his master's footsteps in persecuting sectarians with Pauline zeal, regarding homeopathy as baseless and its founder to be "deceived, next to insane and a deceiver." Of homeopathy, he said "the whole system seemed to me, in my then profound ignorance of the subject, so preposterous, and so far beyond the bounds of human credibility and reason, as that no ordinary thoughtsman could be blamed if he refused to give it even a hearing, far less to take the system into his serious consideration" [48]. In expressing these sentiments, Skinner's words are virtually identical to the diatribes heard from today's opponents of homeopathy. So great was his abhorrence of homeopathy, and so determined was he to put it down, that in 1861 he successfully pursued a campaign to deny staff privileges for homeopaths at Liverpool's main hospital, making sure that rule was codified in the hospital bylaws.

It thus came as a surprise to many when Skinner underwent a *volte-face*. His conversion occurred in 1875 in Liverpool as a result of personal health problems. For over 3 years, Skinner had suffered from insomnia, constipation, acidic stomach, general debility, and "unutterable bodily and mental anguish." Regular treatments having failed to help, Skinner took the recommendation of a Liverpool homeopath, Dr. Edward Berridge, who suggested a few doses of high potency sulfur at the millionth potency. Much to Skinner's amazement, his symptoms were cured. We cannot be certain as to the nature of his illness, although depression seems a prime candidate. But in any event, this personal experience had a salutary effect on Skinner's attitude towards homeopathy, which he increasingly began to embrace in his own practice. Simultaneously, he underwent personal training and, in the remaining three decades of his life, earned a distinguished reputation in the homeopathic world. He brought to homeopathy the same inventive genius that characterized his career as an allopathic physician and invented the "centesimal fluxion machine," also known as the Skinner machine, for preparing high potency remedies. He did much to forge closer links between British and American homeopathy, but at the same time, his pugnacious nature inflamed a large section of the homeopathic community on doctrinal grounds and in some ways had a divisive effect.

Apropos his conversion from orthodox medicine to homeopathy, he wrote an *apologia*, called *Homeopathy and Gynecology*, which had run into four editions by 1903. In this book, Skinner extolled the value of treating gynecological problems constitutionally rather than on the basis of symptoms. Skinner published numerous peer-reviewed articles, initially in orthodox journals, such as the *British Medical Journal*, and later in various homeopathic journals. Ironically, one consequence of Skinner's conversion to homeopathy was the necessity for him to resign from the medical staff of the Liverpool Infirmary – the same infirmary where Skinner had forbidden homeopaths from holding staff privileges: he was hoist by his own petard.

August Bier

August Bier was one of Germany's most distinguished twentieth-century surgeons (Fig. 5.12). He adopted the cause of homeopathy late in his career, although his sympathies had long been attuned to its fundamental tenets. For example, he believed in the self-healing power of the body and its intimate partnership with the environment [49].

Bier is well known for several innovations, some of which still impact medical practice. Early in his career, he pioneered a safer method of intestinal suturing which is still applicable today. Perhaps his most enduring and best-known contribution was the introduction, in 1898, of spinal anesthesia as a way to bypass the risks of ether and chloroform when given as general anesthetics; even though there is some dispute about who deserves credit for introducing spinal anesthesia, Bier is now generally acknowledged worldwide as deserving

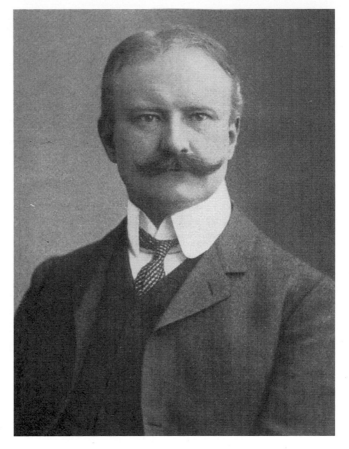

Fig. 5.12 August Bier. German surgeon, anesthesiologist, and champion of homeopathy (Image in the public domain)

the lion's share [50]. Bier also introduced the technique of hyperemia by means of intermittent circulatory occlusion to promote healing of certain types of tuberculosis. While this method enjoyed some success, and brought prestigious awards to its inventor, it is has long since fallen out of use. Another of Bier's innovations which initially fell out of favor due to adverse effects was the application of intravenous regional blockade with local anesthesia, the so-called Bier block, which was first described in 1908. However, as safer local anesthetics were developed, this method experienced something of a renaissance [50] in limb surgery and also in managing certain forms of neuropathic pain.

Bier made undoubted contributions to anesthesia, yet like most of his German contemporaries, he was opposed to the emancipation of anesthesiology as a separate specialty. He preferred to identify himself primarily as a surgeon and considered the two terms he served as president of the German Society of Surgeons in 1910 and 1920 to be among the highlights of his career.

Bier was not one to run away from controversy, and he often adopted unfashionable causes, including homeopathy. In so doing, Bier ran afoul of many colleagues, although it apparently mattered little to him, as he fully acknowledged

Wie sollen wir uns zu der Homöopathie stellen?

Von

Geheimrat Professor Dr. August Bier
Berlin

Sonderabdruck aus der Münchener
Medizinischen Wochenschrift

5. Auflage

J. F. Lehmanns Verlag, München 1925

Fig. 5.13 Title of Bier article "Wie sollen wir uns zur Homöopathie stellen?" (Image by permission, Michael Goerig MD)

their incredulity and hostility [51]. The origins of Bier's interest in homeopathy stemmed from his time at the University of Greifswald, where he was impressed by the prevailing level of cooperation between the various departments; among the many colleagues with whom Bier interacted was the pharmacologist Hugo Schulz, who subscribed to some of Hahnemann's teachings [52]. Specifically, Schulz held with Hahnemann that "weak impulses light vitality, medium ones enhance it, strong ones omit it." During Bier's first academic appointment in Kiel in the 1890s, he had engaged in some research which was relevant to these three principles but had taken it no further. Schulz rekindled Bier's enthusiasm, and over the next several decades, he became increasingly drawn to homeopathy. In 1925, Bier astonished the world of German medicine by publishing a monograph entitled "How Should We View Homoeopathy?" [53] (Fig. 5.13). The thrust of his article was to praise Hahnemann for his "visionary spirit and superior skills of an observing nature that were hidden to less sharp eyes," to report on Bier's own positive experiences with homeopathic sulfur for skin conditions, and to encourage the serious study of homeopathy. Bier went on to found the Society for Examination of Homeopathic Drugs and conducted research on the effects of sulfur, iodine, and ether. Subcutaneous administration of the last mentioned was proposed as a way to prevent postoperative pneumonia, a suggestion which generated considerable interest among the surgical community at the time. "Bier's drops" were manufactured commercially, and for a while, homeopathic medicines were outselling conventional ones in regions of Germany as a result of Bier's influence [51]. However, while Bier managed to revive a nearly moribund profession, and even give it transient academic representation at some major universities, it failed to establish itself on an equal status as other branches of medicine. Furthermore, the homeopathic revival was nipped in the bud with the onset of World War II. In the late 1930s, an ambitious government-sponsored national research program was undertaken to evaluate homeopathy, but firm conclusions were obtained neither for, nor against, homeopathy, and the results were never properly written up.

As Ernst points out, Bier's support of homeopathy did have an impact in Germany, where it prospered in a way that would previously have been unimaginable. His authority and outspokenness narrowed the gap between strongly polarized camps and promoted constructive dialog, out of which homeopathy positioned itself as a potentially useful adjunct to regular medicine rather than as an "either-or" proposition. One measure of Bier's impact, as noted by Ernst, was the appearance of 157 publications on homeopathy in the three leading German medical journals between 1925 and 1935, compared to a total of eight in the previous 5 years. Perhaps Bier's often controversial career typifies the courageous physician who struggles to "understand the complexities of disease, and [sought] the best cures possible, no matter how controversial," and demonstrates that "we must remain open to new ideas and not to assume the conventional wisdom is always correct" [54]. His embracing of homeopathy may be seen in this light, and of all the physicians who have paddled in homeopathic waters, Bier was among the most distinguished.

Summary

In summary, it has been shown that several homeopathic graduates from the Philadelphia and New York colleges played a significant role in the growth of anesthesia as a profession in the first decades of the twentieth century, as well as contributed in other ways. In addition, two distinguished orthodox physicians who had been pioneers in anesthesiology later embraced homeopathy and proselytized on its behalf.

References

1. Lennon R, Lennon RL, Bacon DR. The Anaesthetists' Travel Club: an example of professionalism. J Clin Anesth. 2009;21:137–42.
2. ABIM Foundation, ACP-ASIM Foundation, European Federation of Internal Medicine. Medical professionalism in the new millennium: a physician charter. Ann Int Med. 2002;136:243–6.
3. Wood PM. Thomas Drysdale Buchanan memorial. Anesth Analg. 1941;20:61–3.
4. Northrop HL. A plea for the scientific use of anaesthetics. Hahnemannian Monthly. June 1891;26. p. 1–6.
5. Northrop HL. Reasons for the administration of oxygen with chloroform when the latter is used as an anaesthetic. Hahnemannian Monthly. 1895 Feb;30. p. 1–8.
6. Anonymous. Notabilia: oxygenated chloroform. Monthly Homoeopathic Review. 1896 Mar 2. p. 178.
7. Nicholson TGH. Oxychloroform anaesthesia. BMJ. 1896;ii:233.
8. Nicholson T. Oxychloroform anaesthesia. Br Homeopath Rev. 1897;41:26–30.
9. Reports and analyses. Descriptions of new inventions. Oxychloroform administration. BMJ. 1897;i:666.
10. Anonymous. Surgery as a cure for moral degeneracy. Phrenological J Sci Health. 1908:402–4.
11. Northrop HL. Surgical treatment of kleptomania. N Engl Med Gazette. 1909;43:553–5.
12. Mohr C. The report of the director of provings. Transactions of the 41st Session of the American Institute of Homoeopathy; 1888 June 25–29; Niagara Falls, NY. 1888;45:159–61.
13. Wetchler B. Thomas Drysdale Buchanan or Henry Isaiah Dorr: give credit to both. Anesthesiology. 2001;95:271–2.
14. Vandam LD. Walter M. Boothby, M.D. – the wellsprings of anesthesiology. N Engl J Med. 1967;276:558–67.
15. McNamara O. Generations. A history of Boston University School of Medicine. 1848–1998. Boston: Trustees of Boston University; 1998. p. 153.
16. Tyler E. Presidential address, American Association of Anaesthetists (1924): including some investigations of a newer theory of anesthesia. Anesth Analg. 1924;4:163–7.
17. Barbara Williams. Personal communication. 14 Oct 2011.
18. Rosenberg H, Axelrod JK. Henry Ruth: pioneer of modern anesthesiology. Anesthesiology. 1993;78:178–83.
19. Ruth HS. Postwar planning in anesthesiology. N Engl J Med. 1944;231:669–72.
20. Keown K. Presentation to annual meeting of the academy of anesthesiology, February 13, 1983, personal communication to Patrick Sim, Wood Library Museum of Anesthesiology. 22 Feb 1983.
21. Dressel H. Who killed the queen? The story of a community hospital and how to fix public health care. Montreal: McGill-Queen's University Press; 2008.
22. Bodman R, Gillies D. Harold Griffith: the evolution of modern anesthesia. Toronto: Hannah Institute and Dundurn Press; 1992.
23. Griffith HR. The field of homeopathic remedies in scientific medicine. J Am Inst Homeopath. 1930;23:762–5.
24. Griffith HR, Johnson GE. The use of curare in general anesthesia. Anesthesiology. 1942;3:418–20.
25. Gill RC. White water and black magic. New York: Henry Holt and Co; 1940.
26. Bennett AE. The history of the introduction of curare into medicine. Anesth Analg. 1968;47:484–92.
27. Hunter JM. Antagonising neuromuscular block at the end of surgery. BMJ. 2012;345:e6666.
28. Czarnowski C, Bailey J, Bal S. Curare and a Canadian connection. Can Fam Phys. 2007;53:1531–2.
29. Editorial. Looking back on the millennium in medicine. N Engl J Med. 2000;342:42–9.
30. Rolland J. Whitacre MD. Obituary. Anesth Analg. 1956;35:145–7.
31. Neff WB. Avertin ethylene anaesthesia. Can Med Assoc J. 1932;26:576–8.
32. Calmes SH. Obituary of William B. Neff, M.D., FFARCS. Bull Calif Soc Anesthesiologists. 1997;46:5–9.
33. Neff WB, Mayer H. The sublingual administration of curare. Calif Med. 1953;79:227–30.
34. Neff WB. The study of cyclopropane. Anesthesiology. 1974;41:414–5.
35. Neff WB, Mayer EC, Perales M. Nitrous oxide and oxygen with curare relaxation. Calif Med. 1947;66:67–9.
36. Reves JG. Personal communication. 21 Jan 2013.
37. Siddall J. Personal communication to Patrick Sim. 6 Feb 2007.
38. Rosenberg H, Axelrod JK. Kenneth K. Keown, MD: Pioneer of cardiac anesthesiology. J Cardiothorac Vasc Anesth. 1994;8:577–83.
39. Medicine:gas and needle. Time Magazine. 1953 Oct 19. p. 54.
40. Slatter E. The evolution of anaesthesia. I. Ether in medicine before anaesthesia. Br J Anaesth. 1960;32:31–4.
41. Kirby HA. The history of anaesthetics. Drug Circ. 1916;LX(12):749–51.
42. Information obtained from Helmuth WT. System of surgery. 3rd ed. New York: Boericke and Tafel; 1879. Chapter XLVII: Anaesthesia. p. 970–973.
43. Duncum BM. The development of inhalation anaesthesia. London: Royal Society of Medicine Press Ltd.; 1994. p. 249.
44. Skinner T. Anaesthesia in midwifery; with new apparatus for its safer and more economical induction by chloroform. BMJ. 1862;2:108–11.
45. Bryn Thomas K. The development of anaesthetic apparatus. A history based on the Charles King collection of the association of anaesthetists of Great Britain and Ireland. Oxford: Blackwell Scientific Publications; 1975. p. 250–1.
46. Westhorpe R. Skinner's chloroform mask. Anaesth Intensive Care. 1995;23:3.
47. Skinner T. Ether as an anaesthetic. BMJ. 1875;2:423–4.
48. Obituary: Thomas Skinner M.D. (St. And.) Monthly Homoeopathic Review. 1906 Oct 1. p. 635–9.
49. Goerig M, Agarwal K, Schulte am Esch J. The versatile August Bier (1861–1949), father of spinal anesthesia. J Clin Anesth. 2000;12:561–9.
50. Waas G. To August Bier (1861–1949) on his 120th birthday. Z Arztl Fortbild. 1982;76:72–4.
51. Ernst E. August Bier and German homoeopathy in the early 20th century. Br J Homeopath. 1996;85:49–52.
52. Van Zundert A, Goerig M. August Bier 1861–1949. A tribute to a great surgeon who contributed much to the development of modern anesthesia on the 50th anniversary of his death. Reg Anesth Pain Med. 2000;25:26–33.
53. Bier A. Wie sollen wir uns zu der Homöopathie stellen? Munich: JF Lehmanns Verlag; 1925.
54. Bacon DR. August Bier's legacy: more than just a pioneer in regional anesthesia? J Clin Anesth. 2000;12:501–2.

6

Homeopathy and the Mind: From Alienists to Neuroscientists

Hahnemann's Attitude Towards Mental Illness

Hahnemann was more enlightened than many of his contemporaries when it came to the mentally ill [1]. He described how, in the case of an aristocratic patient who was under his care, he initially spent some weeks in observation before deciding on the best treatment. Hahnemann forbade all kinds of violence, which were common practices in psychiatry at the time, saying "I never allow any insane person to be punished by blows or other painful bodily chastisement….These patients deserve nothing but pity, and are always made worse and not better by such rough treatment" [2]. Today, these principles are taken for granted (although they are still violated too often), but at the time they were rarely followed. Charles Cameron paid tribute to this aspect of Hahnemann's work in saying that "… homeopathy has made contributions to medical progress which have been neglected in the long view …. First, Hahnemann fought vigorously for modification of the treatment of the insane … he wrote and preached of the folly of attempting to overpower psychosis. He pled for an end to the floggings, to solitary confinement, to chains, to starvation rations. He went so far as to set up his own modest sanitarium where the mentally deranged were regarded as the sick people they were, instead of being exorcised." Cameron further acknowledged that Hahnemann was one of the earliest to advocate drug treatment of the mentally ill, "a principle which now – in the past five years – offers the brightest promise yet uncovered for the relief and rehabilitation of the mentally ill" [3]. It is therefore not surprising that Hahnemann's approach to psychiatric illness inspired many of his followers, who created and staffed a national movement of homeopathic mental hospitals that served the US population for over 50 years; seven were still functioning into the 1940s [4]. As will be described below, some solid research, high-quality teaching, and innovative treatment approaches took place in these hospitals. Thus, while Hahnemann shared with Pinel the distinction of being among the first to espouse humane care of the mentally ill, free from enchainment, he went one step further by inspiring a homeopathic asylum movement.

Hahnemann held that mental illnesses could derive from internal (physical) or external (environmental) causes, such as upbringing, beliefs, education, or bad morals; for the former, medicine was usually indicated, whereas for the latter, "sensible advice" was often enough [5]. In the homeopathic canon, utmost importance was placed on the mental influences in illness, for there was no division of body and mind, which were instead viewed as a seamless entity.

Kinship of Homeopathy and Psychiatry

A number of similarities have been noted between homeopathy and psychiatry [6]:

1. Variations of the therapeutic principle *similia similibus curentur*, or the law of similars, play a significant role in some forms of psychiatry, notably in cognitive-behavior therapy (CBT) with prolonged exposure (PE), where the symptoms are repeatedly evoked under controlled conditions in order that they eventually will disappear. In another example, an effective treatment of depression involves inducing deprivation of sleep, that is, a cardinal feature of the illness, in order to enact a cure. Similar to administering the kindred remedy, one "gives the illness" to the patient so that it can be removed by means of the body's adaptation process. Technically, this is most accurately referred to as *isopathy*, rather than *homeopathy*, in that the treatment consists of inducing the exact symptom, akin to treating pollen allergy with a low dose of pollen extract, rather than administering an agent that produces closely similar symptoms.

2. Homeopathy teaches that there is a self-correcting principle referred to as the vital force. So, in psychiatry, it has been posited that some symptoms may represent the body's attempts at self-correction or self-healing. Post and Weiss [7] have suggested that insomnia is less a primary symptom than an endogenous ("from within")

counterreaction and that the same may hold true for certain biological alterations in depression that might be compensatory, like the increases in thyrotropin-releasing hormone (TRH). Post and Weiss characterize some symptoms of depression as the "good guys," emblematic of the body's attempt at self-regulation, and suggest there may be promise in developing treatments that promote internal self-corrective change (i.e., as opposed to treatments that suppress symptoms). This sounds little different from the homeopathic principle of an internal, self-correcting force.

3. Homeopathy holds that "less is more" when it comes to drug dose. Similarly, in psychiatry, the phenomenon of time-dependent sensitization (TDS) echoes this principle. Sensitization refers to the ability of a stimulus, such as a drug, to induce a response that can later be elicited by repeated presentation of the stimulus at a lower dose, or if repeated at the same dose, then the response is amplified. In other words, the system has become more sensitive to the original stimulus over time. Key factors behind TDS appear to include (1) the threatening ("unfriendly") nature of the stimulus and (2) its intermittent application. TDS perhaps can explain how it is possible to obtain a good response to low doses of the remedy when given only intermittently, as some homeopaths advocate. It is also a strong candidate to explain the development of PTSD (posttraumatic stress disorder). Further consideration of TDS is given in Chap. 16, where the work of Iris Bell, a contemporary psychiatrist, neuroscientist, and homeopath, is described.

4. Hering's law teaches that symptoms appear and disappear in a given sequence, with recovery being characterized by symptom disappearance in reverse order of appearance [8, pp. 16–18]. There has been reference to a similar phenomenon in psychiatry by Detre and Jarecki [9]. It is important to keep in mind that these observations were largely made when few treatments were at hand, and they reflect some astute clinical observations on the natural course of illness, many of which are self-limiting. In today's world, the clinical picture is complicated by the fact that patients may have received a treatment that has altered the expression of the illness, by inducing side effects like insomnia or weight gain. The opportunity to confirm such observations is now less likely to occur.

5. In both homeopathy and psychiatry, when a diagnosis is made, it is often according to "whole pattern" recognition, going beyond symptom expression alone. This approach can be contrasted with the use of a biological test, for example, diagnostic x-ray or blood test, or the use of a single measure, as in hypertension.

6. Psychiatry and homeopathy are alike in the amount of time that is set aside for the patient visit. Psychotherapy sessions typically last between 40 and 50 min, while shorter medication management often lasts between 20 and 30 min. As with homeopathy, in psychiatry the doctor spends considerable time listening to the patient. Evidently, both specialties attract professionals willing to give their clients plenty of time to talk and construct a comprehensive life story. This raises interesting questions about the personality traits of psychiatrists and homeopaths. In 1969, Walton [10] found that British students who planned a career in psychiatry were more reflective and had greater complexity (i.e., showed traits of open-mindedness, acceptance of novelty, and tolerance of ambiguity and measured by a 27-item scale) [11]. A person who scores high on complexity is not fixed in his way of viewing events and prefers new ways rather than old ways of doing things; complexity is associated with flexibility and tolerance of unusual conditions. It is therefore striking to find that a study conducted almost 50 years later found identical results among Norwegian homeopaths, in which Rise and colleagues [12] demonstrated a marked increase in openness to new ideas, as well as elevated levels of caring, understanding, and altruism. It is possibly for these reasons that homeopaths were better tolerated, or even welcomed, in American psychiatry during homeopathy's heyday. Noll has commented on the general lack of hostility within psychiatry towards the sect, in contrast to the prevailing attitude of other specialties [13]. The fact that both homeopaths and alienists were stigmatized by orthodox medicine might have also been a factor. Mental hospital professionals were held in low regard by their medical colleagues, and the asylum superintendents tended to keep themselves apart from colleagues in general medicine, while being attacked by neurologists for their lack of interest in medicine as a science. To many neurologists, asylum doctors were no more than custodians.

7. A number of psychiatrists have expressed discomfort in diagnosing patients, which to some is tantamount to labeling. While diagnosis will always be essential to medical practice, the need for individual assessment has also been recognized by leaders such as Adolf Meyer, who espoused the view that "… there is a plurality of causes, and that each case is highly individual and must, therefore, be studied not in the light of some preconceived concept of simple etiology, but rather in the light of the entire life history of the patient" [14]. Such a personal approach approximates the approach of homeopathy. Today, medicine is abuzz with the concept of "personalized medicine" – old wine in new bottles and repackaged in the language of genomics and epigenetics.

In 1961, the famous psychiatrist Sir Aubrey Lewis characterized psychiatry in a manner that could be applied to homeopathy: "Psychiatry, which may in many respects fairly be regarded as in much the same state as medicine was at the end of the eighteenth century, cannot be presented to the medical student as an adequate theoretical system or as body of established and classified facts about causes, pathology, course and treatment of mental diseases." Lewis goes on to say that psychiatry lays itself open to the "system-maker, the empiric and the self-sufficient manipulator" and to somewhat diffuse forms of education and training. While this is less apparent now, it is the case that for much of the twentieth century, the system-making influence of Freudian psychoanalysis predominated in many circles [15]. The same might be said of homeopathy, the product of another system-maker, one who still casts a long shadow.

Influential Individuals

Having broadly compared homeopathy and psychiatry, attention will now turn to individual homeopaths whose professional lives were dedicated to treating the mentally ill. Of those selected, all but one were psychiatrists or alienists to use the nineteenth-century term. The exception was Bayard Holmes, a talented surgeon who spent much of his career searching for a surgical cure of schizophrenia and championing public awareness of the illness then known as *dementia praecox*. The diverse contributions of these men and women encompass the full range of psychiatry: opportunities for African-Americans (Fuller), administrative psychiatry (Overholser, Talcott), neuropathology (Fuller), child and community psychiatry (Klopp), psychiatric nursing (Overholser, Barrus), treatment innovations (Talcott), forensic psychiatry (Talcott, Worcester, Overholser), schizophrenia (Holmes and Boltz), laboratory aids to diagnosis (Fuller, Boltz), medical education (Paine, Richardson, Holmes), clinical practice (Menninger), administration of one of the earliest endowed academic research units in the United States (Richardson and Pollack), administration of state hospitals (Talcott, Williamson, Welch, Patterson), and the ability to overcome amazing odds (Cocke).

Charles Frederick Menninger: An Ambassador-at-Large from the Court of Nature

Dr. Charles Menninger (1862–1953) and his sons are known to almost all psychiatrists and, like the Wesselhoefts, represent one of medicine's more illustrious dynasties. Born in Tell City, Indiana, in 1862, Menninger was the child of German immigrant parents, his father being a lumber manufacturer (Fig. 6.1). His early education prepared him for a teaching position in 1882 on the faculty of Holton College, Kansas, where he was a professor of science and German. In 1887, he embarked on medical training. Partly influencing this choice was Menninger's own frailty, evidenced by his

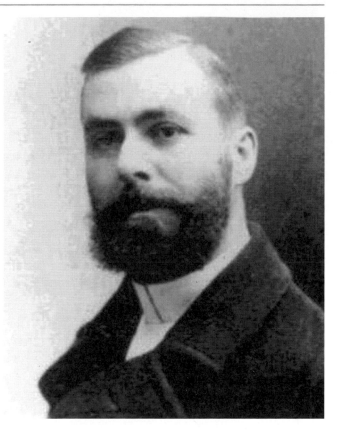

Fig. 6.1 Charles Menninger, founder of the Menninger Clinic (Image in the public domain)

raillike 6′ 2″ physique and 115 lb body weight. A medical friend had told him that he should "get out of the schoolroom because you can't last very long" [16]. In 1887, he enrolled as a student at Hahnemann Medical College in Chicago and excelled so greatly in his studies that he qualified as an MD after 2 years. For approximately 20 years after graduating, Menninger practiced family medicine as a homeopath in Topeka and served first as secretary of the state homeopathic medical society for two terms and then as president. He then served as chairman of the national materia medica section of the American Institute of Homeopathy in 1902 and continued to be a dues-paying member of the institute until 1908 [8, pp. 124–125]. While history remembers Menninger for his contributions to psychiatry, the narrative would be incomplete if it ended there. As noted by Ullman, Menninger was a "Hahnemannian homeopath" of the orthodox faith: he found that the secret of successful homeopathic prescribing lay in careful, precise observation of symptoms and noting the effects of a minimum dose of the single remedy. Homeopathy was more than a brief way station in Menninger's career, for it has been said that he continued to prescribe homeopathic remedies throughout his life [17]. Dr. Menninger would make annual visits to Michigan, often spending several days at the Battle Creek Sanitarium, an eclectically oriented center operated by members of the

Kellogg family, where an array of integrative ("alternative") treatments were provided. Menninger wrote about homeopathy, and an 1897 publication on typhoid fever revealed his position about that system of medicine and why, in his opinion, it was but little better than allopathy in that disease. Among his numerous conclusions were that (1) homeopathy is wholly capable of satisfying the therapeutic demands of this age better than any other system or school of medicine, (2) there is an imperative need to exhaust the homeopathic healing art before trying other methods, (3) prescribing is based on the individual differentiating symptoms peculiar to the person rather than features that are supposedly pathognomonic of the diagnosis, and (4) results were less than optimal on account of a failure to grasp basic homeopathic principles on the practitioner's part [18].

Menninger was a man of wide-ranging scholarship, and his interests included horticulture, mineralogy, conchology, literature, civic affairs, and religion. For his deep understanding of the natural world, Menninger has been characterized as an "Ambassador-at-large from the Court of Nature" [19]. He became interested in psychiatry as the result of his friendship with Dr. B. D. Eastman, superintendent of Topeka State Hospital. From Dr. Eastman, Menninger learnt much about the mentally ill, and this newfound interest soon resulted in Menninger's first psychiatric paper, on *The Insanity of Hamlet*, which he read to his local literary society. In 1908, Menninger paid a visit to the renowned Mayo Clinic, where he met the Mayo brothers, with whom he shared his vision of a group practice akin to the model that had been developed at the Mayo Clinic. He returned home inspired to develop such a place, which would include his sons as partners. Such were the origins of the Menninger Clinic in Topeka, a center that was to achieve worldwide renown for clinical excellence in treating all types of psychiatric patient, including the more difficult ones who had not responded to usual treatments. After an abortive attempt in 1919 to establish a cooperative clinic with other Topeka doctors, Menninger proceeded with his son, Karl, and two other local doctors, to establish the clinic that was ultimately to bear the family name. Dr. C.F. Menninger specialized in internal medicine, his son in neurology and psychiatry, and other staff in general medicine, dermatology, venereal disease, and radiology. Psychiatric patients were at first treated surreptitiously in order not to alienate the local community and were even given disguised diagnoses. In 1925, the Menningers raised sufficient funds to create a psychiatric sanatorium, followed 1 year later by the Southard School for mentally ill children. After encountering initial skepticism in their venture, the Menningers were ultimately able to procure support from many in the Topeka community.

The clinic went from strength to strength, and by the 1950s it had become the largest psychiatric training center in the country. After World War II, Dr. Will Menninger (who was not a homeopath) became well known for his community lobbying on behalf of mental illness and, in the 1960s, provided compelling testimony to the congress and to President Kennedy that society was not doing enough for the mentally ill. Soon afterwards, Kennedy became the first president to speak out for mental health reform. The Menninger Clinic has continued to prosper and today commands great respect in the psychiatric community.

Rudolf Arndt

Rudolf Arndt (1835–1900) was an acclaimed nineteenth-century German psychiatrist who authored papers and a major textbook and who is best known for his observations on the relationship between dose and response, as in the so-called Arndt-Schultz law, a term that still appears in the literature.

Most of Arndt's career was spent at the University of Greifswald, where he attained the rank of professor and served as director of the local state asylum. Among his teachers was Heinrich Damerow, an influential psychiatrist who may have had some mild sympathy towards homeopathy [20, 21]. Arndt has been referred to as "a homeopathic physician" [22], but the actual evidence supporting that is slim [23]. However, unlike most of his colleagues, he was willing to engage in constructive dialog about homeopathy [24, 25]. Because Arndt's main link with homeopathy is his promotion of nonlinear dose effects, an idea later adopted enthusiastically by Hugo Schulz, he is discussed in more detail in Chap. 16.

Selden Talcott

Expert witness at President Garfield's assassination trial; advocate for baseball therapy; prescriber of heat, milk, rest, and a healthy diet; innovator of progressive humane treatments at a time when psychiatry still had one foot in the dark ages; author; hospital administrator par excellence; and a man "of imposing presence … and full beard in abundance" [26] – all of these characterize Selden Talcott, who was one of the most famous of homeopathic psychiatrists (Fig. 6.2).

Selden Haines Talcott (1842–1902) completed 3 years of service in the Union army during the Civil War and then returned to school, where he completed his undergraduate education, and then enrolled as a medical student at New York Homeopathic Medical School. In 1872, he graduated MD as class president and valedictorian. Nine years later, he completed a PhD degree at his old college.

Talcott earned national respect as a leading alienist. In 1877, he was appointed director of the New York State Homeopathic Asylum for the Insane at Middletown, where

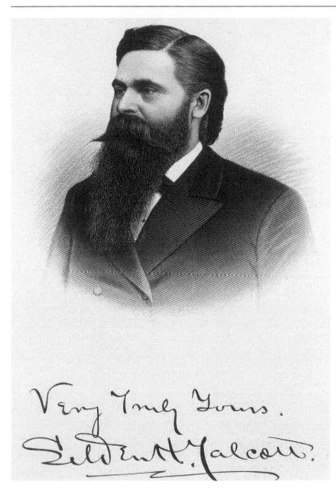

Fig. 6.2 Selden H. Talcott. Superintendent of Middletown State Hospital, New York (Image from National Library of Medicine, who believes the image to be in the public domain)

he remained for 25 years until his death at the age of 60. While homeopathic medicines formed a cornerstone of patient management, Talcott ensured that a broad range of activities was offered to asylum inpatients. He authored a textbook *Mental Diseases and Their Modern Treatment*, which was published in 1901 [27]. Although the book was widely used in the homeopathic community, it received only a lukewarm reception in the main journal of American psychiatry, perhaps because of sectarian tensions or philosophical disagreements. A reviewer commented that the book may be commended to those desirous of greater familiarity with homeopathy, but for the "general student of psychiatry the book has no great value" [28]. The book was written from lectures to medical students. What Talcott writes about mental illness in general would have almost certainly have been found in other books, but the sections on homeopathy are unique.

Whatever one may think of Talcott's book and his eventual place in history, his creativity and reputation were undeniable. One obituary noted that he began his medical career

as a homeopathic practitioner but broadened his practice and was an alienist of high diagnostic skill and fine administrative ability. Talcott was an active member of the American Medico-Psychological Association (a forerunner of the American Psychiatric Association) and was held in high regard as a forensic expert, giving expert witness testimony in the 1881 murder trial of Charles J. Guiteau, the assassin of President James Garfield (see below). Talcott made an interesting proposal for a type of insanity in farmers caused by early rising. In doing so, he took exception to the old adage that "early to bed, early to rise, makes a man healthy, wealthy and wise." Rather than it being the manifestation of insanity, Talcott held it to be the cause, related to disturbed circadian rhythms from occupational demands. His proposal sparked some interest, and a contemporary medical journal made the comment that "Medical psychologists have a true collector's enthusiasm for a new species, and we hope that what we venture to call 'matutinal mania' may find a place in the next classification of mental diseases that may be proposed" [29]. Things have changed little, and today, whenever a new psychiatric diagnostic manual appears, there is the inevitable scramble to include new diagnostic entities. As far as matutinal ("of the morning") insanity goes, the concept has not gained traction. However, occupationally induced disturbance of circadian rhythms can produce unique forms of mental derangement, and there is some merit to Talcott's observation, as recent studies have shown the benefit of treatment that restores routine sleep-wake cycle rhythms [30]. The 4th edition of the Diagnostic and Statistical of Mental Disorders (DSM-IV^{TR}) [31] contains a disorder known as circadian rhythm sleep disorder, which is caused by shift work or jet lag. Other features may include social, work, and family functioning, as well as alcohol and drug misuse. Whether or not it leads to severe forms to "insanity" is unclear. At the least, however, Talcott was farsighted in drawing attention to forms of psychopathology related to disturbances of circadian rhythm and linking them to occupation.

Baseball at Middletown

Middletown Asylum was one of several mental hospitals in the New York state system and remained homeopathic at least until the 1930s. Thereafter, it continued to serve the psychiatric needs of the state, employing conventional psychiatric treatments, until its closure in 2006. During its heyday at the end of the nineteenth century, Middletown was known as a progressive center for treating the mentally ill. One of Talcott's more unusual innovations was the establishment of a semiprofessional baseball team. Baseball had already been incorporated into the therapy programs of some hospitals, but Talcott took it to another level. He was convinced that participating in the national game could arouse a healthy interest in the depressed and mentally disturbed. In 1888, the hospital fielded a team composed of patients, hospital employees, talented local amateurs, and semiprofessionals. Initially, the team called itself the "Asylum Nine" and later "The Asylums." Before long, the team had developed into a "semipro powerhouse in the lower-Hudson River Valley area … and thousands came to see its marquee games" [32]. Each year, the number of games increased, such that by 1890 they played a total of 25, winning 21. Not only did they play more games, but the quality of opposition became progressively tougher, and one notable victory was gained over the Cuban Giants, the first fully professional African-American team in the country. The Asylums team was self-supporting from attendance fees and cost the hospital little or nothing. An 1891 game against the New York Giants ended in a close 4–3 loss for the Asylums, who again played and lost two closely fought contests with the Giants in 1892. Professional squads signed up a number of Asylum players to the minor and major leagues. Perhaps the most famous person to have played in the "Asylum Nine" team was Jack ("Happy Jack") Chesbro, who joined the hospital staff as an attendant in 1894 specifically to play on the team. Chesbro went on to a stellar career in the major leagues, set a record for number of wins in a season which still stands, and was eventually inducted into the Baseball Hall of Fame. Chesbro gained his nickname of "Happy Jack" from a Middletown patient who was impressed by Chesbro's pleasant demeanor.

In due course, mental health policy changes in New York caused overcrowding of the state mental institutions, including at Middletown, and it was no longer possible to devote the resources needed for competitive baseball. Although the game continued on the hospital diamond for some years, a reunion game in 1905 appears to have been the last time the Asylums took the field. One mark of the affection in which Dr. Talcott was held was the decision by Wilbur Cook, the Asylums' team manager, and his wife, who was director of nursing, to name their son Selden Talcott Cook.

In his commitment to organized baseball as therapy for mental illness, Talcott stood out among his peers. It is not unreasonable to regard him as a pioneer in using team sport to engender recovery from major mental illness, and it is of interest that, in the 1930s, a similar program was subsequently developed using rugby football [33]. Recent work has shown how team sports such as football can produce a number of therapeutic benefits in psychotic patients, such as more openness, calmness, and an improved sense of being needed and valued by others in their community [34]. Others have reported how self-esteem and social connectedness, and a sense of safety, trust, and empowerment all improved secondary to the type of sport that Talcott believed in so enthusiastically, when these benefits had not been forthcoming from the use of other treatments [35].

Heat, Milk, and Rest

Dr. Talcott placed the highest importance on healthy diet, rest, and exercise for the mentally ill. In relation to diet, he wrote and spoke in detail about his ideas, advocating warm milk, grains, vegetables, and fruits, with only small amounts of meat. He was not in favor of fish, disagreeing with some other contemporary authorities on this point, believing that it was an inferior source of fat and phospholipids. Epidemiological findings 100 years later have shown that countries with high fish consumption may have lower rates of depression, so Talcott's statement that "Those nations whose component subjects subsist largely upon fish … do not develop great brain power or mental activity" seems wide of the mark, although his comments were quite general in nature [36]. In fact, fish oil appears to have antidepressant effects, as well as possibly protecting against suicide. Warm milk was preferred by Talcott as a source of fat and phosphates and also was used to help promote sleep in his patients. According to need, Talcott would prescribe milk with thick cream or skimmed milk. He said "… the amount of fat to be administered to a given patient may be regulated, by experience, to meet the actual necessities of each individual case" [36, p. 346]. As his patients gained weight from high-fat foods, Talcott instructed them to engage in exercise to build muscle mass. Talcott spoke passionately about his ideas, which he presented at a dietetic program in a meeting of the Association of Medical Superintendents of American Institutions for the Insane in Washington DC in May 1891. It was of the utmost importance, he believed, that state hospitals should budget sufficient funds to provide the best food, the preparation of which "should be made with the anxious care of a mother, the delicate tact of a sister, and the scientific skill of an accomplished chef. Those who prepare food for the use of human beings should be earnest students of physiological effects, as well as adepts in the aesthetics of cookery" [36, p. 348]. He further stated, "I believe that the American Association of Medical Superintendents should declare itself in favor of a generous and effective dietary for the insane, even though it costs much money," and that the diet should be administered by skilled nurses.

A special problem that sometimes occurs in mental institutions is the refusal of food by patients who are psychotic or deeply depressed, rendering it necessary at times to provide food involuntarily. In order to facilitate this difficult and sometimes hazardous task, one of Dr. Talcott's assistants, Dr. Nathaniel Emmons Paine (see below), devised a nasogastric tube for feeding patients in the supine position (i.e., lying on the back), thereby lessening the risk of regurgitation. So it is clear that among the many causes championed by Selden Talcott, the provision of a diet based on the best scientific standards of the time was close to his heart. Diet was individualized in a way redolent of today's personalized medicine and played a crucial part in comprehensive patient care.

Administrator and Educator

Talcott was active in various professional organizations, becoming president of the American Institute of Homeopathy and member of the American Medico-Psychological Association and of the New York Medico-Legal Society. He was awarded honorary membership of the Royal Society of Medicine in Belgium. In 1889, he was appointed to the New York State Board of Medical Examiners. As chair of psychiatry at the New York Homeopathic Medical College for 16 years and lecturer at Hahnemann College in Philadelphia for 4 years, Talcott contributed to psychiatric education, and his textbook became a standard in this respect. According to Emmet Dent, MD, superintendent of the Manhattan State Hospital on Ward's Island, Talcott was one of homeopathy's "most brilliant stars" [37]. Talcott's skill as an administrator and leader quickly put Middletown in a sound financial position. He is believed to have been the first to fully demonstrate the successful application of homeopathy in the treatment of the insane. His successes at Middletown were described as "a showcase to the nation and the world" [38, p. 136]. When the prestigious superintendent's position fell vacant at Utica State Hospital, Talcott's name was on the short list. It is likely that the main reason he was not selected relates to the fact that his appointment would have necessitated a switch from the allopathic to the homeopathic system: a wholesale change that would have proved disruptive and contentious.

Expert Witness in the Trial of Charles Guiteau, Assassin of President Garfield

Charles Guiteau was an unsuccessful attorney and perpetually disenchanted office seeker, who often appeared at the White House and Republican Party gatherings, demanding a high-profile appointment, such as the ambassadorship to France, to which he felt entitled. After repeated rejections, he decided to kill President James Garfield and, on July 2, 1881, carried out his plan. Garfield did not die immediately and almost certainly would have survived the shooting had it not been for poor medical care, even by the standards of the time. After several weeks, however, the president died, and his assassin stood trial for murder.

The case of the United States vs. Charles J. Guiteau began on November 14, 1881. A phalanx of leading authorities was subpoenaed to give testimony as to Guiteau's sanity. Among these individuals were George Beard, a leading neurologist, best known today for creating the diagnosis of neurasthenia, and John Grey, superintendent of the Utica State Asylum, a foremost medicolegal expert and editor of the *American Journal of Insanity* (now the *American Journal of Psychiatry*). Beard was one of the few experts who believed that Guiteau was insane and even met later with President Arthur to appeal the harsh sentence. Among the 30 of so trial experts, at least two were homeopaths, Drs. Selden Talcott and Samuel Worcester (see below).

Talcott was initially subpoenaed by the defense, who were under the impression that Talcott considered the prisoner to be insane. However, after examining the defendant and observing his conduct in court, Talcott became convinced

of the defendant's sanity, holding him responsible for the crime [26]. Having communicated this opinion to the defense team, Talcott thought he was now free to leave Washington and return to his practice, only to be detained with another subpoena, this time from the prosecution. In the witness stand, Talcott testified that Guiteau was sane: he expounded on his own thinking that insanity was a brain disease, the exact nature of which awaited better means of detection with technology that did not exist at the time but which he expected to be eventually developed [39]. Talcott proved more than a match for the weak case made by the defense and gave some instructive explanations as to the finer distinctions about insanity. After he had completed his testimony, Talcott received praiseworthy congratulations from many of the notable experts.

Samuel Worcester

Samuel Worcester (1847–1918) came from a medical family and followed his father into the profession. During the Civil War, he served in the Union army as a medical cadet. After the war, he entered Harvard University Medical School. He graduated MD in 1868 and joined the staff of the Butler Hospital for the Insane in Providence, RI. He later entered private practice in Vermont and held a faculty appointment as lecturer on insanity and jurisprudence at Boston University School of Medicine. He was active in several homeopathic societies and served as associate editor of the *New England Medical Gazette*.

Worcester was one of the first to propose establishing the Westborough Insane Asylum and authored a psychiatric textbook, *Insanity and Its Treatment*, in which he described some illustrative homeopathic approaches to treatment, emphasizing how much the remedy could vary within one diagnosis, based on presenting symptoms. For example, in postpartum psychosis, one remedy (*Aconite*) was indicated for fear of imminent death accompanied by tachycardia. A different remedy (*Hyoscyamus*) was recommended for fear of being poisoned, and yet another (*Lycopodium*) for attempting to escape. He also found room for allopathic remedies when homeopathic ones had failed. Although Worcester's book was well received by the homeopathic community, it was not favorably reviewed by the *American Journal of Insanity*, which described it as containing little of scientific value and as evidence of "how far a devotion to a dogma may lead its votaries" [40]. Worcester also authored a book entitled *Repertory to the Modalities*, based on Hering's condensed materia medica.

After the assassination attempt on Garfield, Worcester was retained by the defense in the ensuing trial. At first, Worcester believed Guiteau to be insane and felt that, as a psychiatric expert, he might be able to "save the American people from the disgrace of hanging an insane man, merely because the man he murdered was our President" [41]. However, as with other defense experts, Worcester changed his mind after observing and examining Guiteau. Worcester subsequently explained that Guiteau's actions were not borne out of delusion, with an inability to distinguish right from wrong, but that "wickedness, and not insanity, stand out as the motive power prompting all his acts" [41, p. 152]. Worcester used the word "fanaticism" in a way that calls to mind the motivating force behind today's terrorists who are driven by the same force in their religious beliefs to justify acts of violence. As described in the *St. Louis Clinical Review* (1882), Worcester and Talcott "showed themselves as learned in their specialties as any of the Old School [i.e., orthodox] experts" [42].

Bayard Holmes

Bayard Taylor Holmes (1852–1924) entered medicine relatively late in life, graduating from the Chicago Homeopathic Medical College in 1884 at the age of 32 (Fig. 6.3). While studying at the college, Holmes showed an early interest in bacteriology and, 1 year after graduating, attached himself to the famous surgeon and bacteriologist in Chicago, Christian Fenger, who had been the first to introduce antiseptic surgery at Cook County Hospital. Fenger was impressed by Holmes' aptitude and amazed at what he had already accomplished in bacteriology (as a medical student) at such an early stage of his career, largely through self-education. Not knowing how to culture bacteria himself, Fenger saw the need for assistance and offered Holmes a prestigious internship at Cook County Hospital upon graduation in 1884, where he remained for 18 months. To be offered such an appointment with a mere homeopathic degree was an impressive feat [43]. While

serving as an intern, Holmes set up a small bathroom laboratory to investigate bacteriology and incurred ridicule from his fellow interns for what they regarded erroneously as high-potency homeopathic research [44]. Subsequently, homeopathy played little or no part in Holmes' career, although towards the end of his life, he published two resumés of his ideas about autotoxicity in the homeopathic literature [45, 46].

In 1887, Fenger and Holmes published a paper on antisepsis in abdominal surgery in the *Journal of the American Medical Association* [47]. At the time of his *JAMA* publication, Holmes was a medical student at the Chicago College of Physicians and Surgeons, from which he emerged with a second MD degree in 1888. Soon afterwards, he was called upon to teach the first bacteriology course in a Chicago medical school.

For many years, Holmes pursued his surgical and bacteriological career as professor at the College of Physicians and Surgeons, but branched out into other areas, including medical education, social reform, and politics. In the area of medical education, he oversaw the construction of a large laboratory building, an expression of his personal commitment to making medical training more laboratory based and less didactic. As secretary of the college, Holmes led its reorganization in 1891 and recruited some outstanding faculty to its ranks.

Chicago had no meaningful medical library, and to remedy this deficiency, in 1889, Holmes created the Medical Library Association. Starting from a small collection that he had assembled, Holmes secured cooperation from the Newberry Library, which pledged to create a medical section. In due course, this collection was taken over by the John Crerar Library, which continues today at the University of Chicago as one of the major American medical libraries.

Holmes as Social Activist

Being moved by the destructive effects of industrialization on health, Holmes took to social activism. He came under the influence of Florence Kelley, and they worked together to improve health conditions of exploited garment industry workers. (It is of interest that Kelley held meetings of like-minded reformers at the Hull House community and that a number of her associates were homeopaths, such as Julia Holmes Smith and Leila Bedell, who gave talks on physiology and hygiene to the clients served by Hull House.) During this time, Holmes adopted ideas not so far removed from Marxism. He was outspoken in his attacks on conditions in the sweatshops, for which he received backing in the Illinois Factory Inspector's 1894 report. Holmes was also instrumental in establishing the National Christian Citizens League, an organization devoted to improving lives of the impoverished. Holmes became well known in Chicago for his activism and was persuaded to run for mayor in the 1895 election, finishing

90

The Medical College Library.

By BAYARD HOLMES, B., S. M. D.,
Professor of the Priciples of Surgery in the College of Physicians and Surgeons, of Chicago.

Six years ago I published an account of an experiment I had made in teaching a class of thirty students to use a medical library. Since that time it has been my privilege to take several classes of students through similar exercises in the Newberry Library and the library of the College of Physicians and Surgeons. This library is known as the "Quine Library," on account of the support which the Dean of the Medical School of the University of Illinois has given it. It has been my duty and pleasure to see to the growth of this library, and I have been able to carry out the provisions of this article in relation to it in a very large degree. A number of other circumstances besides my teaching have led me to give my attention to libraries for medical schools and medical societies. I hope, therefore, that the presentation of this subject, however incomplete it may be, will be found useful to teachers and save some of them much waste of energy in their attempts to organize medical libraries.

Fig. 6.3 Bayard Holmes. Surgeon and advocate for research in schizophrenia. Medical Libraries 1899;2(May):90–94 (Image in public domain)

a distant third. In his campaign, he was supported by followers of Eugene Debs and Henry Demarest Lloyd.

Holmes' ire was aroused by the power monopoly in the American Medical Association, a problem discussed in Chap. 17 in connection with George Simmons. He joined forces with other reformists in the organization who bucked against Simmons' autocratic exclusion of the rank and file from the workings of the AMA. It is of note that, in 1899, Holmes was one of four short-listed candidates for the position of AMA secretary, which was awarded to Simmons: perhaps there had been some lingering hard feelings, although Fishbein does not suggest it in his autobiography [48].

Schizophrenia: Searching for a Surgical Cure

A watershed occurred in Holmes' life when his second son, Ralph, developed schizophrenia while away in Germany in 1905. Holmes' experience in seeking help for Ralph left him disillusioned with psychiatrists, whom he concluded were cold shouldered and had little to offer. After a demoralizing hospitalization, during which Ralph was sedated by "pounds of sedatives" [49, 50], Holmes determined to learn more about psychosis and undertake a personal quest to discover its cause and treatment. Ralph's illness caused Holmes to forsake his academic activities in favor of mental illness research and advocacy. After visiting a number of mental asylums, where the conditions left him appalled, he published about the need for better institutional care of the mentally ill [51, 52]. To familiarize himself with the extant literature, Holmes assembled a bibliography of over 8,000 articles on schizophrenia (*dementia praecox*) and founded *Dementia Praecox Studies*, which is believed to have been the first journal to focus on a psychiatric disorder (Fig. 6.4). He edited the publication from its inception in 1918 until its closure in 1922, which came about because of Holmes' declining health.

In 1915, he obtained funding for a research laboratory and, by 1916, believed he had discovered the cause of *dementia praecox*, which he ascribed to accumulation of a toxin in the gut, perhaps from bacterial infection. The nature of the toxic substance, he thought, was either histamine or indolethylamine, both of which were derivatives of ergot. It was his opinion that accumulation of these toxins in the cecum was responsible and that the indicated treatment was to remove the appendix and leave an opening (appendicostomy or cecostomy) for subsequent colonic irrigation. To put his theories to the test, he began operating on willing subjects. Holmes' first patient, however, was his son Ralph. The outcome could not have been worse. Four days after surgery, Ralph died from abdominal complications. While this personal disaster failed to deter Holmes in his quest, he spoke about it to very few people and in his medical writings glossed over this misadventure by presenting his second patient as though it was his first. All told, Holmes operated on 22 patients between 1916 and 1918, claiming a number of good successes, as well as some fatalities. His record was better than that of Henry A. Cotton, who performed over 600 operations to treat schizophrenia between 1918 and 1932, at the cost of a more than 30 % mortality rate and precious few cures [50].

Bayard Holmes was never accepted by American psychiatry, largely because he was untrained in the discipline and, perhaps more importantly, because he looked askance at his psychiatric colleagues, of whom he wrote scathing essays and editorials. While there was much to admire about Holmes – his undeniable talent, dedication to teaching and research, reformism, and identification with the oppressed – his confrontational manner led to difficult relationships. Sadly, but understandably, he became so enmeshed with his son's situation that it affected his scientific objectivity and academic career. As far as his approach to schizophrenia

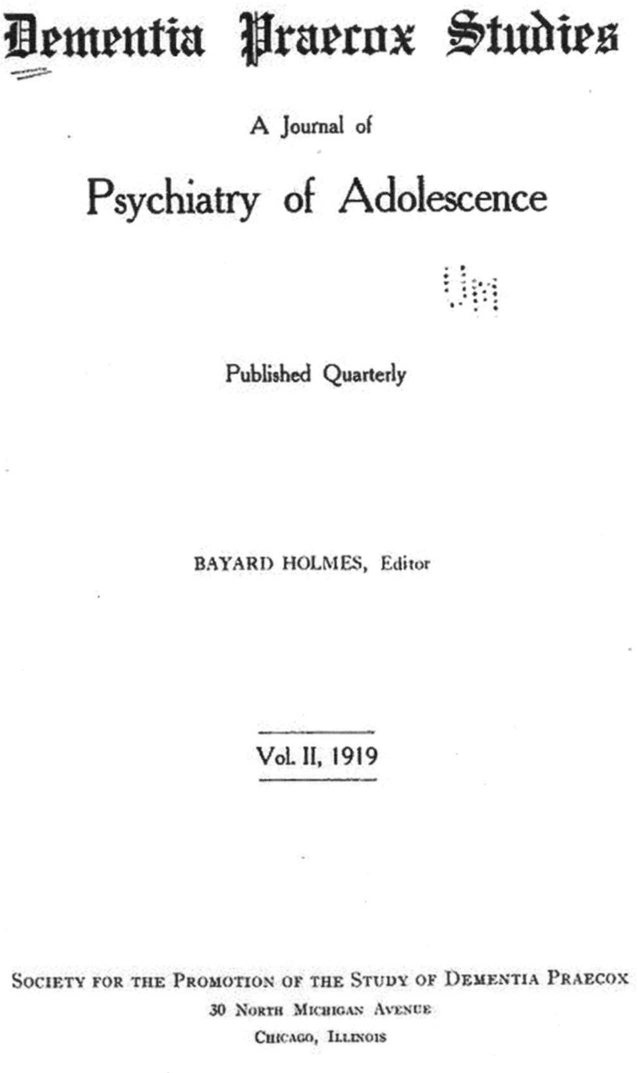

Dementia Praecox Studies

A Journal of

Psychiatry of Adolescence

Published Quarterly

BAYARD HOLMES, Editor

Vol. II, 1919

SOCIETY FOR THE PROMOTION OF THE STUDY OF DEMENTIA PRAECOX
30 NORTH MICHIGAN AVENUE
CHICAGO, ILLINOIS

Fig. 6.4 Bayard Holmes. Editor of *Dementia Praecox Studies*. 1919 (Image in the public domain)

goes, it must be said in fairness that his belief in autointoxication was consistent with contemporary medical thinking – many famous surgeons in America and Europe were removing body parts to cure various diseases with the presumption that by so doing, a focal toxic cause was being removed. Even the venerable Emil Kraepelin, who delineated the features of *dementia praecox*, thought it could be caused by a toxin. In England, one of the most celebrated surgeons of the day, Sir Arbuthnot Lane, removed the colons of many patients on the unproven assumption that colonic infection gave rise to myriad conditions. As late as the mid-1920s and beyond, the British psychiatric establishment was very ready to accept the focal sepsis theory, to which it gave considerable attention in its journals and who fêted Cotton at its main meetings [53].

Although the outcome was not as he would have wished, Holmes may still be seen as a pioneer in biological psychiatry and early advocate for improved care and more accepting public attitudes towards schizophrenia: the need to stand up for these causes is no less today. Bayard Holmes is appropriately remembered in the words of a well-known contemporary social reformer, Graham Taylor, as a man who "had the courage not only of his convictions, but also of his sympathies. He was unafraid and not ashamed to think ahead of his time … or to stand alone and dare to fail … He served his generation by seeking the coming of the better day, and died not until he saw its early dawning" [43].

Before casting Holmes' ideas into the wilderness, we should keep in mind that schizophrenia takes a dreadful toll of people in the prime of life and remains challenging to treat. Autointoxication and focal sepsis are far from having been the only discarded explanations of the disorder. Since Holmes' time, other theories and treatments have come and gone. These include the application of brain surgery (leucotomy), insulin coma, dialysis, vitamins (orthomolecular treatment), and the taraxein theory. Even the psychotherapists had their field day of mistaken theories, such as the double bind. In case we rest satisfied that the antipsychotic drugs, which are today's standard of care, are the final answer, there is concern that their benefit-to-risk ratio is not as favorable as was once believed [54].

Was there some truth in Holmes' theories? The surprising answer is "maybe." Perhaps he will yet be vindicated, for in 2007, a team of Japanese doctors stumbled on the fact that minocycline, a tetracycline-related antibiotic, resulted in the improvement of schizophrenic symptoms in two patients who received the drug for concomitant infection. Upon stopping the drug after the infections had healed, psychotic symptoms returned, only to disappear again when the drug was reintroduced [55]. Further studies have confirmed this finding, and a large multicenter trial of the drug is now underway. It is not yet known how minocycline could work. Although it is believed to be related to the anti-inflammatory or neurotrophic effects of the drug rather than its antibiotic

properties, Sir Robin Murray has opined that "infection or inflammation might be involved in a minority of people with acute psychosis and minocycline might counter this" [56]. The last word on sepsis in schizophrenia has not been written.

To the victor goes the spoil, while the loser may fade away ingloriously. But as was said of Holmes, he dared to fail. While his journey met with personal tragedy and he failed to reach the goal, his approach was courageous; the trail he blazed and the causes he championed remain alive today.

Emmons Paine

While not attaining the prominence of his teacher, Dr. Talcott, Emmons Paine (1853–1948) deserves mention in his own right. He was yet another homeopathic psychiatrist who became a respected member of the American Psychiatric Association, was active in education, researched the extent of psychiatric teaching in the US medical schools, and served on the Boston University Medical School faculty from 1887 to 1925. His knowledge about the history of the Association of Medical Superintendents of American Hospitals for the Insane was comprehensive, and he was much appreciated for his encouragement of younger generation psychiatrists. At the time of his death, Paine was the oldest member of the American Psychiatric Association and was eulogized as a "gentleman of the old school … progressive … socially minded … devoted to high standards in the care of patients, in education," and that "to have known him is an inspiring privilege" [57]. Noll has described Paine as one of the leading psychiatry teachers of his time, saying "Paine may have been one of the most enlightened instructors of psychiatry in 1893 … it is doubtful if medical students in other North American colleges received a better education in psychiatry" [13]. Paine was instrumental in creating a rotation for Boston University medical students at the outlying Westborough State Hospital, something of a rarity in those days, but which established a precedent that was eventually followed nationwide. His modification of the Nélaton rubber catheter, in 1879, to create a nasogastric tube with less risk of aspiration has been mentioned; this tube, which was widely used, was known as Paine's naso-stomach feeding tube [58].

Frank C. Richardson

Frank Chase Richardson (1858–1918) was raised in Boston; attended the BU Medical School, where he graduated in 1879; and earned a second degree 1 year later from the Hahnemann College of Philadelphia. Further training followed in New York and Vienna and twice at Harvard: impeccable credentials to be sure. He was then appointed to the faculty at BU, where he served as professor of neurology and electrotherapeutics. Like many neurologists of the time, he practiced psychiatry and was known as one of Boston's most prominent neurologists and alienists. He was active in the American Institute of Homeopathy for many years, being a founder in 1905 of the section on neurology and mental diseases, serving as its president for a number of years. At one of the meetings, as conference chair in 1908, he presented a paper entitled *Prevalent Psychic-Therapeutic Quackery*: *A Menace to the American Intellect*.

An interesting publication by Richardson appeared in 1909 on the subject of executive stress, entitled *The Problem of American Business Neurosis* [59]. In coining a new term, Richardson drew attention to executive burnout – a problem that still arises today and which then, as well as now, results in excessive use of alcohol and tobacco, lack of exercise, and a diet overly rich in meat with saturated fat. His eminently sound prescriptions advocated emotional and physical balance, a healthy diet, exercise, relaxation, and taking control of one's work schedule. Richardson's report, which was originally presented at a regional neurology meeting, attracted attention of the mainstream medical press, being abstracted in journals such as *Medical Times* and *Western Medical Review*.

Perhaps Richardson's most significant achievement was as clinical director of the Evans Memorial Research Center, founded in 1910 with an endowment from Mrs. Maria Antoinette Evans. The Evans (as it is often called) was one of the country's earliest medical school research departments (Fig. 6.5). The center has grown over time and now occupies over 100,000 square feet of floor space as headquarters of the BUSM Department of Medicine. Its endowment, built up over 100 years from the initial Evans bequest, has grown into a multimillion dollar fund which currently serves as the school's research engine, supporting the mission of clinical investigation, and has turned out thousands of trainees and internationally recognized physician scientists. As intended by Mrs. Evans, the center continues to perform high-quality clinical research, teaching, and care. Richardson was its first director, holding office for 6 years until his death from neuritis at the age of 58.

How Richardson came to be appointed first director of the Evans Memorial Department of Clinical Research and Preventive Medicine is of interest. Richardson numbered some of Boston's wealthiest families among his patients, including Mr. and Mrs. Evans. After Robert Evans was thrown from a horse and sustained fatal injuries, Mrs. Evans was so impressed by the care she received at the Massachusetts Homeopathic Hospital that she arranged through Dr. Richardson to establish the new foundation.

Of homeopathy at the Evans, Richardson had this to say: "no effort had been made scientifically to investigate the merits or mistakes of homeopathy until it was taken up at the Evans Memorial. In that institution, efforts are being and

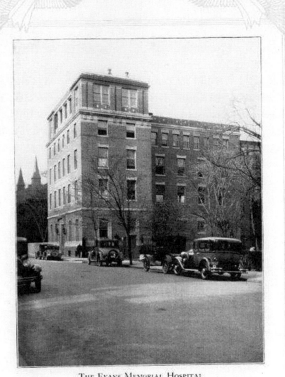

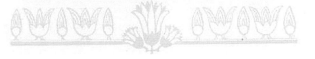

Fig. 6.5 Evans Memorial Institute, Boston University Medical Center

have been made to determine the limits and efficacy of the therapeutic principle of homeopathy. It has been rather disheartening to find that the members of the homeopathic profession have displayed so little active interest in the very suggestive and constructive work which has already been done along those lines." Richardson believed that members of the Evans staff were "just as loyal to homeopathy as any members of this society [American Institute of Homeopathy]." He went on to state that "it is essential that the fallacies shall be cleared out in order that we may rid ourselves of deadwood and delusion" [60].

Richardson was a valued teacher and mentor, who had a profound influence on Winfred Overholser and Conrad Wesselhoeft (see below for both).

Henry M. Pollock

Following the death of Frank Richardson, Henry Pollock (c. 1875–1954) was appointed director at the Evans Institute. Pollock was trained in homeopathy at the University of Minnesota, graduating in 1897. In 1899, he was appointed assistant physician at Fergus Falls State Hospital, which was one of the homeopathic psychiatric hospitals in the United States. He was promoted to the assistant superintendent position and, in 1904, left to become superintendent of the Norwich State Hospital in Connecticut, before joining Boston University Medical School in 1916 and becoming director of the Massachusetts Homeopathic Hospital. His term of office as director of the Evans Institute lasted from 1916 to 1930. He published an article in the *Boston Medical and Surgical Journal* entitled *Success in Medicine*, where he outlined the four main criteria behind success in the profession: good work habits, courage, knowledge/wisdom, and personality of the doctor. Much that is in the article is of a timeless quality which repays rereading, as it embodies fundamental principles relevant to the practice of medicine [61]. Later, Pollock became associate commissioner in the Massachusetts Department of Mental Disease and was well respected as a psychiatric and public health administrator.

Clara Barrus

Clara Barrus (1864–1931) is best known to posterity as the literary executrix of John Burroughs, essayist, naturalist, and early American conservationist, who was friendly with Walt Whitman, John Muir, and other eminent people of the time. Barrus met Burroughs in 1901, when she was 37 and Burroughs 64. Barrus became the love of Burroughs' life and eventually moved into his home upon the death of his wife. Less well known is Barrus the psychiatrist and her importance in the developing role of women in academic psychiatry. Her life and contributions to medicine are considered in Chap. 3 on women and homeopathy.

Henry I. Klopp

Dr. Henry Klopp (1870–1945) graduated from Hahnemann Medical College in Philadelphia in 1894 (Fig. 6.6). Deciding upon a career in mental health, he joined the staff at Westborough Homeopathic State Hospital, where he remained from 1895 to 1912. As a young psychiatrist, Klopp must have made quite an impression on the leaders of Boston psychiatry, for, along with his colleague Solomon Carter Fuller, he was invited to a major meeting at Clark University, held to commemorate the university's 20th anniversary. Klopp appears in the now iconic photograph of the psychology department's conference, standing next to Fuller in the back row at the far right of the picture. The meeting was a landmark in American psychiatry, as it was the first (and only) time Sigmund Freud visited the United States, and also drew other European luminaries such as Carl Jung, Ernest

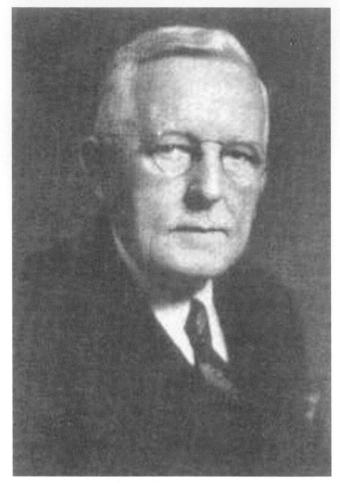

Fig. 6.6 Henry I. Klopp. Child psychiatrist and hospital administrator (Image by permission of The Historical Society of Berks County Museum and Library, Reading, PA)

Jones, and Sandor Ferenczi, all of whom feature prominently in the photograph.

In 1912, Klopp accepted a position as superintendent of the new Homeopathic State Hospital in Allentown, PA. Many of its medical staff had been recruited from the homeopathic ranks, with Drs. Charles Trites and CB Reitz having graduated from Hahnemann and Dr. Sara Adelman from Boston University. Allentown was to be the last of several psychiatric asylums that operated on homeopathic principles, bringing to an end the 38-year span of construction for these facilities. There were seven homeopaths and two allopaths on the staff. Under Klopp's direction, the hospital developed a strong reputation, particularly for its innovations in child psychiatry.

At Allentown, Klopp initiated programs of occupational therapy, physical therapy, music therapy, general medical and surgical care, and a research and pathology laboratory. He created a special department for tuberculosis patients, a network of community mental health clinics, and established productive contacts with the school and court systems. As an academician, Klopp published in major psychiatric and homeopathic journals. He was professor of mental diseases at Hahnemann and received an honorary D. Sc. degree from Muhlenberg College in 1927. In 1937, he earned board certification from the American Board of Psychiatry and Neurology, later being elected as Fellow of the American Psychiatric Association, and served on the APA council. In addition, he was president of the Pennsylvania State Homeopathic Society.

Klopp is perhaps best remembered for the Mental Health Institute for Children. This was one of the first such units in the country and filled a vital need at a time when the only option for severely disturbed children in need of hospitalization was to admit them to the adult wards of large state mental asylums, scarcely the most therapeutic environment. Klopp's unit opened in 1930 and rapidly attracted the attention of some the world's leading child psychiatrists. For example, in 1932, Dr. Mildred Creek visited the Allentown Children's Institute on a Rockefeller award to learn about new developments in child care, as she set about creating similar services in the United Kingdom. In a review of twentieth-century influences on the development of child psychiatry services, Klopp is mentioned both for setting up his unit and for publishing his first paper in 1932 [62, 63]. At its peak, the institute cared for around 140 children and remained a significant part of the hospital's mission for a long time, before closing its doors in 1992.

Klopp's publications were by no means restricted to his work with children, and they will be reviewed briefly here.

In 1912, Klopp coauthored a publication with Solomon Carter Fuller, a rising star of the homeopathy community (see below). In this paper, the authors described a case of dementia that did not fully conform to the classical picture of Alzheimer's disease, and they discussed the variations of its presentation [64]. Fuller became internationally acclaimed as a pioneer researcher in dementia, while Klopp's career went in other directions, but the two men maintained contact, and Klopp appointed Fuller as consultant pathologist at Allentown.

In 1915, Klopp published a report on the need to create special teaching positions for occupational and recreational therapy in mental institutions. He used the term "occupational teacher," which would broadly correspond today to occupational therapy, recreational therapy, and vocational rehabilitation. He recognized that traditionally this had been the domain of the psychiatric nurse, an overworked figure who would often be pulled away from this task by other more pressing duties. However, Klopp urged that the occupational teacher work very closely with nurses and that in their training, each nursing student should be exposed to "a period of instruction in diversional occupation," thereby enabling her to continue playing a role in the delivery of these activities, under the supervision of the teacher [65].

In one report, Klopp addressed the important need to provide for the large numbers of patients in mental hospitals who suffered from tuberculosis [66]. In his paper, Klopp identified four groups of hospitalized psychiatric patient: acute care, severe cases needing custodial care, able-bodied with some capacity for rehabilitation, and, lastly, those with tuberculosis. He described the results of a national survey that he had conducted, finding that 3.1 % of all patients in 106 mental hospitals were diagnosed with the disease, as well as another study of 286 necropsies at Allentown in which the hospital pathologist found tuberculosis was the cause of death in 17 % of all patients. Klopp concluded his paper with some general thoughts about the therapeutic needs for patients with tuberculosis, including separate pavilions for housing of these patients. He surmised with good reason that the death rate from tuberculosis in mental hospitals had not declined in parallel with the national decline and that more concerted efforts were required by the local authorities, public, and legislators to deal with the problem.

Integral to Klopp's vision was the forging of links between the mental health sector and local academic facilities. Klopp saw Allentown as a place that could offer itself as a regional teaching and clinical resource for the large nearby communities. He arranged with the psychology department at Lehigh University for their students to attend lectures and clinics at the hospital and expanded this collaboration to include a rotation for pupil teachers attending the university extension summer school course. The Lehigh student teachers would spend 20 h attending lectures by Dr. Harry Hoffman on mental deficiency, psychosis, the role of nutrition in development, and the assessment and treatment of the main psychiatric syndromes. The students were also allowed to observe and learn in the clinic. Further connections were forged with biology students at Muhlenberg College and with the Allentown High School civic students. Klopp placed high priority on broadening awareness of mental health issues among school principals, students, and local education board, which he saw as part of an effort to prevent the development of more serious problems [67].

Klopp and War-Related Disorders

With his experience in clinical practice during and after World War I, Klopp was well positioned to describe the psychological problems that result from combat. In 1922, he wrote a penetrating report based on the examination and treatment of many World War I veterans [68]. In content and tone, it would hold its own against the many scholarly papers that appear in today's psychiatric literature about posttraumatic stress disorder. From reading his main paper, it is clear that Klopp deeply understood the disorder. He doubted that there was one single type of war neurosis or "shell shock," but acknowledged a subgroup with what is today called mild traumatic brain injury (mTBI), where blast injury played a part, a possibility that has again been raised in recent times and for which there is some evidence [69]. He understood the historical continuity of PTSD, realizing that different generations tended to focus on different aspects of the condition and thus give it different names, such as "nostalgia" in the Civil War and "shell shock" in World War I. But all in all, he held that posttraumatic neurosis from civilian life and from war had much in common: "This group of functional nervous diseases presents no problems that are different from those which have been studied for many years. They do not differ in any essential from those met with after railroad or other accidents." He outlined four main groups of traumatic neurosis: concussion, neurasthenia (i.e., mental or physical fatigue after minimal effort), anxiety, and hysteria (more dramatic presentations such as deafness, paralysis, muscle contracture, stupor). Klopp was fully aware of the problems caused by compensation and its effect on the self-image of many veterans; he wrote on the characteristic symptoms that might be seen in "compensation neurosis."

For the treatment of traumatic neuroses, Klopp advised a multimodal approach, which began with a thorough evaluation "following the homeopathic mode of treatment," by which he meant not only to elicit the chief symptoms but also to understand their timing and nature of onset. He stated that for neurosis especially, "… no detail, however trivial, should be ignored." In addition, Klopp instructed that a full physical and neurological examination be performed. From this information, the physician could then pick the most suitable homeopathic remedy. He then provided a list of 18 of the more useful remedies. Other interventions included psychotherapy, recreational therapy, hydrotherapy, and work rehabilitation when possible. Even with the above, Klopp knew that the outcome remained variable: some cases recovered better than others. He concluded that careful assessment led him to the impression that he was "not always treating a disease but a personality – many of these cases of neuroses and psychoneuroses are due to lack of adaptation to life …. In treating the personality, one must adjust the individual to life in such a way that he can lead a healthy existence." These challenges remain the same today as we deal once more with the reintegration into society of those who have served in military combat.

Klopp wrote little about homeopathic prescribing in his papers, and it is unclear to what extent homeopathy was used at Allentown, although it did form part of his own practice approach. No doubt this reflected the age, for, as the twentieth century progressed, not only were more treatment options becoming available, but the image of homeopathy grew increasingly tarnished as its status sank lower and lower. We do know, however, that as late as 1929, many homeopathic remedies were prescribed at Allentown: there were a total of 2,295 different prescriptions given between June 1, 1928, and May 30, 1929. The most common were *Bryonia, Belladonna, Nux vomica, and Gelsemium*, with 3X, 1X, 6X, and 2X beginning the most frequent potencies – all low potency doses [38, p. 132].

Psychiatrists at Fergus Falls State Hospital

In 1885, the Minnesota state legislature commissioned a third hospital to alleviate overcrowding at the state's two extant institutions. This hospital, which was to be run as a homeopathic facility, opened its doors in 1890, under the direction of Alonzo Williamson. It gained a strong reputation for innovative and liberal approaches to treating the insane and, many years later, was a center of research at the dawn of psychopharmacology and modern psychiatry. The hospital was closed in 2005, but for over 100 years, it served the state of Minnesota in providing assessment and care to those with serious mental illness, drug and alcohol problems, and developmental disorders. Throughout most of its history, from 1890 to 1965, its clinical directors were all trained homeopaths. When it opened, Fergus Falls was considered to be something of a showcase asylum. The first director stated, "The entire theory and practice of this institution will be based on the fact that these [patients] are not criminals … but sick people – brain sick … They are just as much the subjects of disease as one who has (tuberculosis), and the treatment will be directed not to restraint and punishment, but to cure" [70]. While this now sounds trite, such views about mental illness were uncommon at the time. Even into the 1930s, American psychiatry was quite resistant to seeing psychosis as amenable to biological treatment [71]. Williamson further explained that "Good food, exercise, regular hours and habits – all these play as important a part in the cure of lunacy as they do in the cure of other diseases" [70]. The hospital went from stride to stride, and in 1901 the Fergus Falls Weekly Journal proclaimed that "Of the 15 or more public institutions in the state, the greatest, the most complete … is the state hospital for the insane in Fergus Falls" [70]. Despite eventually succumbing to overcrowding and its attendant consequences, the hospital generated some impactful research in the 1950s and 1960s, while it was still under the direction of a homeopathically trained superintendent. During the twentieth century, the hospital leaders were in the forefront of treatment innovation, for example, occupational therapy and shock treatment [72], and *Life* magazine featured the hospital's treatment program in an article on progress in the nation's state hospitals [73]. The department of clinical psychology developed instruments to measure behavior, to predict outcome from neurosurgery, to acquire normative data for the Minnesota Multiphasic Personality Inventory (MMPI), to assess the hospital's "total push" program for schizophrenia, and to test the effects of the first monoamine oxidase inhibitor antidepressant drug. The first placebo-controlled trial of reserpine in disturbed chronic patients was conducted at Fergus Falls. Behind this very productive team was the administrative support of the hospital's third director, *William Patterson*, a homeopathic graduate of Boston University Medical School who was in charge of the hospital between 1927 and 1968. During his long administration, the hospital transitioned from the age of homeopathy and hydrotherapy into the era of Metrazol convulsive therapy, insulin shock, leucotomy, then into electroconvulsive therapy, and later still into the age of neuroleptic and antidepressant drugs, as well as the community psychiatry movement. According to Ralph G. Hirschowitz, a staff psychiatrist at Fergus Falls in the early 1960s, by that time, homeopathy had completely disappeared from the scene, and he has no recollection of any staff member ever discussing it. It was his recollection that by then Dr. Patterson had become something of a "shadow figure" [74], but his half century of service set the stage for many accomplishments.

Preceding Patterson were two other homeopathic doctors. The first, as noted above, was *Alonzo Williamson*, a graduate of Hahnemann in Philadelphia, who stayed a brief 2 years, before leaving for Minneapolis and then California. His approach was progressive, and like his teacher Selden Talcott, he adhered to the belief that hot milk was a key part of the diet: "Milk is the main special diet in this hospital and we prefer to give it hot … Next in importance is rest. All new patients are immediately placed in bed on admission. Through the complimentary forces of rest and milk, we have been able to largely dispense with every kind of physical restraint and we have not used one grain of any narcotic or chemical restraint whatever" [70]. In addition to his psychiatric qualification, Williamson obtained a doctor of law degree from the University of Minnesota, where he held a faculty position in the law department. Williamson affirmed that voluntary admissions should be permitted into state hospitals since it would allow for intervention at an earlier point in the disease process and render a better prognosis. Some years after his departure, in 1910, the law was indeed changed [75]. The second superintendent was *George Oakes Welch*, an 1887 homeopathic graduate of Boston University. Welch's term covered 35 years, from 1892 to 1927. During his administration, Welch had to deal with hospital overcrowding, but kept the ship afloat at a time when there were few major innovations in the management of serious mental illness. He presided over a period of expansion, during which the hospital grew from one building for 200 patients into a large community of 1,683 patients and specialized services. Following Welch, the four-decade long administration of Patterson took place.

After a period of downsizing, the hospital eventually closed in 2005. It is not known when the practice of homeopathy ceased at Fergus Falls. A great deal of what was achieved at there can be credited to the progressive philosophy and administrative skills of its first three superintendents, in partnership with state support, most notably of Luther Youngdahl, the state's reformist governor in the 1940s, and David Vail, director of medical services in the state department of public works.

The Life and Career of Solomon Carter Fuller: America's First African-American Psychiatrist

Solomon Carter Fuller (1872–1953) is remembered today chiefly for his research into the neuropathology of dementia and for opposing discrimination against African-American physicians (Fig. 6.7). However, these bare details conceal a remarkable story of triumph over adversity. Proper recognition of Fuller's work came late – long after his death in fact – and his critical and formative connections with homeopathy have been entirely overlooked. Today, Fuller is rightly honored as one of the great twentieth-century figures in psychiatry. In 1974, the Black Psychiatrists of America created the Solomon Carter Fuller Program for aspiring young African-American psychiatrists to complete their training. In the same year, his alma mater, Boston University School of Medicine, dedicated the Dr. Solomon Carter Fuller Mental Health Center, which forms a major element in that facility's training and service programs. Fuller's portrait now hangs in the headquarters of the American Psychiatric Association (APA), where a senior officer in the APA has described Fuller as "way ahead of his time" [76], a phrase that has been

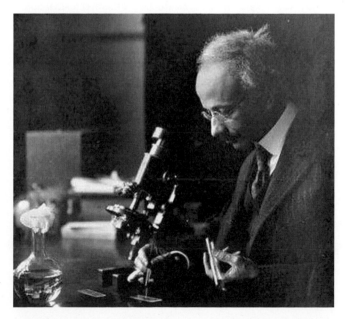

Fig. 6.7 Solomon Carter Fuller. Early leader in study of Alzheimer's disease (Image by courtesy of Boston University Alumni Medical Library Archives)

used in connection with others mentioned in this book. In 1969, the APA created an annual award named for Dr. Fuller, to honor contributions by an African-American that have benefited the quality of life for African-Americans.

Fuller's ability to overcome great odds through quiet determination and focus and to produce work of the greatest quality is inspirational. Strident protest and public militancy were not Fuller's style, although he could well have been justified in expressing himself in that manner: on countless occasions, he endured racial discrimination in his professional life. As Kaplan has expressed it, "Unlike his wife, Meta, Solomon had never been an outspoken activist for injustice and social change. His battles against prejudice were fought quietly and through academic excellence" [77, p. 18].

Fuller was born in Liberia, where in 1852 his grandfather, John Fuller, had emigrated after purchasing his freedom from slavery. The family prospered and established themselves in the upper echelons of Liberian society. Solomon's father, also named Solomon, owned large tracts of land and a coffee plantation. He died in 1889, when his son was 17. Three months afterwards, Solomon Jr. journeyed to the United States to pursue his life goal of becoming a physician. Fuller enrolled as a student in Livingstone College, North Carolina, graduating in 1893. The next year, he was accepted as a medical student at Long Island College Hospital, but later in that same year transferred to Boston University for reasons that remain unclear. At all events, it proved a good move, and he found Boston to be a stimulating place. He impressed his teachers, one of whom was Elmer Southard, a leader in the infant specialty of neuropathology and who inspired Fuller to follow the same path. This eminent Harvard neuropathologist paid tribute to Fuller as early as 1912, when saying at the opening of the Evans Memorial Institution: "In my annual reports [for the State board of Insanity] I find much to commend publicly in the Westboro work, and particularly the work of Dr. S.C. Fuller, pathologist at Westboro. No better enthusiasm prevails than that found in Fuller's laboratory" [78]. Southard, who was in charge of neuropathology training at Harvard, would later rotate his entire class to Fuller's laboratory at Westborough State Hospital. Another teacher, Dr. Edward Colby at Boston University, was equally impressed by Fuller's potential and, upon Fuller's graduation in 1897, recommended him for a position as intern in the new laboratory at Westborough, an appointment that Fuller took up eagerly. One of the duties of this laboratory was to complete postmortem specimens of brain tissue, acquired from patients who had died insane, mainly from syphilis, schizophrenia, manic-depressive insanity, dementia, alcohol poisoning, pernicious anemia, and other less common conditions. By then, the search to understand physical changes in the brain and relate them to clinical features of disease was an area of intense scientific activity. Thus began in 1897

Dr. Fuller's association with Westborough, a relationship that was to continue in one form or another until 1933. Fuller took to his responsibilities so well that when the laboratory director left Westborough only a few months later, Fuller was appointed to replace him just 1 year out of medical school. Two years later, Fuller was made an instructor in neuropathology at Boston University Medical School, thus becoming one of the first African-Americans to be appointed to any medical school faculty outside of the established Black institutions at Meharry and Howard Universities. To further his professional growth, Fuller took leaves of absence in 1900 and 1905, the former in New York and the latter in Munich, at the laboratory of Emil Kraepelin and Alois Alzheimer. As might be imagined, postdoctoral fellowships with these eminent psychiatrists were much sought after, and it speaks to Fuller's excellence that he was one of five foreign students selected to study in Alzheimer's laboratory. In making the selection, Alzheimer was influenced by Fuller's prior experience in the Westborough pathology laboratory. Fuller's sojourn in Germany lasted from November 1904 to August 1905.

Alzheimer's Disease or Fuller's Disease?

Alzheimer was the only neuropathologist in his laboratory; he had no funds to support his research and depended entirely on his students to perform the lion's share of the work. Alzheimer was self-effacing and ill at ease socially, but he established cordial relationships with his students, who were deeply appreciative of the experience and teaching he offered. Fuller found Alzheimer to be "a delightful, unassuming person who was a poor lecturer, but when you spent time with him in the laboratory and on the wards, you learned the stuff" [79]. Fuller was a conspicuously hardworking student, and it has been suggested that he examined more brain specimens than anyone else in the lab, apart from the chief himself. The extent of Fuller's contributions in Alzheimer's lab may never be known, but they are likely to have been substantial [77, p. 38] and Berrios has more than rhetorically posed the question of why the disease was eponymously named after Alzheimer and not Fuller or perhaps Oskar Fischer, a contemporary who observed the presence of plaques in senile brains [80].

Berrios' case may be briefly summarized. At a scientific meeting in Tübingen, November 1906, Alzheimer presented the case of Auguste Deter, a patient who showed a rapidly developing dementia in her late 40s, leading to death at the age of 51. Besides the many clinical features that are associated with dementia, postmortem findings showed nerve tangles in the brain (the so-called neurofibrillary tangles). Such tangles were already known to be a key characteristic of senile dementia, but were not believed to occur in younger adults. Alzheimer published the case in 1907 [81] and later described a second case. By 1910, more cases had been described, leading Alzheimer's boss, Emil Kraepelin, to name this supposedly new condition after Alzheimer. Even Alzheimer was reluctant to give his full support to such a move. It is still unclear why Kraepelin took this step, apart from reasons having to do with academic prestige or professional rivalry vis-a-vis other European departments of psychiatry. Today, the term "Alzheimer's disease" refers to a type of dementia regardless of when it develops and not simply to early-onset dementia.

To appreciate the importance of Fuller's early work, we may note that in June of 1906, 5 months *before* Alzheimer's Tübingen presentation, Fuller presented certain findings at the annual meeting of the American Medico-Psychological Association. These findings were later published (April 1907) in the leading American psychiatric journal, under the title *A Study of the Neurofibrils in Dementia Paralytica, Dementia Senilis, Chronic Alcoholism, Cerebral Lues, and Microcephalic Idiocy* [82]. For many years, Fuller remained in no rush to jump on board the "new disease" train, as he was well aware of the preliminary and somewhat confused understanding about dementia. As Berrios noted, even by 1912, the 17 reports of cases referred to as having Alzheimer's disease showed many inconsistencies in their symptoms and postmortem abnormalities. Fuller's caution was well placed.

Fuller was the first to translate Alzheimer's work into English. He also made a number of original contributions, including a 1912 publication of the first American case of Alzheimer's disease, and reviewed the world literature of 12 cases [83]. In this review, Fuller stressed the many variations in mental symptoms and microscopy findings, as well as the small overall sample base, rendering it premature to confirm Alzheimer's paradigm. A second case of Alzheimer's disease from Westborough also did not entirely fulfill the criteria laid down by Alzheimer, leading Fuller and Klopp (1912) [84] to discuss further the divergence that existed in the field. In his publication with Klopp, Fuller again expressed doubt that Alzheimer's (presenile) disease was a separate clinical condition. Fuller did not believe that arteriosclerosis was the cause of the disease, as some had thought, and he also debated the significance of plaques and tangles as peculiar to Alzheimer's disease.

Further Contributions

Fuller's legacy reaches beyond his work in neuropathology. As noted above, he was invited to attend the Clark University psychology conference in 1909 and appeared in the iconic photograph of attendees at that gathering (Fig. 6.8). What was Fuller doing there, and how did he come to be at such a prestigious meeting? Fuller had previously come to the attention of the conference organizer, Stanley Hall, from one of Hall's departmental colleagues, Clifford Hodge, who was impressed by Fuller's autopsy work. Since the Clark faculty had worked

only with animals, they requested Fuller to give lectures at Clark on his work with human pathology. It has been noted that Fuller gave a presentation at the meeting, entitled *Cerebral Histology, with Special Reference to Histopathology of the Psychoses* [77, p. 51], and a biographical sketch from Boston University indicates that "Because of his own stature in the field of psychiatry, Fuller was invited to present a lecture at Clark alongside Sigmund Freud and Carl Jung" [85]. However, the Clark records do not provide any support for Fuller giving a talk at the meeting, and it is perhaps more likely that he gave his talk on another occasion [86].

Fuller, Psychiatry and Psychoanalysis

For all his inclinations to neuropathology, Fuller identified enthusiastically with early developments in psychoanalysis. Although his abiding fascination with structural change in the brain did not diminish, Fuller readily took to the ideas of Freud, Meyer, and others, and for some years after the Clark conference, he continued to exchange ideas with Jung, Adler, and Meyer. In fact, Meyer recommended Fuller for a faculty position at Johns Hopkins Medical School, which at the time was arguably the leading center in the country. Sadly, the application was rejected because Fuller was a "colored man" [87]. Fuller embraced the ideas of Freud, Meyer, and Jung and incorporated them into his clinical practice, which he developed parallel to his career in neuropathology. In 1919, Fuller became America's first African-American psychiatrist. At this stage in Fuller's career, a typical workday would see him at the Westborough lab in the mornings, at Boston University in the afternoons, treating patients at home into the late evening, and then reading until sleep at 2 am [88]. Fuller and Hall also shared affinities, and Fuller became Hall's personal physician as well as, perhaps, his personal therapist [89].

Fuller was a man of eclectic tastes. Not only was he an active participant in homeopathy (as described later), but he attended William James' lectures at Harvard on spiritualism. The manner in which he practiced psychiatry serves as a model for all aspiring psychiatrists: he thought about brain disease in neuroanatomical terms and applied careful scientific observation and reasoning in the clinical setting when he saw his patients. At the same time, Fuller was attentive to the life stories that made each patient a unique individual and realized that many symptoms were brought about as the response to environmental stress, including shell shock, which had become a topic of special interest to Fuller during and after World War I. He attracted patients from all walks of life and would never turn anyone away for lack of money, class, or color.

Fuller's Academic Career in Boston

From 1897 to 1919, Fuller was on the staff at the Westborough Insane Asylum, where he developed the pathology laboratory. He resigned to take up an appointment at Boston

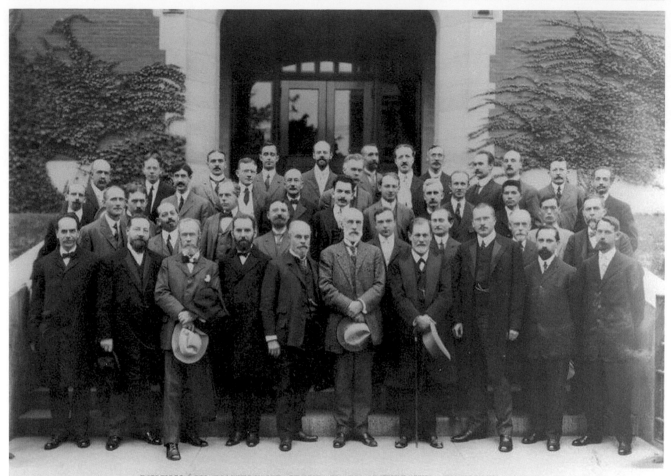

PSYCHOLOGY CONFERENCE GROUP, CLARK UNIVERSITY, SEPTEMBER, 1909

Beginning with first row, left to right: Franz Boas, E. B. Titchener, William James, William Stern, Leo Burgerstein, G. Stanley Hall, Sigmund Freud, Carl G. Jung, Adolf Meyer, H. S. Jennings. *Second row:* C. E. Seashore, Joseph Jastrow, J. McK. Cattell, E. F. Buchner, E. Katzenellenbogen, Ernest Jones, A. A. Brill, Wm. H. Burnham, A. F. Chamberlain. *Third row:* Albert Schinz, J. A. Magni, B. T. Baldwin, F. Lyman Wells, G. M. Forbes, E. A. Kirkpatrick, Sandor Ferenczi, E. C. Sanford, J. P. Porter, Sakyo Kanda, Hikoso Kakise. *Fourth row:* G. E. Dawson, S. P. Hayes, E. B. Holt, C. S. Berry, G. M. Whipple, Frank Drew, J. W. A. Young, L. N. Wilson, K. J. Karlson, H. H. Goddard, H. I. Klopp, S. C. Fuller

Fig. 6.8 Fuller and Klopp (*end of top row at right*) at the famous 1909 Clark University Conference attended by Sigmund Freud and Carl Jung (in *front row*) (Image in the public domain)

University School of Medicine (BUSM), where he continued his research and taught pathology to neurology and psychiatry students. He was the only African-American on faculty and drew no salary apart from a small stipend for teaching. Although Fuller served as acting chair of the Neurology Department for 5 years at the mid-level rank of associate professor, he was never formally given the title of chair nor was he promoted to full professor. In 1933, when a white assistant professor was promoted over Fuller's head to run the department, he decided to retire, saying "I thoroughly dislike publicity of that sort and despise sympathy. I regard life as a battle in which we win or lose. As far as I am concerned, to be vanquished, if not vaingloriously is not so bad after all" [88, p. 35a]. Fuller was eventually recognized with the title of emeritus professor of neurology at the place he had served with such distinction for 34 years. He continued the private practice of psychiatry at his home until the end of

his life. Very belatedly, on the occasion of its centenary, BUSM recognized Fuller by the commission of a bronze sculpture (by Fuller's wife, Meta). One year later, in 1974, BUSM opened the Mental Health Center named for him through an act of the state legislature.

African-American Psychiatry

Fuller's work to advance the cause of African-American psychiatrists deserves as much recognition as his contributions to neuropathology. His personal life represents a triumph over racial discrimination yet, as he correctly yet understatedly characterized it, "With the sort of work that I have done, I might have gone farther and reached a higher plane had it not been for my color" [88, p. 35b]. A lower salary than white counterparts at Westborough, no regular faculty salary at BU, and job rejection at Johns Hopkins on account of his race – these were just a few examples of the discrimination with which Fuller had to contend. It is astonishing that for such a distinguished person, the only award he received during his lifetime was an honorary Doctor of Science degree at his alma mater, Livingstone College.

Fuller encountered blatant discrimination when he offered his services to help in the war effort. During World War I, the surgeon-general's office created a neuropsychiatry division to assess and treat soldiers who were returning from battle with neuropsychiatric problems. Fuller was a member of Advisory Board 17, Boston Society for Psychiatry and Neurology, a regional component of this program. There continued to be pressing need for qualified civilian and military psychiatrists to assess the large numbers of veterans with psychiatric problems, and Fuller indicated his readiness to help in the cause. In response to his application, Fuller, who was by then well known, was told that because of his race, there was virtually no chance of promotion higher than captain but that, under those terms, the surgeon-general's office would be glad to put forward his name. Not surprisingly, Fuller declined.

Fuller devoted himself to creating opportunities for African-Americans in medicine. His involvement with the Tuskegee hospital is perhaps the best known in this respect. By way of background, the 400,000 African-Americans who had served in the US Armed Forces during World War I returned home to find themselves excluded from the new veterans' medical facilities that catered to whites. In response to pressure from black veterans, the Harding administration developed a plan to provide for the health needs of disabled black veterans and in 1921 established a VA facility in Tuskegee, Alabama. At first, the main role of this center was to treat patients with tuberculosis or neuropsychiatric disorders. The National Medical Association and the NAACP lobbied successfully for the hospital to be staffed by African-Americans. With an extremely short-time deadline, the government required a cadre of African-American doctors to be appointed to run the hospital. Qualified staff was scarce, due to discriminatory practices within the medical profession. Fuller was approached by the director of the Veterans Administration to serve as director of the Tuskegee VA. After declining, he was then asked if he would train a group of physicians in neuropsychiatry. Fuller engaged the cooperation of his colleagues at BU, particularly John P. Sutherland, professor of anatomy and dean of BUSM, and by November 1923, he had overseen the successful training of five graduates from the two African-American medical schools. These doctors duly took up their positions at Tuskegee, and some gained prominence in their own right. Dr. Toussaint Tildon became director of a facility, which, by 1929, had earned national recognition as "one of the best managed veterans hospitals in the country, both as to administration and to the scientific work done" [77, p. 65]. Dr. George Branche supervised training of several doctors

who went on to provide psychiatric services to the African-American community. At Tuskegee, Branche became chief of neuropsychiatry and earned fame for discovering the value of quartan malaria to treat syphilitic patients who had generally been resistant to tertian malaria therapy. His paper on this matter at the 95th Annual Meeting of the American Psychiatric Association was hailed by Walter Bruetsch, a leader in the treatment of syphilis, as "one of the best contributions which has been made in recent years in the treatment of neurosyphilis" [90]. Branche's success in part was due to Fuller's inspiration and lifelong passion "both to teach and search out the causes of things" [91]. Specifically, Fuller's knowledge about syphilis had helped his trainees to diagnose the disease in veterans, a matter of great importance because it had been the custom of military doctors to misdiagnose syphilitic individuals as having behavior or personality disorders, which often led to dishonorable discharge and denial of military benefits.

Fuller and Homeopathy

Very little information can be found in the main literature about Fuller's contacts with homeopathy, which were in fact quite significant. In 1894, Fuller was accepted into Boston University School of Medicine, which had been founded as a homeopathic institution in 1873. Initially, Fuller had enrolled at the Long Island Medical College, but, perhaps for reasons of ambition, he visited Boston hoping that perhaps he could gain acceptance into Harvard. During the course of that visit, "as he strolled through the city, he found himself at Boston University, where he made his way to the administrative offices and introduced himself to the Dean" [77, p. 18] (Fig. 6.9). Either deans were not so busy attending meetings or fund raising in those days, or perhaps it just happened to be Fuller's lucky day, but whichever the case, the dean apparently recognized talent when it stood in front of him and offered a scholarship provided that Fuller would return to his native country for medical mission work. Fuller refused to enter the program on those terms and convinced the university to accept his personal note of payment, which he was able to honor by employment as an elevator attendant in the evenings and at weekends, while he worked his way through medical school.

Because of its orientation, the medical school at Boston University would have been connected to a national network of homeopaths, homeopathic societies, and professional opportunities. Given Fuller's strong interest in neuropathology, it is no surprise that he accepted an offer from the nearby homeopathic state psychiatric hospital at Westborough. One of Fuller's first publications, in 1901, appeared in a homeopathic journal, the *New England Medical Gazette*; it described four cases of pernicious anemia with insanity. Five years later, Fuller published a detailed account of the homeopathic proving of belladonna in animals [92]. This laborious study took over one year and was performed gratis. It may well have been the first placebo-controlled homeopathic proving in animals and formed part of the larger report by Bellows of the entire belladonna proving project. Although it is unclear what lasting scientific payoff came out of the project, historically it was an important exercise for homeopathy and for clinical trials in general. The protocol required clear inclusion criteria, a double-blind placebo control, and agreement on the part of investigators at different sites on following a common procedure. In many ways, it was a forerunner of modern multisite clinical trials. The study also gave notice that homeopaths were prepared to conduct good-quality scientific research, the avoidance of which had often been charged against them by their opponents and also resisted from within. Fuller's significant participation in this study has largely gone unnoticed. Fuller joined the Massachusetts Homeopathic Medical Society, presented at a number of its meetings, published in the journal (a talk he gave on the clinical value of urine analysis in common diseases [93]), and provided service on the society's committee on dermatology, syphilology, and genitourinary disease. He retained a connection with the society throughout his life, attending its annual meetings until 1952 when, because of declining health, he wrote a letter to the society's president, Dr. Burt, on April 12, apologizing for his absence and expressing appreciation for the society's positive influence on his medical career [85]. It has to be concluded that homeopathy continued to exert an influence in Fuller's life, and he did not sever his ties with the homeopathic community, even if his participation remained under the surface, at least as his life and work are described in the literature.

Winfred Overholser: The Dean of Forensic Psychiatry

Dr. Winfred Overholser (1892–1964) studied medicine at Boston University (BU) and graduated with a homeopathic medical degree (MB) in 1915 and with a regular MD degree in 1916 (Fig. 6.10). As a student, Overholser was strongly influenced by two homeopathic psychiatrists at BU, Frank Richardson and N. Emmons Paine, especially the former, who played a significant mentoring role. This "outstanding" doctor (Richardson), as characterized by Moore, offered Overholser a 1-year residency position at the Evans Memorial Hospital [94]. Arguing for the progressive nature

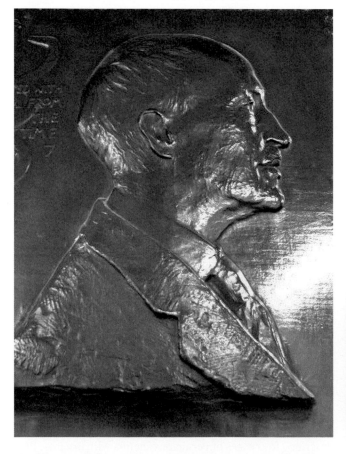

Fig. 6.9 John Sutherland, dean of Boston University Medical School 1899–1923, who recruited Solomon Carter Fuller as a medical student. Bas-relief by Frederick Warren Allen (Image by permission of Christina Abbott (www.fwallen.com))

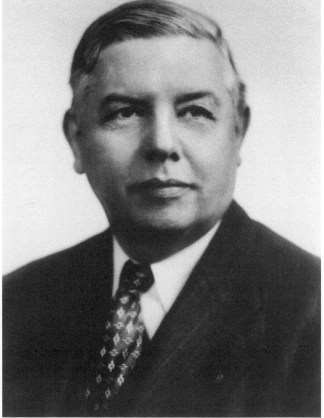

Fig. 6.10 Winfred Overholser. Psychiatrist and president of the American Psychiatric Association. Superintendent of St. Elizabeth's Hospital, Washington, DC (Image courtesy of National Library of Medicine)

of homeopathic training, Moore makes the point that BU was one of the earliest medical schools to send its students to the local state hospital for a psychiatry training rotation, a practice that was "emulated many years later by some other medical schools." Like Fuller, Overholser accepted a position at Westborough State Hospital, beginning duties there in 1917 and remaining on staff until 1924, with a 1-year leave of absence in 1918–1919 while he served in France as part of the US Army Medical Corps' neuropsychiatry section. At Westborough, Overholser gave notice of his creative approach to treating the mentally ill when he organized the first state hospital orchestra in Massachusetts. On his return, he was appointed assistant superintendent of the Gardner State Hospital in Massachusetts, while keeping his Westborough position. Overholser published a report on the cerebrospinal fluid in 108 cases of poliomyelitis [95]. For some years, Overholser remained active in the homeopathic community, presenting papers at homeopathic meetings and holding an associate editor position of the *New England Gazette*. He was an elected officer (secretary) of the homeopathic fraternity Alpha Sigma in 1920 [96]. In 1926, he spoke on the topic of sanitary science (public health) and preventive medicine at the 63rd session of the Homeopathic Society of Pennsylvania, held on September 14–16 at Bedford Springs [97]. He published a paper on nervous and mental phenomena of hyperthyroidism, in which he offered a comprehensive description of the physical and mental manifestations of the disorder, making the interesting observation that the stress of war could bring on Graves' disease (hyperthyroidism) in both veterans ("war neurosis") and civilians who were in fear of death or who had to be confronted with the corpses of dead family members [98].

Subsequently, Overholser's career took him into public health, forensic psychiatry, religion, and administration. He became assistant commissioner of the Massachusetts Department of Mental Diseases in 1924, a post he retained until 1934, as well as directed the Division for the Examination of Prisoners between 1924 and 1930. In these posts, Overholser had the opportunity to play an important part in implementing the Briggs law, which was passed in Massachusetts in 1921, the first legislation in the United States to mandate psychiatric examinations of certain criminal defendants, for example, those charged with capital offenses or repeat violators. Throughout his time in Boston, Overholser held a faculty appointment at BU as professor of psychiatry and lecturer at the BU School of Law. During 1933–1934, Overholser was president of the Massachusetts Psychiatric Society.

Controversy: Ezra Pound and the CIA

After 22 years in Boston, Overholser was appointed superintendent of St. Elizabeth's Hospital, a high-profile government-run institution in the capital city and the nation's largest civilian mental hospital. At its peak, it accommodated around 8,000 patients and employed 4,000 men and women. Among its more famous patients were Ezra Pound, who had been charged with treason in World War II, Mary Fuller (an early screen star), and William Chester Minor, a former Civil War soldier, who after release from hospital subsequently found his way to England, where he was incarcerated for murder, and who in jail helped create the Oxford English Dictionary. Three presidential assassins, or would-be assassins, have also been hospitalized at St. Elizabeth's: Richard Lawrence (Andrew Jackson), James Guiteau (Garfield), and John Hinckley (Reagan). St. Elizabeth's had a close relationship with the National Institute of Mental Health (NIMH) which, as an arm of the federal government, administered the facility until 1987, when it was taken over by city administration. NIMH continued its research at St. Elizabeth's, incubating an important program of basic and clinical research in schizophrenia. Under Overholser's leadership, much progress was made in this respect. However, his reign was not without controversy. Overholser's management of Ezra Pound has been characterized as "one of the earliest and most flagrant examples of the ongoing abuse of psychiatry in the American criminal justice system" [99, 100]. In essence, it was alleged that, because Overholser was an admirer of Pound's poetry, he disagreed with the supposedly clear-cut absence of psychotic features, thereby circumventing the justice system and protecting Pound from a potential death sentence. By judging Pound to be insane, it was possible to assure him a comfortable, even privileged, life in St. Elizabeth's, which is precisely what happened. Whether there is merit to this argument or whether Overholser simply had an honest difference of opinion from his colleagues is a question that may never be resolved, but the charges are serious ones. On the one hand, it may have been an instance of purposefully misdiagnosing someone as psychotic because of political or other reasons; on the other hand, it could be seen as a humane approach based on firm clinical opinion, albeit one that was not shared by others.

There was also the issue of Overholser's involvement in work with the Office of Strategic Security (OSS) and the Central Intelligence Agency (CIA). During World War II, the Office of Strategic Services (OSS), forerunner of the CIA, worked with Overholser to evaluate the effects of the so-called truth sera. The OSS had become aware that drugs like mescaline facilitated the ability of subjects to disclose information that would otherwise have been kept quiet, and they desired to pursue more extensive research into the use of drugs for this purpose. As reported by Stevens, "Under the guidance of Winfred Overholser, the director of St. Elizabeth's, Washington's famous mental hospital, an OSS drug squad had field tested a number of compounds, including mescaline and scopolamine. Their best luck had come with concentrated liquid marijuana … which they had injected into cigarettes…. But its most rigorous test came in a program designed to cleanse the armed forces of suspected communists." Overholser's team was able to break almost every soldier they examined [101].

Forensic Psychiatry

Forensic psychiatry was a defining part of Overholser's life, and he was sometimes known as the "dean of forensic psychiatry." Overholser was an influence behind the DC Circuit Court ruling known as the "Product Rule" or "Durham Rule" [102]. This ruling liberalized the more restrictive McNaughten insanity defense, which required that to be judged legally insane, the accused must have been unable to either know the nature and quality of the act or know that it was wrong *at the time of committing the crime* [103]. The intent of the Product Rule was to liberalize the definition of insanity, which was then defined as being the result ("product") of mental disease or defect, thereby taking into account long-term factors, like the effects of chronic mental illness, rather than only the state of mind at time of the crime. Although hailed at the time as progressive, the rule was problematic to implement and was eventually removed from the statutes in 1972, except for New Hampshire, where it had been originally introduced in 1871.

Religion

Honors accorded to Dr. Overholser included presidency of the American Psychiatric Association in 1947–1948, doctoral degrees from George Washington University and St. Bonaventure University, as well as the French Legion of Honor. Overholser was a man of deep religious commitment, being an active member of the Unitarian Church, which elected him to its highest post, moderator of the American Unitarian Association, in 1946. He was interested in how religion and mental illness were related and proposed that sometimes religious conflicts were an outgrowth of mental illness. In this respect, he presaged American psychiatry's renewed attention to the overlap of religion and mental illness, with its later inclusion of a category known as "religious or spiritual problem" in the diagnostic manual. Beyond this of course, religious preoccupations can be symptomatic of other mental illnesses. One product of Overholser's religious writings was a collaborative venture with Albert Schweitzer on the psychology of Jesus, in which Overholser wrote an introduction to the English translation of Schweitzer's refutation against books claiming Jesus to be mentally ill and which had misquoted an earlier work by Schweitzer in support of these claims [104]. (Parenthetically, one little-known fact about Albert Schweitzer concerns his use of homeopathy. It has been reported [105, 106] that, in the 1950s, Schweitzer repeatedly purchased remedies from Laboratoires Homeopathique de France, through his French homeopathic colleague Leon Vannier, to treat malaria and other tropical diseases at his African hospital. Personal com-

munication from Dr. Walter Munz, colleague of Schweitzer's and director of the Lambaréné Hospital, indicated that, although he had no direct knowledge about this, he stated that Schweitzer was always open-minded about different forms of medical practice and that he used the available medicines of his day.) [107]

Overholser died in 1964 at the age of 72 after a distinguished career. Every psychiatrist probably has his or her own prescription for mental health. For Overholser, it was "Don't take yourself too seriously. Be tolerant of the peculiarities of others. Try to do something worthwhile in your life and observe the Golden Rule."

Oswald Boltz: From Psychiatry to Homeopathy

Oswald Boltz (1895–1975) was trained as a conventional doctor and specialized in psychiatry. He was appointed to the staff at Binghamton State Hospital in New York, serving as director of Clinical Psychiatry. Extensive experience brought him face to face with the limitations of usual treatment, which he attempted to remedy by teaching himself homeopathy. As he said: "I soon discovered on reading a number of different homeopathic *Materia Medicas* that in many cases there was sharp relationship between the drug provings as described in the *Materia Medicas* and the clinical manifestations, which I observed in the varieties of schizophrenias, over many years" [108].

Boltz was well known for introducing the Boltz test to diagnose general paresis (neurosyphilis) [109]. Originally, he had developed this test to measure cholesterol but found that in patients with the aforementioned diagnosis, the fluid turned a characteristic lilac color which, he believed, was strongly suggestive of that condition; the more advanced the disorder, the more positive was the reaction. For the next decade, the test was used widely in the United States and Europe and stimulated a number of critical appraisals, which gave mixed results ranging from concluding that the test was valueless to being worthy of more investigation and carrying some utility [110–112].

Boltz was reputed to have been one of the earliest psychiatrists in the United States to use Metrazol™ convulsive therapy and insulin therapy for schizophrenia, both of which became extremely popular at the time [113]. In 1937, 59 cases of schizophrenia had been treated with insulin at Binghamton [114]. He was also interested in the concept of recovered schizophrenia [115]. Although schizophrenia usually carries a guarded to poor prognosis, full recovery can occur. Sometimes in retrospect it becomes clear that the original diagnosis was faulty, but not in all cases. Boltz was not alone in his interest in recovered schizophrenia: in 1924, Strecker and Willey [116] reported on 187 patients with the diagnosis, finding that 13 % made a good recovery. The authors studied these 20 cases and reported that intact personality, a precipitating stressor that continued to influence the illness, and an acute stormy onset all predicted good outcome. It was due to the difficulties in treating schizophrenia that Boltz turned to homeopathy and reported his experiences many years later in 1968. His paper describes six cases who responded well to homeopathy, and it seems that these patients did indeed suffer from a condition that would be regarded today as schizophrenia-spectrum cases. Boltz was impressed at the ability of remedies like *Hyoscyamus, Pulsatilla, stramonium, sulfur, and Natrum muriaticum* in doses ranging from 3X to 200X, but mainly at the low potency end, that is, doses that had pharmacological activity. Remedies were generally selected on the basis of either the target organ or the patient's constitution. All patients had undergone conventional treatments before they received homeopathy. Although Boltz was well aware that recovery could have been quite unrelated to the use of homeopathy, he remained of the opinion that it was due to the remedies, a possibility that deserves more investigation.

James Cocke

James Richard Cocke (1863–1900) may have been one of the most remarkable physicians in nineteenth-century medicine. Cocke became completely blind at the age of 3 months (or possibly 3 days, according to source), after some acid had been administered to his eyes. This handicap did not prevent him from entering medical school at Boston University and graduating top of his class in 1892. Cocke is believed to have been the first blind person to qualify as a medical doctor. Although he was associated with homeopathy for a time, Cocke is best known as a practitioner of hypnotherapy and author of the book "*Hypnotism: How It Is Done; Its Uses and Dangers.*" He wrote other papers on the subject, as well as authored an autobiographical novel entitled "*Blind Leaders of the Blind: The Romance of a Blind Lawyer.*" Cocke was an accomplished musician, who composed a comic opera and played the piano. As a physician, he treated a large number of clients, including 1350 to whom he had given hypnosis by the time his book was published in 1894 [117]. Cocke was quite celebrated, and articles about him appeared from time to time in the main newspapers.

Cocke encountered considerable discouragement from friends and acquaintances to whom he shared his plans to become a doctor, yet this did not deter him. He paid his way through college, earning money by testing tobacco products for the Lorillard Company, as well as by conducting a massage practice in Boston. Cocke's stormy life was punctuated by bigamy, bankruptcy, three marriages, institutionalization for psychosis in a Boston psychiatric hospital, and eventual suicide by gunshot at the age of 30. This enterprising and remarkable man defied expectations, and his all-too-brief life was tragically cut short before he could unfold his astonishing potential.

Conclusions

The formative role of homeopaths upon psychiatry is more than a minor historical footnote. As this account demonstrates, the growth of psychiatry has been enriched by men and women who were trained as homeopaths. At least two (Fuller and Holmes) were acknowledged as "ahead of their time." Not many of the selected individuals actually practiced homeopathy, other than those employed in the asylums and the universities prior to World War I. This is hardly surprising as the old remedies inevitably gave way to newer approaches, and pressure to distance oneself from homeopathy was always there, especially as the homeopathic power base eroded. Nonetheless, as eminent a psychiatrist as Fuller continued to be an active member of his state homeopathic medical society to the end of his life, and Klopp was prescribing homeopathically well into his career; the same is true for Charles Menninger. As a presence in the history of psychiatry, homeopathy has punched above its weight, reaching into the following areas: child, adult, inpatient, forensic, community, training, research, rehabilitation, occupational therapy, the use of the laboratory for diagnosis, and the emerging field of biological psychiatry.

References

1. Rampes H, Davidson JRT. Images in psychiatry: Samuel Hahnemann, 1755–1843. Am J Psychiatry. 1997;154:1450.
2. Stapf E, editor. Lesser writings of Samuel Hahnemann, vol. 11. Arnold Dresden; 1829. p. 239–46.
3. Cameron CS. Homeopathy in retrospect. Trans Stud Coll Physicians Phila. 1959;27:28–33.
4. Davidson JRT, Dantas F. Senator Royal Copeland: the medical and political career of a homeopathic physician. Pharos Alpha Omega Alpha Honor Med Soc. 2008;71:5–10.
5. Perez CB, Tomsko PL. Homeopathy and the treatment of mental illness in the 19th century. Hosp Comm Psychiatry. 1994;45: 1030–3.
6. Davidson JRT. Psychiatry and homoeopathy: basis for a dialogue. Br Homoeopathic J. 1994;83:78–83.
7. Post RM, Weiss SRB. Endogenous biochemical abnormalities in affective illness: therapeutic versus pathogenic. Biol Psychiatry. 1992;32:469–84.
8. Ullman D. Discovering homeopathy: medicine for the 21st century. Berkeley: North Atlantic Books; 1991.
9. Detre TP, Jarecki HG. Modern psychiatric treatment. Philadelphia: JP Lippincott; 1971. p. 53–4.

10. Walton HJ. Personality correlates of a career interest in psychiatry. Br J Psychiatry. 1969;115:211–9.
11. Walton HJ, Hope K. The effect of age and personality on doctors' clinical preferences. Br J Soc Clin Psychology. 1967;6:43–51.
12. Rise MB, Langvik E, Steinsbekk A. The personality of homeopaths: a cross-sectional survey of the personality profiles of homeopaths compared to a norm sample. J Altern Compl Med. 2012;18:42–7.
13. Noll R. American madness and the rise and fall of dementia praecox. Cambridge: Harvard University Press; 2011. p. 383–5.
14. Bowman KM. Modern concept of the neuroses. J Am Med Assoc. 1946;132:555–7.
15. Lewis A. Undergraduate Teaching of Psychiatry and Mental Health Promotion. World Health Organization Technical Report Series. Geneva, 1961. No. 28.
16. Townsend N. The story of "Doctor C.F." The Menninger Quarterly. 1952;Summer Ivssue:2–7.
17. Winslow W. The Menninger story. New York: Doubleday; 1956. p. 105.
18. Menninger CF. Some reflections relative to the symptomatology and materia medica of typhoid fever. Trans Am Inst Homeopath. 1897;52:427–31.
19. Maine H. A man who has never grown old. Menninger Quarterly. 1952;Summer Issue:8–14.
20. Damerow H. Paracelsus über psychische Krankheiten. In: Wissenschaftliche Annalen der gesamten Heilkunde 10(1834): 389–427.
21. Eric Engstrom. Personal communication. 6 Feb 2012.
22. Calabrese EJ, Baldwin LA. U-shaped dose-responses in biology, toxicology, and public health. Ann Rev Public Health. 2001;22: 15–33.
23. Eric Engstrom. Personal communication to the author. 30 Jan 2012.
24. Arndt R. Das Nervenerregungs-beziehentlich biologische Grundgesetz und die Therapie Berliner. Klin Wochenschr. 1889;26:949–53.
25. Tischner R. Geschichte der Homöopathie, vol. 4. Leipzig: Wilmar Schwabe; 1939. p. 694–5.
26. Anonymous. Selden H. Talcott, MD. The Medical Call. 1882;2:47–9.
27. Talcott S. Mental diseases and their modern treatment. New York: Boericke & Runyon; 1901.
28. Anonymous. Book Review, Mental diseases and their modern treatment. Am J Insanity. 1901;58:347–50.
29. Editorial. Cincinnati Lancet and Clinic. 1896;36:173.
30. Frank E, Swartz HA, Kupfer DJ. Interpersonal and social rhythm therapy: managing the chaos of bipolar disorder. Biol Psychiatry. 2000;48:593–604.
31. American Psychiatric Association. Diagnostic and statistical manual for mental disorders. 4th ed. Washington: American Psychiatric Association; 1994.
32. Overmyer JE. Baseball for the Insane. The Middletown State Homeopathic Hospital and its "Asylums". NINE: J Baseball Hist Cult. 2011;19:27–43.
33. Mahieu E. L'Argentine, entre la psychoanalyse et le football: le rugby [Internet]. Cercle d'etudes, psychiatriques Henri Ey de Paris. 2 Feb 2005 [Cited 2012 Nov 12]. Available from: http://eduardo.mahieu.free.fr/2004/rugby.htm.
34. Nolot F, Védie C, Stewart A. Football and psychosis. The Psychiatrist. 2012;36:307–9.
35. Mason OJ, Holt R. A role for football in mental health: The Coping Through Football project. The Psychiatrist. 2012;36:290–3.
36. Talcott SH. Dietetics in the treatment and cure of insanity. Am J Psychiatry. 1892;48:342–9.
37. Dent EC. Selden Haines Talcott, MD. Proc Am Medico-Psychol Assoc. 1902;9:322–7.
38. Winston J. The faces of homoeopathy. Tawa: Great Auk Publishing; 1999.
39. The United States vs. Charles. J. Guiteau. The Guiteau Trial. Am J Psychiatry. 1882;38–39, 303–448.
40. Book reviews and notices. Insanity and its treatment. Am J Insanity. 1882;39:93–5.
41. Worcester S. A review of the Guiteau case. New Eng Med Gazette. 1882;17(114–22):148–58.
42. Editors' drawer. St. Louis Clinical Review. 1882;4(Jan 15):417.
43. Bonner TW. A forgotten figure in Chicago's medical history. J Illinois State Historical Society (1908–1984). 1952;45:212–9.
44. Holmes BT. Medical education in Chicago in 1882 and after. Medical Life. 1921;XXVIII:409.
45. Holmes BT. Dementia praecox studies – the origin of toxic substances in the body and a method of extruding them. N Am J Homeopath. 1921;69:238–42.
46. Holmes BT. The pathogenesis of dementia praecox. N Am J Homeopath. 1921;69:243–7.
47. Fenger C, Holmes B. Antisepsis in abdominal operations; synopsis of a series of bacteriological studies. J Am Med Assoc. 1887;IX: 444, 470–2.
48. Morris Fishbein MD. An autobiography. Garden City: Doubleday & Company; 1969. p. 36–7.
49. Noll R. Infectious insanities, surgical solutions: Bayard Taylor Holmes, dementia praecox, and laboratory science in early twentieth-century America. Part I. Hist Psychiatry. 2006;17:183–204.
50. Noll R. Chicago's Dr. Bayard Taylor Holmes: a forgotten pioneer in the history of biological psychiatry. Chicago Med. 2006;106:28–32.
51. Holmes BT. The friends of the insane, the soul of medical education and other essays. Cincinnati: The Lancet-Clinic Publishing Company; 1911.
52. Holmes BT. The insanity of youth and other essays. Cincinnati: The Lancet-Clinic Publishing Company; 1915.
53. Occasional Note. Chronic sepsis and mental disease. Br J Psychiatry. 1923;69:502–4
54. Morrison AP, Hutton P, Shiers D, Turkington D. Antipsychotics: is it time to introduce patient choice? Br J Psychiatry. 2012;201:83–4.
55. Miyaoka T, Yasukawa R, Yasuda H, et al. Possible antipsychotic effects of minocycline in patients with schizophrenia. Prog Neuropsychopharmacol Biol Psychiatry. 2007;31:304–7.
56. Laurence J. Scientists shocked to find antibiotics alleviate symptoms of schizophrenia [Internet]. The Independent. 2 Mar 2012 [Cited 2012 Aug 15]. Available from: http://www.independent.co.uk/news/science/scientists-shocked-to-find-antibiotics-alleviate-symptoms-of-schizophrenia-7469121.html#
57. Overholser W. In memoriam. N. Emmons Paine. Am J Psychiatry. 1949;105:719–20.
58. Talcott SH. New methods in the treatment of the insane. N Am J Homeopath. 1901;XLIX:528–31.
59. Richardson FC. The problem of American business neurosis. New Engl Med Gazette. 1909;43:533–9.
60. Societies. The Boston District of the Massachusetts Homoeopathic Medical Society. February 1, 1917. Evans Memorial. New Engl Med Gazette 1917;52:169–70.
61. Pollock HC. Success in medicine. Bost Med Surg J. 1925;193: 867–71.
62. Wardle CJ. Twentieth-century influences on the development in Britain of services for child and adult psychiatry. Br J Psychiatry. 1991;159:53–68.
63. Klopp HI. The Children's Institute of the Allentown State Hospital. Am J Psychiatry. 1932;88:1107–18.
64. Fuller SC, Klopp HI. Further observations on Alzheimer's disease. Proceedings of the 68th Annual Meeting, American Medico-Psychological Association; 1912; Atlantic City, NJ, USA. Am J Insanity 1912;12:321–37.
65. Klopp HI. Is an occupational teacher desirable? Proceedings of the 71st Annual Meeting, American Medico-Psychological Association; 1915; Old Point Comfort, VA, USA. Am J Insanity 1915; 22:329–33.
66. Klopp HI. The care of tuberculosis patients in mental hospitals. Am J Psychiatry. 1927;83:641–59.

67. Klopp HI. How a state hospital cooperated with a university to meet a community need. Am J Psychiatry. 1922;1:159–65.

68. Klopp HI. War neuroses in general practice. The Hahnemannian Monthly. 1922;Feb: 91–100.

69. Bazarian JJ, Donnelly K, Peterson DR, Warner G, Zhu T, Zhong J. The relation between posttraumatic stress disorder and mild traumatic brain injury acquired during Operations Enduring Freedom and Iraqi Freedom: a diffusion tensor imaging study. J Head Trauma Rehabil. 2013;28:1–12.

70. Hoglund L. The Asylum [Internet]. East Otter Trail Focus [Cited 2012 Jul 22]. Available from: http://www.eotfocus.com/event/article/id/13362/.

71. Lebensohn Z. The history of electroconvulsive therapy in the United States and its place in American psychiatry: a personal memoir. Comp Psychiatry. 1999;40:173–81.

72. Cartwright RL. Fergus Falls State Hospital [Internet]. Minnesota Historical Society, MN Cyclopedia Minnesota Encyclopedia. 6 Jun 2012 [Cited 2012 Jul 23]. Available from: http://www.mnopedia.org/structure/fergus-falls-state-hospital.

73. Maisel AQ. Scandal results in real reforms [Internet]. Life Magazine. 12 Nov 1951 [Cited 2012 Jul 23]. Available from: http://discussions.mnhs.org/collections/2008/03/fergus-falls-state-hospital-papers/comment-page-1/#comment-16499.

74. Hirschowitz RG. Personal communication. 24 Jan 2013.

75. Gardner DP. Minnesota treasures: stories behind the state's historic places. St. Paul: Minnesota Historical Society; 2004. p. 164.

76. In celebration of Black History Month: African-American left indelible mark on both psychiatry and Alzheimer's research [Internet]. US Department of Health and Human Services. National Institutes of Health, National Institute on Aging. 1 Mar 2008 [Cited 2012 Jan 24]. Available from: http://www.nia.nih.gov/alzheimers/features/celebration-black-history-month-african-american-left-indelible-mark-both.

77. Kaplan M. Solomon Carter Fuller: where my caravan has rested. New York: University Press of America; 2005.

78. Southard EE. The significance of a homeopathic foundation for clinical research and preventive medicine. Boston Med Surg J. 1912;166:585–7.

79. Kaplan M, Henderson AR. Solomon Carter Fuller, M.D. (1872–1953): American pioneer in Alzheimer's disease research. J Hist Neurosci. 2000;9:250–61.

80. Berrios GE. Alzheimer's disease: a conceptual history. Int J Geriatr Psychiatry. 1990;5:355–65.

81. Alzheimer A. Uber eine eigenartige Erkrankung der Hirnrinde. Allgemeine Zeitung Psychiatrie. 1907;64:146–8.

82. Fuller SC. A study of the neurofibrils in dementia paralytica, dementia senilis, chronic alcoholism, cerebral lues and microcephalic idiocy. Am J Insanity. 1907;LXIII:415–62.

83. Fuller SC. Alzheimer's disease (senium praecox): The report of a case and review of published cases. J Nerv Ment Dis. 1912;36:440–55, 530–57.

84. Fuller SC, Klopp III. Further observations on Alzheimer's disease. Am J Insanity. 1912;69:17–29.

85. Mary Kaplan. Personal communication. 11 May 2012.

86. Mott R. Linn, D.A., C.A., Head of Collections Management, Clark University, Worcester, MA. Personal communication, 21 Mar 2012.

87. Bowman KM. President of the American Psychiatric Association (1944–1946). From C. Prudhomme and D.F. Musto. Historical Perspectives on Mental Health and Racism in the United States. Paper presented at the conference on Mental Health and Racism, Syracuse University, April 1971. Cited in Kaplan, 2005, p. 52.

88. Hayden R. Eleven African American Doctors. New York: Twenty-first Century Books; 1992. p. 27–8.

89. Ross DG. Stanley Hall. In: Gifford Jr GE, editor. Psychoanalysis, psychotherapy and the New England medical scene, 1894–1944. New York: Science History Publications; 1978. p. 181–95.

90. Branche GC. Therapeutic quartan malaria in the treatment of neurosyphilis among Negroes. Am J Psychiatry. 1940;97:967–78.

91. Graves J. Dr. Solomon Carter Fuller. Bostonia. 1995;Fall:22–25, 81

92. Fuller SC. The effects of belladonna upon animal tissues. In: Bellows HP, editor. The test drug-proving of the "O.O. & L. Society": a re-proving of belladonna. Boston: The O.O. & L. Society; 1906. p. 628–38.

93. Fuller SC. The clinical value of a urinalysis in some of the common diseases. Proceedings of the Massachusetts Homeopathic Medical Society; 1901, vol. XV; published 1902. p. 240–7.

94. Moore M. Winfred Overholser, M.D., Sc. D. President 1947–1948. A biographical sketch. Am J Psychiatry. 1948;105:10–4.

95. Overholser W. The cerebrospinal fluid in anterior poliomyelitis. Report on 108 cases. Bost Med Surg J. 1917;177:480–1.

96. Delta Alumni notes. The Alpha Sigma Semi Annual. 1920;(May)3:37.

97. The Indiana Evening Gazette. 1926 Aug 31;12.

98. Overholser W. Nervous and mental phenomena of hyperthyroidism. The Hahnemannian Monthly. 1920;55:401–5.

99. Franklin BA. Hospital once 'home' for Ezra Pound [Internet]. The New York Times. 23 June 1982 [Cited 2012 Feb 8]. Available from: www.nytimes.com/1982/06/23/us/hospital-once-home-for-ezra-pound.html?.

100. Carlson P. A life dedicated to helping the mentally ill [Internet]. The Los Angeles Times. 16 Apr 2001 [Cited 2012 Feb 8]. Available from: www.articles.latimes.com/print/2001/apr/16/health/he-51593.

101. Stevens J. Storming heaven: LSD and the American dream. New York: Grove; 1987. p. 79–80.

102. Lescouflair E. Winfred Overholser: Psychiatrist 1892–1964 [Internet]. [Cited 2012 Feb 7]. Available from: www.harvard-squarelibrary.org/unitarians/overholser.html.

103. Slater E, Roth M, editors. Mayer-Gross, Slater and Roth clinical psychiatry. 3rd ed. London: Baillière, Tindall & Cassell; 1970. p. 769.

104. Schweitzer A, Joy CR, Overholser W. The psychiatric study of Jesus: exposition and criticism. Boston: The Beacon Press; 1948.

105. Young S. Albert Schweitzer [Internet]. Sue Young Histories; 2010 [Cited 2012 Feb 12]. Available from: www.sueyounghistories.com/archives/2010/04/22/albert-schweitzer-1875-1965.

106. Young S. A homeopathic history of malaria. Sue Young Histories; 2010 April 10 [Cited 2013 Apr 21]. [Internet]. Available from: http://sueyounghistories.com/archives/2010/04/22/a-homeopathic-history-of-malaria/

107. Munz W. Personal communication to the author. 1 Nov 2012.

108. Boltz OH. Some original investigations on the treatment of schizophrenia and associated symptoms due to a functional disturbance of integration in the diencephalon using the principle of similia similibus curentur. J Am Inst Homeopath. 1968;61:218–35.

109. Boltz OH. Studies on the cerebro-spinal fluid with an acetic anhydride-sulphuric acid test. Am J Psychiatry. 1923;80:111–9.

110. Walker BS, Sleeper FH. The Boltz (A.A.S.) test in cerebrospinal fluid. Am J Psychiatry. 1930;87:229–35.

111. Brice AT. The Boltz test in urinalysis. Arch Intern Med. 1930;46:778–81.

112. Nicole JE, Fitzgerald EJ. Further results with the Boltz acetic anhydride test. Br J Psychiatry. 1931;77:321–31.

113. Bernaldo Merizalde, M.D. Personal communication to author. 16 July 2012.

114. News of state institutions. Noteworthy occurrences. Psychiatric Quarterly. 1938;12:106–24.

115. Boltz OH. A report of spontaneous recovery in two cases of advanced schizophrenic organismic stagnation. Am J Psychiatry. 1948;105:339–45.

116. Strecker EA, Willey GF. An analysis of recoverable "dementia precox" reactions. Am J Psychiatry. 1924;81:593–679.

117. Cocke JR. Hypnotism: how it is done; its uses and dangers. Boston: Arena Publishing Co; 1894.

A number of homeopathically trained physicians have specialized in public health. Cities or territories that once appointed homeopaths to positions of responsibility include Washington, DC (Tullio Verdi); New York City (Royal Copeland and Marcus Kogel); New York State (Eugene Porter and Hills Cole); San Francisco (James Ward); Los Angeles (Geraldine Burton-Branch); Rochester, New York (Charles Sumner); and Puerto Rico (Pedro Ortiz). In Victorian England, John Drysdale and John Hayward were prominent in the domestic sanitation movement.

Tullio S. Verdi

Tullio Suzzara Verdi's (1827–1902) most famous patient was William Seward, the secretary of state in President Lincoln's cabinet (Fig. 7.1). Without Verdi's care, it is doubtful whether Seward would have survived the assassination attempt that took place in his home simultaneous to the fatal assassination of President Lincoln on April 14, 1865. A week before this tragedy, Seward had been injured in a runaway horse accident and Verdi devised a metal collar to protect his patient's injured neck. At the time of the assassination attempt, it was this collar that protected Seward from being mortally stabbed in the neck by his assailant. Without the care that Seward received from Verdi, he may not have survived to purchase Alaska from Russia ("Seward's Folly") and influence history [1]. Verdi had been Seward's personal physician and it was logical that he was on the scene treating Seward's injuries on April 14. But for Surgeon-General Joseph Barnes, a prominent allopathic surgeon who came to assist in Seward's treatment, the incident nearly turned into a professional disaster as the American Medical Association (AMA) seriously considered censuring him for consulting with a quack, which they deemed Verdi to be. The AMA stopped short of this step only due to fear of public condemnation.

Verdi was born in Italy and served in the Sardinian army, where he fought to drive the occupying Austrians out of Italy.

Following the Sardinian defeat at the Battle of Novara, he fled to England in 1849. Soon after, and with only $5 in his pocket, he came to the United States and befriended Garibaldi, who helped find him employment as a language teacher on the faculty at the University of Rhode Island. In 1852, he became the chair of Modern Languages at Brown University. It was there that Verdi was introduced to homeopathy, and in due course, he enrolled at the Hahnemann Medical College of Pennsylvania, graduating in 1856. Verdi

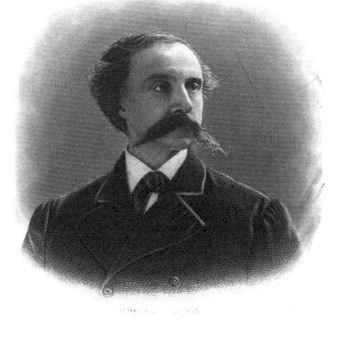

Fig. 7.1 Tullio Verdi. President of Washington DC Board of Health (Image in the public domain)

J. Davidson, *A Century of Homeopaths*,
DOI 10.1007/978-1-4939-0527-0_7, © Springer Science+Business Media New York 2014

settled in Washington, DC, where he rose to prominence. He secured congressional approval to charter the Washington Homeopathic Medical Society, which was granted authority to issue medical licenses. Unlike its counterpart allopathic medical society, the homeopathic society accepted black doctors to membership.

In 1871, President Grant appointed Verdi to the DC Health Board, which he served for 7 years (five as health officer and two as president). Because of his scientific accomplishments and mastery of languages, Verdi was selected to visit Europe as Special Sanitary Commissioner, carrying letters of introduction from the governor of DC to US consuls and ministers in England, France, Germany, and Italy (Fig. 7.2). Verdi was to bring back information on the rules, regulations, and legislations believed to underlie European success at reducing the risk of epidemics and public health threats. It was intended that the lessons brought back would be applied to the DC community and that "With his report for its guidance, it will be the fault of our Legislature if the sanitary regulations of Washington are not more perfect than those of any other American City" [2]. The board was well pleased with Verdi's report, which they called "able and excellent" [3] (Fig. 7.3).

Given the hostility that existed towards homeopathy, one may ask how Verdi obtained supervisory power on the DC Board of Health. The answer lies partly in his influence in the local community. When he heard of the allopaths' plans to create this board, Verdi ensured that he was to be included, despite knowing that it would rankle the medical establishment. As health officer, Verdi was to receive reports of all infectious disease cases from doctors in the district. Despite vigorous protest by the DC Medical Society, who demanded Verdi's removal on the grounds that he was not a regular practitioner of medicine, the board stood its ground. In answering the DC Medical Society's charge that Verdi was an "irregular practitioner [who] was not recognized by the American Medical Association" [4, p. 296], the board replied that "an educated homeopathic physician is fully as competent to judge of and direct the rules of hygiene as a graduate of any other school of medicine and that Dr. Verdi held a high position in this community for intelligence and zeal in promoting the interests of the same" [4, p. 396].

As health officer for the District of Columbia, Verdi made his mark, opening new dispensaries, enforcing regulations for smallpox vaccination, and subsequently being chosen as president of the board in 1875 and then reelected in 1876. Perhaps his biggest challenge as health officer occurred during the yellow fever epidemic in 1878. The manner in which Verdi handled this crisis was recognized in congress and led to higher appointment on the newly formed National Board of Health in 1879. Yellow fever had spread from New Orleans up the Mississippi valley, leaving thousands of deaths in its wake. Joseph Woodward, then the US surgeon-general,

DOCUMENTS AND CORRESPONDENCE.

UNITED STATES OF AMERICA,
DISTRICT OF COLUMBIA.

To all whom it may concern :

Know ye, that reposing confidence in the ability, integrity, and judgment of Tullio S. Verdi, M. D., a member of the Board of Health of the District of Columbia, I hereby appoint him Special Sanitary Commissioner, to visit the principal cities of Europe for the purpose of investigating their sanitary laws and regulations, with the view of obtaining information to assist in perfecting a sanitary system for the District of Columbia.

In testimony whereof, I have hereunto set my hand and caused the seal of the District of Columbia to be attached.

Done at the city of Washington, this eighth day of April, A. D. 1873.

H. D. COOKE,
Governor.

By the Governor:
    EDWIN L. STANTON,
        Secretary of the District of Columbia.

Fig. 7.2 Announcement of Verdi's mission to Europe. From 2nd Annual Report, Board of Health of the District of Columbia, 1873 (Image in the public domain)

To this report I add one hundred and fifty documents, viz., reports, regulations, laws, ordinances, blanks, statistics, maps, &c., regarding practical sanitary science, collected from various governments and municipalities in Europe, for the use and information of the Board of Health.

All of which I respectfully submit.

TULLIO S. VERDI.

———

DISTRICT OF COLUMBIA, BOARD OF HEALTH,
        WASHINGTON, *Nov.* 4, 1873.

Resolved, That the able and excellent report of Dr. T. S. Verdi, as Special Sanitary Commissioner to the principal cities of Europe, addressed to his Excellency the Governor of the District, and by him referred to this Board, be published as an appendix to the forthcoming annual report of the Board, and that we tender to its author our thanks for the valuable suggestions therein contained, and for the many important documents he has presented.

Passed November 4, 1873.

———

All of which is respectfully submitted.

C. C. COX,
T. S. VERDI,
JOHN MARBURY, JR.,
JOHN M. LANGSTON,
D. W. BLISS,
    Board of Health of the District of Columbia.

Fig. 7.3 Acknowledgment and praise for Verdi's report. From 2nd Annual Report, Board of Health of the District of Columbia, 1873 (Image in the public domain)

appointed a commission to investigate the causes and prevention of yellow fever, a commission from which Verdi and any other homeopaths were excluded. In response, Verdi obtained funding to set up a parallel homeopathic commission, but with an interesting and subtle difference. Whereas the Woodward Commission was tasked with reporting on the causes and prevention of the disease, the homeopathic commission was concerned with its treatment using homeopathic remedies and the statistics of practice. The cause of yellow fever was then in dispute. While the American Public Health Association claimed that yellow fever was imported on ships into the United States, and could therefore be adequately contained by quarantine measures, a homeopath and former port physician in Savannah, Dr. Louis Falligant, insisted that it was endemic in the south and that other measures would be needed in addition to quarantine. The homeopathic commission held a number of meetings, obtained information from over 60 homeopathic practitioners, and concluded that yellow fever was caused by a specific germ that was both indigenous and imported. To bring it under control, the commission continued, it would be desirable to establish a permanent sanitary commission, drain the city (referring to New Orleans), burn garbage, flush the streets, and use limited quarantine. The American Public Health Association, on the other hand, continued to insist that yellow fever was exclusively imported and that quarantine should be the main form of containment. The New Orleans Press was more favorably inclined to the homeopathic commission's findings, and congress was impressed with 5–7 % mortality rate in those treated homeopathically, compared to 16 % with conventional measures [4, p. 302]. These findings were followed in 1879, by the creation in congress of a joint committee to investigate the previous year's epidemic: among its members was the homeopath Dr. Falligant. As part of its findings, the committee ordered that the homeopathic commission's findings be included in the report. Although orthodox physicians eventually accepted most of the homeopaths' recommendations, apart from certain remedies, the committee adhered to the belief that yellow fever was acquired from outside the United States and could be excluded by rigid quarantine. Falligant dissented from this opinion.

For his efforts to control yellow fever, the French government awarded Verdi a gold medal. More honors were as follows: President Rutherford Hayes, acting on the recommendations of the American Public Health Association, invited Verdi to serve as one of the ten distinguished members of the newly created National Board of Health. Verdi owed this honor to his work with the yellow fever committee, and it was to be his last major involvement in public health. As Verdi explained, he was appointed at the request of about 30 senators and representatives, who "singled me out by name as their proper representative on said board" and thereby snuffed out any potential resistance from allopaths [4, p. 303]. Among his other achievements on the National Board was a report on diseases in food-producing animals and recommended legislation in this area.

Verdi's health began to worsen and he decided to return to his native country, where he spent the remaining years of his life practicing homeopathy in Florence. Besides his work in public health, Verdi wrote books and articles on women's and children's health, among which were *Maternity, Mothers and Daughters; Infant Philosopher*; and *Popular Diagnosis and Treatment of Diseases*. He was the president of the Homeopathic Medical Society of DC and of the Washington Homeopathic Hospital. In 1890, he was knighted by King Umberto of Italy, who awarded him the honorific title of *Cavaliere della Corona d'Italia* [5].

Coulter notes that Verdi's work was an important milestone for homeopathy in the public health arena. Verdi showed that homeopaths could perform at a high level of competence in a field which, in the 1870 s, was beginning to emerge as an important medical specialty. It was not long before homeopaths were appointed or elected to prominent public health positions in many parts of the United States. In the proceedings of the 35th Session of the American Institute of Homeopathy [6], 25 homeopaths were listed as holding public health office, including as surgeon-generals of Rhode Island (J.C. Budlong, who served in that capacity for 19 years, being reelected three times) and New York State (William Henry Watson), and examining pension surgeon to the Creek and Seminole Nations (Nathaniel V. Wright). Later homeopathic stars in public health include Royal Copeland, Jacob Gallinger, and, described elsewhere, Geraldine Burton-Branch and James Ward, who both performed important work in the Los Angeles and San Francisco communities.

Charles Sumner

Charles Sumner (1852–1928) received his medical training at NYHMC, graduating in 1877 (Fig. 7.4). He returned to his hometown of Rochester to join his father in medical practice. Between 1894 and 1900, Sumner was a health commissioner for Rochester and the president of the Rochester Academy of Medicine from 1902 to 1905. He remained actively involved with the Rochester Homeopathic Hospital until 1926, serving as vice-president and later president of the hospital medical staff [7] (Fig. 7.5).

Eugene Porter

Eugene Porter (1856–1929) graduated from the New York Homeopathic Medical College in 1885, where he subsequently became professor of physiological *materia medica*, medical chemistry, and sanitary science (public health). He served as general secretary of the American Institute of Homeopathy for 7 years and editor of the *North American Journal of Homeopathy* for many years. He was also a member of the American Public Health Association and the New York Academy of Sciences. In 1905, Porter was appointed as

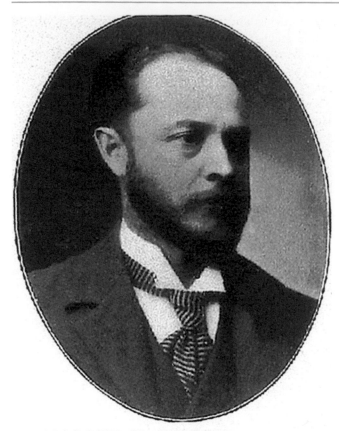

CHARLES R. SUMNER, A.M., M.D

VISITING PHYSICIAN

TO ROCHESTER HOMEOPATHIC HOSPITAL

Fig. 7.4 Charles Sumner. Public health commissioner, Rochester, and president of the Rochester Homeopathic Hospital medical staff. Image in the public domain. In: William F. Peck. History of Rochester and Monroe County, New York. New York. Pioneer Publishing. 1908 (By courtesy Robert Dickson)

the second state commissioner of health by Governor Higgins and remained in office through six administrations before retiring in 1913.

New York's allopaths objected to Porter's appointment. As the *New York Times* stated, "One man who had some knowledge of the appointment explained … that there had been spirited opposition to the appointment by the allopaths, and that the Governor had disregarded that opposition, deciding that the time had come to recognize homeopathy" [8]. The resistance had little to do with Porter's competence, however, for his 8 years as commissioner were well regarded. He supported the establishment of county tuberculosis hospitals, reduced the mortality rate from typhoid to its lowest level in the history of New York State's records, created a special commission that recommended new responsibilities for the State Health Department, and established the New York State Health Council [9]. Other achievements included the attack on water pollution in New York State and general education work in public health.

Porter fought repeatedly, and ultimately successfully, to change legislation regarding stream pollution. In 1911, the Bush Bill was passed and was the first legislative change in this class since 1903. The most important provision of the Bush Bill was to empower the health commissioner, in cooperation with the governor and attorney-general, to order to any municipality to remove sewage or provide for its treatment if investigation had shown that such discharge was a danger to public health. Porter recognized that this was only a start and that further legislation was needed, for example, to ensure cleanliness of water in the state barge canals [10].

Yet, another of Porter's achievements related to his persistent attempts to ensure that all births, deaths, and stillbirths be recorded. In 1913, new registration laws were passed in the state legislature that made this a mandatory procedure, with the state commissioner being granted powers of enforcement (outside of New York City). The commissioner was also required to provide local registrars with a list of those contagious diseases that were deemed a public health hazard, so that local disease precautions could be taken [11]. Wide-ranging recommendations were made by a governor's commission in 1913, as reported in *JAMA*. Although the Porter administration drew criticism, particularly with regard to the state of affairs in rural areas, it was acknowledged that New York "has probably one of the most effective health departments in the country" [12]. (Of some interest is the fact that Elliott's boss, Governor Sulzer, was impeached 10 months after election – the only time this has happened to a governor of the state.)

On the academic front, Porter was among the participating faculty in an inaugural public health course offered at Cornell University in 1908. Indeed, the advent of this course was the outcome of a cooperative effort by the university and the state public health department, of which Porter was the director. The Cornell Alumni News of November 4, 1908 reported that Porter gave an address on the history of public health and an overview of modern conditions and future needs. He believed the course to be a harbinger of a new epoch in sanitary science [13]. Porter continued to lecture at Cornell for several years. He served on the organizing committee of the 15th International Congress on Hygiene and Vital Statistics, held in Washington, DC, September 1912 [14]. In 1913, Syracuse University awarded him an honorary doctorate in public health.

He also was responsible to determining that "Typhoid Mary," whose real name was Mary Mallon, need not remain in perpetual quarantine, but that she could be released provided she did not return to employment as a cook. Mary Mallon had become a *cause célèbre* because of her status as a symptomless carrier of typhoid, which she had transmitted to over 50 people as a cook who never washed her hands. Three of her victims died. For this, the health authorities quarantined her on an island, where she remained until Porter authorized her release under the conditions described above. Typhoid Mary was placed back in quarantine after she

Fig. 7.5 Nurses at the Rochester Homeopathic Hospital, 1910 (Image by permission from the Collection of the Local History Division, Rochester Public Library)

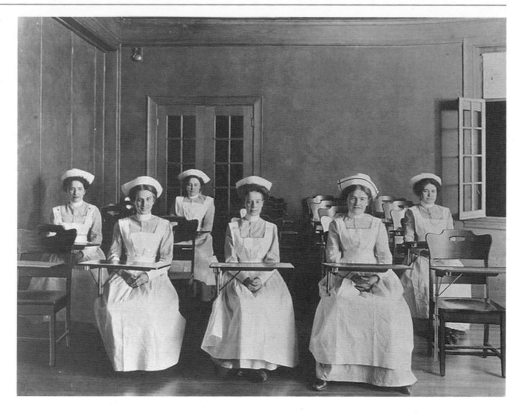

violated the terms of release and returned to employment as a cook under another name.

Following retirement, Porter pursued his avocation of dairy farming. He became actively involved in local farming societies and perfected a strong regional organization of farmers. In 1917, he was appointed commissioner of farms and markets in the state's newly created Department of Foods and Markets. In this capacity, he was responsible for the efficient distribution of food throughout the state. He held his position until the end of 1922.

Charles V. Chapin

Charles Chapin (1856–1941), a leading light in American public health, is famous for showing that certain contagious diseases like diphtheria and typhoid were not airborne but spread through contact. He was the president of the American Public Health Association (APHA) in 1926 and first president of the American Epidemiological Society in 1927. In 1930, he was the first recipient of the Sedgwick Medal, the APHA's highest honor. Although Chapin's connection with homeopathy is tenuous, it does exist and will therefore be described.

Chapin spent most of his life in Providence, Rhode Island, where his father had been a family doctor and owner of a pharmacy. After completing his undergraduate study at Brown University, Chapin apprenticed for a year with a well-known homeopath in Providence, George D. Wilcox. This experience prepared him for entry into Columbia College of Physicians and Surgeons. While homeopathy played no further part in Chapin's career [15], his year with Wilcox would have exposed him to some training in that method. Wilcox was sought out by others who were about to embark on a medical career, and Chapin was not the first of Wilcox's pupils to enter Columbia. Since Chapin could have trained with any number of allopaths in town, one can only speculate why he sought out Wilcox. It could be that his father held Wilcox in high regard as a teacher and clinician, regardless of Wilcox's affiliation. It could also be that the Chapins were favorably disposed towards homeopathy. Thus, although Chapin's exposure to homeopathy was limited, it marked the beginning of his medical career [16]. Given that medical schools would often require apprenticeship as a precondition of admission, a 1-year attachment of this type was analogous to first year in medical school today. Chapin's year of homeopathy may therefore have been more than a trivial footnote.

Rebecca Lee Dorsey

Rebecca Lee Dorsey (1859–1954) graduated from Boston University Medical School in 1883 and became a well-known Los Angeles surgeon. Her achievements in public health included a forceful presence in bringing cleaner drinking water, better streets and playgrounds, and improved food inspection in her community. Other aspects of Dorsey's career have been described in Chap. 3.

Hills Cole

Dr. Hills Cole was born in England in 1868 and immigrated to the United States after completing high school in London. He graduated with a homeopathic MD degree from New York College in 1894 and became a career public health official. While a medical student, Cole was awarded second prize for his coursework grades over the entire 3 years of study. After graduation, he was in practice for a period of time before entering public health as director of the Bureau of Publicity and Education under Dr. Eugene Porter in the NY State Health Department. Thereafter, he followed Porter to the newly created Food and Market Division, of which he was the secretary. In addition, he was responsible for editing the division's pamphlets, circulars, and other publications [17]. He was the secretary of the National Society of Electro-Therapeutics and assistant managing editor of the *North American Journal of Homeopathy* for many years [18]. Cole was the chair of the American Institute of Homeopathy's Insurance Committee and represented that body at a national conference on medical benefits and insurance [19].

James W. Ward

James Ward has been described in the chapter on surgery, but his term as health commissioner of San Francisco was an important part of his professional record. As noted, he effectively handled the health issues that arose from the 1906 San Francisco earthquake.

Royal Copeland

The manifold medical and surgical accomplishments of Royal Copeland (1868–1938) are presented in Chap. 4. As health commissioner for New York City during the 1918 influenza epidemic, Copeland was responsible for limiting the spread and damage from this disease. In order to maintain morale and educate the public, Copeland insisted that the city's movie theaters remain open (Fig. 7.6). Copeland believed that public education about influenza and its prevention could be furthered through this medium, and he urged managers to give brief talks before the movie about basic health practices such as the avoidance of coughing, sneezing, and expectoration and forbidding smoking during the show. Copeland also suspected that keeping movie theaters open would lessen the likelihood of panic and hysteria. His instincts were sound: the state commissioner claimed that New York City's mortality rate from the flu was the lowest of any large east coast city.

"I am interested in the problem of obesity because it is becoming a public health problem.... The worst of it is that when the scales show an increase of weight beyond a certain point, we have decreased the expectation of life," so wrote Copeland in his 1922 book *Over Weight? Guard Your Health* [20] (Fig. 7.7). In this book, Copeland offered practical, comprehensive, and specific recommendations, nearly all of which has been repeated in today's books on how to remain healthy. He used his position as New York City health commissioner to emphasize the importance of preventing obesity, and for 1 month before the American Public Health Association's meeting in New York, he conducted a campaign in which a class of 50 women underwent a weight reduction course, at the end of which the group had cumulatively lost half a ton of weight and reduced their waistlines by 7 ft.

Although Copeland was responsible for much good, he did not always make the right calls, most notably in the case of Henry Cotton, a psychiatrist-surgeon at Trenton State Hospital. Cotton was the subject of an inquiry into his monomaniacal and harmful removal of teeth, tonsils, colons, cervices, and other body parts in the mistaken belief that focal sepsis underlay psychotic and neurotic disorders. As was noted in Chap. 6, the fatality rate of Cotton's procedures was over 30 %. During the inquiry, Copeland came down firmly on Cotton's side, saying that "we commend [the hospital's] work in every way possible." He even turned against the interrogators, claiming that the problems at Trenton were caused by lack of state funding rather than malpractice by Henry Cotton [21].

Pedro Ortiz

Pedro Ortiz (1887?–1949) graduated from Boston University in 1919 and joined the AIH as member that same year. He then received training in tropical medicine at Columbia before taking up an appointment as health commissioner for Puerto Rico. During his administration, Ortiz instituted several changes, including the inauguration of a new leper hospital, expanding the state psychiatric hospital, and a productive collaboration with Columbia University and the Rockefeller Foundation. Although the leper hospital was new and more spacious, it failed to bring about any improvement in the life of its residents [22]. Another initiative during Ortiz' term was the creation of a bureau for the prevention and treatment of hookworm, to carry on the work that had been started earlier by Bailey Ashford, MD, of the US Army Medical Corps [23]. Ortiz' department collaborated with the school system to introduce basic hygiene principles into the school curriculum. Under his administration, the health department limited the growth of *barrios*, or shanty towns, which had no sanitation. As a result of the department's action, a health permit was required before new construction could start [24]. Ortiz was also the editor of the *Porto[sic]*

Fig. 7.6 Letter from Dr. Copeland, health commissioner, New York City concerning movie theaters in the 1981 influenza epidemic (Image by permission of Bentley Historical Library, University of Michigan, Box 11, folder "Correspondence, December 1918 (1)")

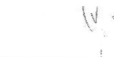

DEPARTMENT OF HEALTH
CITY OF NEW YORK
139 CENTRE STREET
NEW YORK

OFFICE OF THE COMMISSIONER
ROYAL S. COPELAND, M. D.
COMMISSIONER

December 17, 1918, ACK._____

National Association of the Motion Picture Industry,
Times Building, City.

Gentlemen:-

      I am pleased to comply with your request to furnish you with my observations regarding the relation of the theatre, and the motion-picture theatre in particular, to the recent epidemic of influenza in New York City. As you know, I was steadfastly of the opinion that in a city like New York it would be folly to expect to obtain relief through the closing of moving-picture theatres, when crowded transportation lines and other densely packed places of assembly were permitted to operate. There never was any doubt in my mind regarding the status of the well-ventilated, sanitary theatre, but I did have serious objection to allowing the insanitary, hole-in-the-wall theatre to continue. Every place of the latter sort which our inspectors found was closed immediately and was not allowed to reopen until the necessary alterations and improvements in operation were made.

      In view of our experience in New York City, where the death rate from influenza was the lowest of any large city on the coast, we are convinced that our decision to keep the theatres open was wisely made.

      The moving-picture theatre was of great assistance to the Department of Health in furthering the work of public health education during the epidemic. Managers of the various theatres gave brief talks before the opening of each performance, advising their patrons of the requirements of the Board of Health regarding sneezing, coughing and expectorating. In every moving-picture theatre in the City messages were flashed on the screens with appeals from the Board of Health for the co-operation of the public in stamping out the epidemic. Managers limited their audiences to the number of persons that could be seated and prohibited smoking for the period of the epidemic. Wilful or careless coughers and sneezers were excluded from these houses.

      My principal purpose in keeping open the theatres in New York City was to prevent the spread of panic and hysteria, and thus to protect the public from a condition of mind which would predispose it to physical ills.

      Properly operated theatres were valuable factors in maintaining the morale of the City, and New York City was notably free from a hysterical sense of calamity during our epidemic, and I am firmly convinced that it would have ... very unwise to have closed them.

      Very truly yours,

R. S. Copeland

Commissioner.

Rico Health Review and a sought-after speaker in the United States on public health and tropical diseases.

In the mid-1920s, discussions were held between Columbia University, the Puerto Rico government, and the University of Puerto Rico (UPR) to establish a School of Tropical Medicine, which became operational in 1926. It was run as a joint venture with Columbia until 1948, when it was subsumed under the UPR School of Medicine; the UPR School of Tropical Medicine was the first such institution in the Americas. Ortiz was a member of the Towner Commission, which had been set up to plan the initial Columbia/Puerto Rico venture, and served on the interim board of directors in its first year. Ortiz held an appointment as professor of hygiene and transmissible diseases and played an integral part in the teaching curriculum, giving lectures to students on public health administration and research and laboratory or clinical lectures and demonstrations on plague and leprosy.

Other academic positions held by Ortiz included an instructorship in Spanish at Boston University [25] and clinical and advisory posts in tropical disease at New York's Mount Sinai Hospital.

Marcus Kogel

Marcus D. Kogel (1903–1989) was born in Austria and immigrated to the United States as a child. He obtained his homeopathic training at NYHMC, qualifying there in 1927. For 2 years thereafter, he served as chief resident physician

Fig. 7.7 Cover of Over Weight?
Guard Your Health. 1922 (Image
in possession of author)

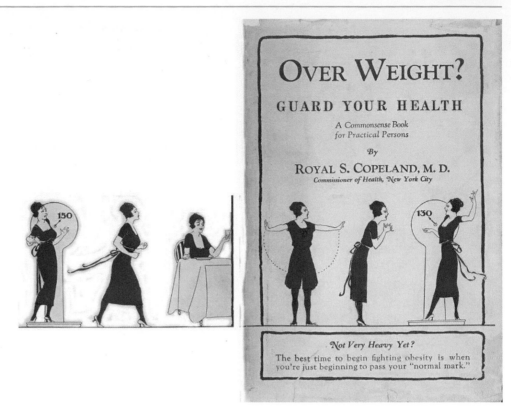

at the affiliated Metropolitan Hospital. During World War II, he served as director of military sanitation (public health) at the Medical Field Service School and later as chief of preventive medicine in China, where he was awarded the Legion of Merit for his efforts in combating a cholera epidemic [26].

Kogel was considered to be one of the nation's foremost authorities in public health and hospital administration [27]. Between 1949 and 1953, he served as New York City's Commissioner of Hospitals, leaving behind a solid reputation for rebuilding and modernizing hospitals, as well as forging closer contacts between city hospitals and medical schools. He was a tireless advocate of research, which was promoted as a result of his efforts. He was responsible for saving from closure the nation's first voluntary interracial hospital, Sydenham Hospital.

Kogel had to wrestle with the problem of overcrowded and obsolescent hospitals, many of which were used as long-term holding facilities. He articulated his plans for modernization, rebuilding and improving efficiency in a 1950 paper, as well as the need for rehabilitation programs, changes in the management of cancer, tuberculosis, mental illness, home-based care, and structuring of outpatient departments [28]. His article concluded that the huge New York City hospital system was stirring itself in response to expanding community needs and changing health and social patterns. He recognized that a community should be judged by its compassion for the poor and disabled.

Kogel was rewarded for his performance as hospital commissioner in 1954 when he was appointed founding dean of Albert Einstein Medical College, which opened its doors in 1955. Under his leadership, the college rapidly established itself as one the country's top-tier medical schools. A contemporary described Kogel as "a feisty, insightful, get-things-done leader who got a new medical school off to a running start.… He attracted such an outstanding faculty that we were prestigious from Day 1. For a medical school, that's phenomenal" [26]. Kogel also held the chair of epidemiology and social medicine at Einstein and was a fellow of the American Public Health Association.

In his 1927 class book, *The Fleuro-O-Scope*, Kogel was described by his classmates as quiet, unassuming, and inclined to side with the dissenting minority, but with a keen sense of humor, albeit sarcastic and cynical and able to laugh off his worries. He was "always the outstanding figure in our class … a brilliant scholar" [29]. Whimsically playing on Kogel's initials, the profile ended with the statement: "Possessed of such enviable characteristics no one can question his right to carry an MD both before and after his name. Here's to our future great internist, M.D. Kogel, M.D." Kogel's personal attributes were to serve him well, and it is interesting to see how he was described in his obituary, which emphasized his "strong and stocky [of] nature," his skill as a master builder and outstanding teacher, and described him as a "superb administrator who studied people carefully and rarely made judgmental mistakes" [30].

Geraldine Burton-Branch

Geraldine Burton-Branch (born 1908) served as medical examiner and district health officer for the Watts section of Los Angeles, and her accomplishments in public health are outlined in Chap. 3.

The Domestic Sanitation Movement

In the latter part of the nineteenth century, a movement began in Britain, which was to spread around the English-speaking world, advocating the need for improved architectural design. This medically driven movement held that the spread of disease was enhanced by poor home design and inadequate airflow or ventilation. Moving beyond a concern with the house in relation to its external environment, proselytes of the sanitation movement gave attention to the internal design, holding the home as analogous to the human body, in that it could be sick or it could be well. Focus moved beyond simply a preoccupation with drainage and sewer systems, to embrace the notion of "healthy buildings." To this extent, one may view the Victorian domestic sanitation movement as a forerunner of today's concern about "sick buildings," with their poor airflow and presence of environmental toxins, mold, etc. The medical profession's involvement in domestic sanitation partly arose from the observations made by physicians from their domiciliary visits, where they saw at firsthand the relation between health and home design. The effect of the domestic sanitation movement in Britain and North America was considerable, including its effect on the practice of architecture [31]. Two physicians who featured prominently in the movement were the Liverpool homeopaths, John James Drysdale and John William Hayward.

John James Drysdale and John William Hayward

John James Drysdale (1816–1890) was well known to British homeopaths in the nineteenth century, serving as coeditor of the *British Journal of Homeopathy* between 1846 and 1884. For much of his life, he practiced in Liverpool. From the many home visits to his patients, he became convinced that poorly designed homes were a factor in the spread of disease, because of either inadequate space apportionment (diseases were known to spread more easily when people were in close proximity) or poor ventilation. He therefore took the leap into architecture and designed a suburban house (called Design #1) which included a single airflow system, rather than the customary separate ventilation for each room. Drysdale's design was later adapted to

an urban site by his colleague *John Hayward* (1833–1918), who produced Design #2. Both of these homes were lived in and the health of their occupants (one of whom was a physician) was followed for 10 years by Hayward and Drysdale. The occupants of both homes claimed that their health had improved compared to their time in previous residences. The two homeopaths saw physicians as primary agents of change in regard of home design and argued that architects had forsaken health considerations for aesthetic ones. Hayward and Drysdale wrote a book entitled long-windedly *Health and Comfort in House Building: Or, Ventilation with Warm Air by Self-Acting Suction Power, with Review of the Mode of Calculation of the Draught in Hot-Air Flues; and with Some Actual Experiments*, which was published in 1890. Hayward contributed to the design of the Liverpool Hahnemann Homeopathic Hospital, being responsible for its hydraulic lifts and an innovative heating system: the first of their kind in British hospitals. Many years later, in 1898, Hayward also wrote a booklet entitled *The Construction of Hospitals for Consumption and Other Infectious Diseases*, which gave detailed information on how to incorporate thorough ventilation and a continuous supply of warm or cold air. Measures were described on how to achieve disinfection, perfuming, or medication of air before its passage through the building, and attention was given to positioning for sunlight. A review of this book noted that 26 years had passed since Hayward and Drysdale's first book on the subject and praised Dr. Hayward for having "kept up, during the intervening years spent in active practice of his profession, with the ever growing requirements of sanitary house building" [32].

Hayward was a man of many talents, and his work on snake venom is described in Chap. 9. He wrote on other topics, including malaria, the African trade in Liverpool in relation to malaria, cachexia in children, causes of deafness, and books contrasting homeopathy and allopathy. He published in homeopathic and major medical journals, such as the *Lancet*.

References

1. Scafetta J. Washington Doctor: Tullio Verdi, MD. [Internet]. Italian Americans; 2010 Oct 1 [Cited 2012 Aug 10]. Available from: http://www.readperiodicals.com/201010/2166957391.html#b.
2. Personal. The American Observer. 1873;X:397.
3. Second Annual Report of the Board of Health of the District of Columbia. Washington: Gibson Brothers; 1873. p. 206.
4. Coulter HL. Divided legacy: The conflict between homoeopathy and the American Medical Association. Science and ethics in American Medicine 1800–1914, vol. III. Berkeley: North Atlantic Books; 1982.
5. Eminent and representative men of Virginia and the District of Columbia of the nineteenth century. Madison: Brant & Fuller. p. 1905;333–4.

6. Report on the Committee of Medical Legislation. Trans American Inst Homeopath. 1882;XXXV:82–3.

7. Charles R. Sumner [Internet]. Rochester General Hospital System. The Genesee Hospital Archives. 2012 [Cited 2012 Oct 12]. www. rochestergeneral.org.

8. McMackin Out, Sherman In. Child Labor Committee Wins Fight – Homeopath For Health Board [Internet]. The New York Times; 1905 May 4 [Cited 2012 Sep 26]. Available from: www.query. nytimes.com.

9. State Health Commissioners: 1901-Present [Internet]. New York State Documents. Call No. HEA-302-4 DEPHN 202-3551. New York State Department of Health 1901-2001: a century of building healthy communities: commemorative journal, 2007 Mar, page 9 [Cited 2012 Sep 21]. Available from: http://128.121.13.244:8080/ awweb/main.jsp?flag=browse&smd=1&awdid=1.

10. Thirty-Second Annual Report of the State Department of Health of New York [Internet]. Albany: The Argus Company; 1912. p. 1–67 [Cited 2012 Sep 20]. Available from: http://books.google.com/boo ks?id=c34XAQAAIAAJ&pg=PA1003&lpg=PA1003&dq=eugene +porter+control+of+tuberculosis+in+new+york+state+1910&sour ce=bl&ots=Esy53KQYfu&sig=1yW3AiQjY5MlmcNeOr_Jt8P- nmI&hl=en&sa=X&ei=w65cUMGUH5OE8QSvz4CYDw&sqi=2 &ved=0CCUQ6AEwAg#v=onepage&q&f=false.

11. Porter EH. The new vital statistics law of New York State. Am J Public Health. 1914;4:125–9.

12. Anonymous. Governor Sulzer's special message on public health. JAMA. 1913;60:835–6.

13. New Course A Success. Cornell Alumni News. 1908 Nov 4.

14. Cornell Alumni News. 1912 Oct 2.

15. Lee Teverow. Reference Librarian, Rhode Island Historical Society Library, Providence, RI. Personal communication to the author. 2 October 2012.

16. Kemble H, Salotto L, Charles V. Chapin Papers [Internet]. Rhode Island Historical Society Manuscripts Division 1983 and 2001 [Cited 2012 Sep 28]. Available from: www.rihs.org/mssinv/ Mss343.htm.

17. Foods and Markets. State of New York: Department of Farms and Markets. 1918;1:21.

18. Hills Cole. History of homoeopathic biographies. Sylvain Cazalet; 2003 [Cited 2012 Sep 22]. Available from: www.homeoint.org/his- tory/bio/h/hillsc.htm.

19. U.S. Department of Labor. Bureau of Labor Statistics. Proceedings of the Conference on Social Insurance. Washington, DC: Government Printing Office; 1917. p. 725–6.

20. Copeland RS. Over weight? Guard your health. New York: Cosmopolitan Book Corporation; 1922.

21. Scull A, Madhouse A. Tragic tale of monomania and modern medi- cine. New Haven: Yale University Press; 2005. p. 187.

22. Levison JH. Beyond quarantine: a history of leprosy in Puerto Rico, 1898-1930s. Hist Cienc Saude Manguinhos. 2003;10:225–45.

23. Deaths. Pedro. N. Ortiz. Science. 1949;110:224.

24. Perez MA. Report of the conference of district medical inspectors of Porto Rico [Internet]. Porto Rico Health Review. 1926;II:14–8 [Cited 2012 Aug 31]. Available from: http://libraria.rcm.upr. edu:8180/jspui/bitstream/2010/300/1/Conference%20of%20 Medical%20Inspectorsd.pdf

25. Ettien A. Personal communication to the author. 3 Sept 2012.

26. Obituaries. Dr. Marcus David Kogel, 86, Dies; Headed Einstein Medical College. The New York Times. 1989 Nov 29.

27. Einstein College Dean Arrives Here From NY. The Palm Beach Daily News. 1966 Feb 16. p. 29.

28. Kogel MD. New horizons in hospital planning. Am J Public Health. 1950;40:1118–24.

29. Marcus D. Kogel – Graduated NYMC 1927. The Fleur-O-Scope. 1927;88.

30. In memoriam: Dr. Marcus D. Kogel. Einstein Quart J Biol Med. 1990;8:37.

31. Adams A. Architecture in the family way: doctors, houses and women: 1870-1900. Montreal: McGill-Queens University Press; 1996.

32. Hospital construction. Monthly Homoeopathic Review 1899;XLIII:32–43.

The Early Days of Radiation: Homeopathic Shadows

8

Roentgen's discovery of x-rays in 1895 and Curie's discovery of radium in 1898 caused great excitement in medicine. Within months, doctors in Europe and America were experimenting with these new tools for diagnostic and therapeutic purposes. A flood of papers appeared in medical journals and presentations were given at congresses. Expectations of radiation were high. Amidst this gadarene rush, doctors and patients were unaware of the immense harm that could be caused by such promising treatments which seemed capable of treating otherwise fatal cancers. Eventually, recognition of the risks was impossible to deny as patients developed serious complications, and many doctors and laboratory personnel – the so-called martyrs of medicine – acquired serious burns, limb disfigurement, and tumors from excessive amounts of radiation. Death was not unheard of, as graphically illustrated in the case of Mihran Kassabian, an Armenian immigrant who was one of the first to use x-rays in medicine. Kassabian died at the age of 40 from metastatic cancer in his hands caused by radiation exposure when he served as a military doctor in the Spanish-American War. Another example is the case of Emil Grubbé (*vide infra*), who endured over 90 operations for cancerous burns from heavy exposure to radiation. Despite serious disfigurement, Grubbé at least lived to the age of 85, although paying a high price.

There were many pioneers in the early days of radiotherapy, including Kassabian and Piffard in the United States, Freund and Schiff in Austria, and Finsen, Stenbeck, and Sjögren from Scandinavia, to name a few. Among the contributors, four homeopaths can be counted: Emil Grubbé, Francis Benson, William Dieffenbach, and John Mallory Lee.

Emil Grubbé: First to Use X-Rays in Medicine or Teller of Tall Tales?

The contradictions of Emil Grubbé are evident in the following characterizations: "a reputation for accuracy and honesty which were characteristic of his life throughout" and "vain, boastful, incompletely truthful" (Fig. 8.1).

Who was the real Emil Grubbé? What were his contributions to medicine? In its obituary column, the *British Medical Journal* (*BMJ*) wrote that Grubbé "soon gained a reputation for accuracy and honesty which were characteristic of his life throughout" and enumerated several prestigious awards and the offices he held [1]. By contrast, other authoritative sources have described Grubbé as "difficult and often mean-spirited … [a man of] relentless bitterness and contentiousness … vain, boastful [and] incompletely truthful … personally despicable, given to confabulation" [2, 3]. Grubbé was nothing if not a self-promoter and wrote on one occasion, "From a purely historical standpoint, I promise that [my next] paper will be one of the most momentous in X-Ray literature" [4]. In another publication that same year, Grubbé (retroactively) asserted a series of claims in radiology [5]. An article in *Science* refers to him rather cautiously as being "probably the first American to treat a patient with x-rays" [6].

Such inconsistency gives reason to pause and ask about the real person behind the mask. Among homeopaths, it is accepted that Grubbé was the first person to treat cancer with radiation, and this is likely true, although there is enough doubt that the true facts demand critical appraisal.

Emil Grubbé was born in Chicago in 1875 and the son of German immigrants. He went to work at the age of 13 as a bottle washer and errand boy in a local drug store and then left to work at Marshall Field's department store, where Mr. Fields was impressed enough with Grubbé to urge that he pursue his interests in science and medicine. To prepare for medical school, it was necessary for Emil to obtain further education, so he enrolled at a local normal school, supplementing his income by night watchman work. At the age of 20, in 1895, Grubbé entered the Chicago Hahnemann Medical College, where he was simultaneously given a faculty appointment in physics and chemistry. Grubbé completed his medical training in 1898 and remained on the Hahnemann faculty for several decades, holding the titles of professor and chair of the departments of electrotherapeutics and radiography until 1919 [7]. According to Orndorff,

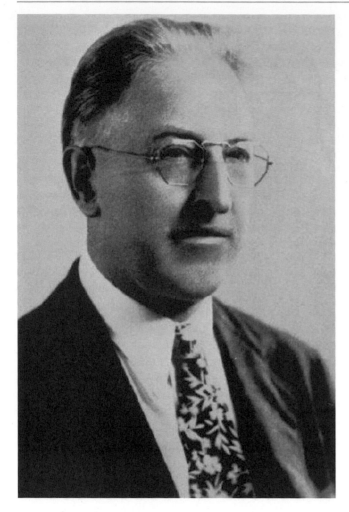

EMILE HERMAN GRUBBE
1875–1960

Fig. 8.1 Emil Grubbé. First to use radiation in medicine (Image by permission of Radiological Society of North America. Author Benjamin H. Orndorff [8])

Grubbé's laboratory at the Hahnemann Hospital formed the nucleus of the first medical school department to teach radiology [8]. Grubbé also founded the first radiation clinic in Chicago and may have been one of the first to establish a continuing medical education (CME) program when he created 2-week courses in radiation physics and the therapeutic use of radiation. He claimed to have taught over 7,000 physicians how to use x-rays over the course of his career. He conducted a busy private practice of radiology and published nearly 100 papers. With increasing age, Grubbé suffered severely from the effects of radiation-induced dermatitis and anemia sustained from his early experiments, and he endured over 90 operations to remove skin cancers and damaged tissue; eventually, he lost his left arm and part of his jaw and face and died from metastatic skin cancer in 1960. Grubbé's

severe disfigurement resulted in divorce and social isolation: it would not be unusual for him to greet visitors from behind a screen to block his disfigurement from view. For his professional accomplishments, Grubbé was recognized with honorary membership of the Institute of Medicine, the Walter Reed Society, and the American Cancer Society, as well as presidency of the National Society for Physical Therapeutics.

The Discovery of X-Rays and Its Impact on Grubbé

By the time of Roentgen's discovery in 1895, Grubbé had already gained experience (or so he claimed) with gases and manufacture of the Crookes' vacuum tube, from which radiation could be generated by the passage of electricity through the tube. So when Roentgen took the first x-ray picture in November 1895 and reported it one month later, the medical community was abuzz with interest and for Grubbé it presented a special opportunity, even before he had completed his medical studies. From previous work with the Crookes tube, Grubbé had already sustained severe dermatitis by putting his arm too close to radiation from the tube. On January 27, 1896, he sought advice from Dr. Cobb, a Hahnemann faculty member, who examined him in the presence of three other colleagues, Drs. Gilman, Ludlam, and Helphide, each of whom gave different suggestions. Dr. Gilman had no particular remedy in mind but, in accordance with the homeopathic principle of *similia similibus curentur*, commented that "any physical agent capable of doing so much damage to normal cells and tissues might offer possibilities, if used as a therapeutic agent, in the treatment of pathologic conditions in which pronounced irritative, blistering, or even destructive effects might be desirable," such as cancer, lupus, and ulcer [5]. Thereupon, Drs. Ludlum and Halphide referred two patients to Grubbé for radiation treatment. The first patient, Mrs. Rose Lee, had incurable breast cancer and the second patient, Mr. A. Carr, had advanced lupus vulgaris. Both patients were treated immediately, on January 29 and 30, respectively, with Grubbé noting that he used a lead shield to protect his patients from harmful effects of x-rays in other parts of the body, a precaution he introduced as the result of his own x-ray-induced burns. So rapidly was treatment undertaken that it had not been possible to set up a suitable office and the radiation was administered in a factory, but by the end of February 1896, Grubbé (who was still a medical student) opened a "properly equipped laboratory for the diagnostic and therapeutic use of x-rays and electric currents." This facility was fully operational, ironically enough, by April Fool's Day (April 1) 1896. Of course, this proved the beginning of a very prosperous (if not preposterous) radiological career for Grubbé. While Grubbé's claim to be the first to use radiation for treating cancer is probably valid, there is a need to account for some puzzling gaps.

Firstly, it is odd that neither he nor his faculty supervisor made any effort to present or write up such epochal results, although in 1902 he did publish a series of seven treated cases [9]. (It is of interest that Grubbé stated in his paper that he was seeing 70 patients a day, "which we believe to be the largest number of daily x-ray treatments yet reported by any individual.") He opened his 1902 report as follows: "Realizing that the reporting of immature results … has been the bane of current medical literature, we have deferred giving for publication our experience with the x-rays in the treatment of malignant diseases because we wished to give the remedy the test of time." Grubbé elaborated further by pointing out that (1) the first patients both died within a few months, (2) he was still a medical student, and (3) he had no access to medical journals. Even if one grants some validity to these reasons, it is surprising that he failed to capitalize academically on Mrs. Lee and Mr. Carr as he obtained further encouraging findings in the ensuing months. It is perhaps even stranger that Grubbé's faculty colleagues failed to pursue an opportunity that could have brought credit to an establishment that had been described as a "third-rate medical school." It makes one wonder exactly what kind of relationship the medical student Grubbé had with his teachers. By failing to claim credit at the time, Grubbé left himself open to a rival claim from Dr. H. P. Pratt, another Chicago physician, who asserted that in April of 1896, he was the first to apply x-rays for treating cancer. It was not until 1933 that Grubbé came forth, explaining that his long silence in this regard was due to the fact that he could furnish no supporting documentation in the form of referral letters or patient notes, all of which he thought had been destroyed in a fire [4]. In 1933, however, Grubbé discovered the two referral letters in a partially burned container that he thought had been completely destroyed. It was in the wake of this discovery that Grubbé published a paper and a book claiming priority in applying x-rays for cancer therapy [10]. While some literature accepts this claim [11], other reports are more circumspect. For example, the above cited *BMJ* obituary asserts that Grubbé "probably" was the first, and a biography published by the Chicago Radiological Society describes him as "one of the earliest radiation therapy specialists in this city and perhaps in the United States" [7]. The most exhaustive account comes from Paul Hodges [12], a former chairman of the Radiology Department at the University of Chicago, and himself a distinguished radiologist, who was commissioned to write Grubbé's biography. For this, Grubbé himself can be thanked, since he bequeathed his estate to the University of Chicago with the stipulation that the university publish his life story. It is likely that what was written differed from what Grubbé had in mind, but Hodges' biography is well regarded and considered frank yet fair [3, 13]. Hodges asked the FBI to analyze the two referral letters from Ludlam and Halphide

to Grubbé; their analysis showed that the handwriting was authentic, leading Hodges to conclude that Grubbé was the first to employ x-rays for therapeutic purposes, but others are still unconvinced [14, 15].

It can be concluded that Grubbé was an early enthusiast of radiation and that even before completing medical training, he had acquired requisite skills that allowed him to seize an opportunity provided by his Hahnemann colleagues – perhaps he *was* the first to apply radiation for treating cancer. Whether he was the first to use protective lead shielding is not proven, although that too is one of his claims. There is little doubt that Grubbé was a leader in the emerging field of radiation therapy. But some of his claims were far-fetched, such as alleged worldwide travelling when he was a medical student, his supposed discovery of platinum in Idaho (where only traces have ever been found), his manufacture of synthetic diamonds, and his claim to be first with fluoroscopy and likewise with the therapeutic use of radioisotopes all are "palpably erroneous" according to Hodges. Perhaps Grubbé's initial use of radiation was based on homeopathic reasoning, but it is sadly ironic that Grubbé had already been exposed to excessive and destructive doses of radiation from which he eventually died. It is not known whether he ever used homeopathy in his practice or if he followed homeopathic dosing guidelines in the use of radiation.

Francis Benson

Francis Colgate Benson (1870–1941) was a senior surgeon at Hahnemann where, in 1894, he had obtained his medical degree. He developed an interest in radiation as it gained a foothold in American medicine, was one of the first to use radium in the United States [16], and became known as "a pioneer in the adaptation of radium to medical purposes," as well as for "organizing this country's first separate [general hospital] department for the use of radium in medicine and surgery" [17]. He also gave the first complete course in the use of radium at a medical college.

Benson was a man of other interests, including the collection of medieval manuscripts and early bibles, which still appear from time to time on the auction market. Unusually for an American, he was also an aficionado of cricket, writing a collection of verses in praise of the game [18]. In reference to the cricket field at Haverford College, Benson wrote in his poem *The Field*:

> Could you imagine this whole earth could yield
> A spot more beautiful than our old cricket field?
> Ring'd round with immemorial elms it lies
> A fair green lawn.

An unsung figure nowadays, Benson deserves a spot in the history of medicine for his pioneering work with radium.

William Dieffenbach

Although he was once well known in New York circles and beyond, William Hermann Dieffenbach is now largely forgotten (Fig. 8.2). Dieffenbach (1872–1937) trained at the NYHMC, received his medical degree in 1900, and remained on the faculty throughout his career, holding variously professorships of mechanotherapy, bacteriology, and hydrotherapy. He became known for his work in radiotherapy, hydrotherapy, ultrashort wave therapy, electrotherapeutics, mechanotherapy, and the homeopathic proving of radium.

Dieffenbach spent many years in medical administration. In 1918, he was the president of the Medical College and Hospital for Women under turbulent circumstances, which resulted in his suing of four female doctors for slander and libel [19]. The women concerned had made allegations that Dieffenbach eliminated the women's medical college in order to procure the building for the NYHMC. In reality, the women's college had been unable to recruit adequate numbers of students due to World War I and was barely viable. Other offices to which he held included membership of the board of trustees of the Community Hospital, presidency of the medical board and acting president of Broad Street Hospital, vice-president of the New York Homeopathic Medical College, and president of the American Institute of Homeopathy. In 1927, Dieffenbach served as chairman of the endowment committee at a critical time in the history of the New York Homeopathic College and led a successful $1,000,000 fund-raising effort that staved off financial disaster [20].

Dieffenbach quickly achieved fame for his leadership in using radium for nonoperative cancer. His interest in x-ray therapy began shortly after Roentgen's discovery of x-rays. Under the direction of William H. King, dean of the New York Homeopathic College, the first public x-ray therapy clinic was opened at NYHMC in 1900. Encouraging results with x-rays for intractable skin diseases had been reported by Freund and Schiff in Vienna, which caused Dieffenbach to try this approach in the treatment of uterine fibroma. He published the case as the first x-ray-induced cure of fibroma in 1904 in the *North American Journal of Homeopathy*. His 1925 description about this publication is of interest: "The case was published in Dr. E. H. Porter's *North American Journal of Homeopathy* twenty years ago, but being from homeopathic sources has never secured the credit due as the first case of fibroid treated by means of the x-ray. With improvement of apparatus the therapeutic results from many countries soon developed an extensive literature" [21]. As a good homeopath, Dieffenbach stressed in this review the necessity of individualizing the radiation dose and was opposed to the giving of radiation at a standard dose as some were doing. He said that "all these … methods are fallacious, if not dangerous, for they fail to take into consideration the

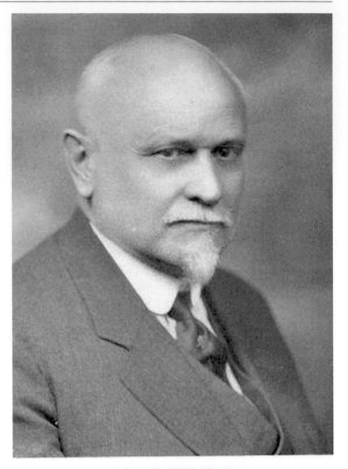

WM. H. DIEFFENBACH, M.D.
1872-1937

Fig. 8.2 William Dieffenbach. New York homeopath and radiation specialist (Courtesy of Sylvain Cazalet, Homeopathe International, Montpellier, France)

personal and biological equation of the individual patient and tissues treated." He then gave examples of different factors to take into account. He thought that the administration of x-rays should be in accordance with the Arndt-Schulz principle (see Chap. 16), just as some had claimed for drugs, and gave several examples of medical conditions that responded to low-radiation doses. Dieffenbach was critical of the use of "knockout doses" of radiation in cancer, as they sometimes proved too much for the patient. Other points of interest in his 1925 review include reference to Dieffenbach's special method of treatment for rectal cancer and of the fact that in 1910 his group had reported on the first ten cases of inoperable bladder cancer treated successfully through an incision with a dose of 2,200 mg hours of radium exposure.

Dieffenbach reported in 1904 that he had cured five cases of cancer with radium coatings on celluloid rods inserted directly into the affected parts: this work gained publicity in the national press [22]. The use of gelatin-radium rods was introduced to Dieffenbach by William King in 1902, but initial results were unsatisfactory and produced dangerous cardiac arrhythmia. Improvements were obtained when a celluloid material was used to enhance the diffusion of radium into diseased tissue [23].

Although Dieffenbach worked in a homeopathic college and published mainly in the homeopathic literature, he interacted with allopathic colleagues, including Henry Piffard, a prominent authority who had begun his own experiments in 1902 and who made important suggestions to Dieffenbach on the delivery of radium. One measure of Dieffenbach's stature can be gauged by the fact that he was invited by President Roosevelt to represent the United States at the First International Congress on Radiology and Ionization, held in Liege, Belgium, in 1905. This invitation had been extended by the Belgian government [24]. Another national representative was Ernest Fox Nichols, a world-famous physicist and future president of Dartmouth University who, with Gordon Hull, conducted experiments to measure the radiation pressure of light. It has been said that the Nichols-Hull experiments are one of the most significant experiments of all time in American physics [25]. Dieffenbach, who served as vice-president of that congress, was in exalted company. He was one of several physicians who presented their experiences with the therapeutic use of x-rays and radium, and his talk was published in full in the *North American Journal of Homeopathy* [23]. Apparently, Dieffenbach's presentation led to greater uptake in radium therapy among European than American doctors [26]. It is of interest that on the same panel, Mihran Kassabian, from Philadelphia, gave a talk in which he drew attention to his disfigurements from years of exposure to radiation. Dieffenbach was fortunate to escape the predations that had affected Grubbé and Kassabian. Whether it was related to Dieffenbach's greater caution or greater awareness of the danger is a matter of conjecture, but as pointed out below, his homeopathic proving study had warned him that doses higher than the 6X dilution were unsafe.

In describing the history of the Flower Hospital Cancer Clinic, Helmuth gave all the credit to Dieffenbach for the use of radium in treating nonoperative malignancies. "I want to state before you all, that the whole credit of this discovery or original research belongs to Dr. Dieffenbach and I have been only the man who has practically given the injections, done the mechanical part of the work," said William Tod Helmuth. He went on to explain that the two men had been deluged with enquiries, but "that, as you know, this is absolutely new and original, and as a consequence we are not yet prepared to give any great or positive statistics" [27].

In 1914, Dieffenbach reported on 16 cases treated with radium, x-rays, and/or surgery [28]. The paper was summarized by Steinke in the *International Abstract of Surgery*, which noted that Dieffenbach had owned to more failures than cures and urged for greater cooperation between surgeon, physician, and radiologist, with more use of postoperative radiation [29].

Other innovative work included the administration of x-rays to chicken eggs, which gained wide coverage in the press and in popular publications [30]. In these studies, Dieffenbach claimed that short-term radiation resulted in many more chicks hatching out as females, which could therefore increase egg-laying yield. However, when x-rays were given for several hours, deformities appeared which, Dieffenbach said, normally require many generations over the course of evolution. Although enthusiastic about his findings, it is not known how much further Dieffenbach took them.

Dieffenbach put radium to the test in the form of homeopathic proving; in this venture, he was joined by two homeopaths who are mentioned elsewhere, Copeland and Crump, and by others. The test methodology was considered to be rigorous by the standards of the time and was undertaken using 30x, 12x, and 6x potencies. Even at such low doses, all subjects reported joint and muscle symptoms as well as increased white blood cell counts. The homeopathic 6x dose produced such severe symptoms that the authors warned against its medical use. Concurrently and independently in Europe, Professor William His and many others began to use radium to treat arthritis and gout, bearing out the findings in Dieffenbach's proving [31].

Other Activities

Hydrotherapy was a fashionable form of treatment for all kinds of medical disorders, especially for neurosis, where it formed a prominent part of the programs offered at health spas. Dieffenbach placed high value on the benefits of this treatment, which he used in his practice and taught to medical students. His book, *Hydrotherapy: A Brief Summary of the Practical Value of Water in Disease for Students and Practitioners of Medicine* [32], was well reviewed [33, 34]. Dieffenbach served on the hydrotherapy committee of the American Electrotherapeutic Association. One of Dieffenbach's students was Benedict Lust, the father of naturopathic medicine, who was already a believer in hydrotherapy as a student and who transmitted this enthusiasm to his teacher. The growth of hydrotherapy and physiotherapy in hospital practice was in part influenced by these two individuals [35]. Although hydrotherapy is rarely used in medicine today, one measure of how it was seen a century ago can be illustrated by the fact that Professor Emil Kraepelin, one of the foremost psychiatrists in the world, attributed the successful treatment of agitation to use of continuous baths [36].

In 1903, Niels Finsen became the first and so far only dermatologist to win the Nobel Prize for his therapeutic work with ultraviolet irradiation in treating lupus vulgaris.

UV light therapy quickly gained popularity and was applied more broadly for a range of conditions. In the 1920s, it became a well-established treatment of psoriasis, with reports by Alderson in 1923 [37] and Goeckerman in 1925 [38] generating much interest. This form of treatment, albeit with modifications, remains part of the armamentarium against psoriasis today. Dieffenbach also made early contributions to the literature about UV phototherapy, with a paper in 1925 recounting his experiences, which were by then extensive [39]. He was already using UV rays by 1915, including in tuberculosis as a means of preventing surgical amputation. Dieffenbach provided a long list of skin diseases as being amenable to this treatment, with detailed mention of a new technique for treating psoriasis at the special clinic he had set up at the Broad Street Hospital in New York. He noted how psoriasis often worsened in the winter and would respond well to UV light. Also, perhaps ahead of his time, he recommended a vegetarian diet for his psoriasis patients, saying "we strongly urge this technic to the profession." Of interest, modern medicine acknowledges the benefit of a vegetarian diet for psoriasis, as reported in 1983 by Lithell and colleagues [40]. It is believed that such a diet works by lowering the levels of proinflammatory arachidonic acid [41]. In 1936, Dieffenbach authored a book on ultraviolet wave therapy, under the somewhat grandiloquent title *Ultra Short Wave Therapy: A New and Important Medical Discovery* [42].

John Mallory Lee

For 50 years, the town of Rochester, New York, was a hive of homeopathy, boasting four homeopathic hospitals and the patronage of wealthy families, including the Sibleys and Watsons, founders of the Western Union Telegraph Company. As mentioned in Chap. 7, Charles Sumner held the position of a city health commissioner. Among the more entrepreneurial of the city's homeopaths was John Mallory Lee (1852–1926), who graduated from the University of Michigan Homeopathic Medical School in 1878 (Fig. 8.3). He settled in Rochester where, for the next 9 years, he practiced general medicine and rose to prominence in the local homeopathic community. Between 1889 and 1894, Lee attended the New York Polyclinic and Postgraduate School in order to be a surgeon. As a surgeon, physician, and expert in radiation therapy, Lee was unusually well trained, but besides his technical proficiency, he gained a reputation as a fine physician who was "distinguished by the degree of time and emphasis spent on careful listening and other factors that contributed to a relationship of sympathy and trust between doctor and patient" [43]. In short, he would have been seen as an outstanding example of what homeopathy stood for. In addition, Lee was remembered as a generous mentor.

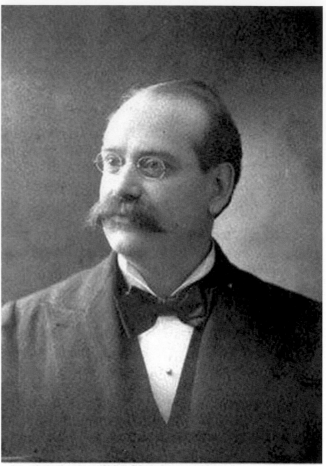

John M. Lee - c. 1880
Courtesy of Rochester Images, Rochester Public Library

Fig. 8.3 John Mallory Lee. Entrepreneur, early pioneer in radiotherapy, and second president of American Radium Society (Image by permission of Central Library of Rochester & Monroe County)

Lee was part of the group that founded the Rochester Homeopathic Hospital in 1887, and in 1898, he established the Lee Private Hospital and Training School for Nurses (Fig. 8.4). This hospital, which survived until 1962, was to become famous for its radiation program, developed by Lee. The facility prospered, expanding in bed capacity from 7 in 1898 to 51 in 1903. While it provided the community with medical, obstetric, and surgical care, it was as a center of radium and x-ray therapy that the hospital became best known. Lee envisioned a time when surgery would become "free from the knife." He set off in a new direction when he installed state-of-the-art equipment for delivering radium to treat cancer and forged an association with Dr. Gioacchino Failla, a New York physicist who had spearheaded the use of radium and deep-therapy x-ray for cancer. Failla was subsequently to become a world-renowned biophysicist and radiobiologist who made very significant contributions to the relation between radiation and cancer, both as treatment and cause. He also set up the first research program to develop

Fig. 8.4 Lee Private Hospital, Rochester, NY. Watkins Publishing Company, 1911 (Image by permission of Central Library of Rochester & Monroe County)

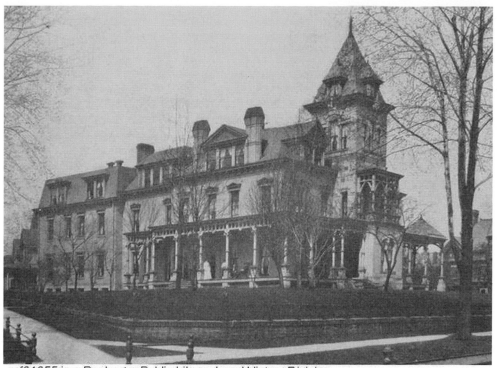

rpf01255.jpg Rochester Public Library Local History Division

the medical applications of radiation, created the first radon generator, and led the way in determining the correct dose of radiation to apply. In 1922, the Lee Hospital was one of the 12 hospitals nationwide to install a new radiation emanation plant and deep x-ray therapy equipment. Dr. Failla assisted Dr. Lee in this venture. Lee designed special glass tubes (known as capillaries) to inject radium fluid into the tumor, and within a few years, these capillaries were being used across the nation [43].

As Dickson noted, with Lee being so widely respected as a physician, surgeon, homeopath, and radiotherapist, his hospital began to attract physicians for residency training. Lee was generous to his trainees and would facilitate their spending time with Dr. Failla in New York [43]. In 1918, Lee was elected as the third president of the American Radium Society in recognition of his accomplishments in the emerging field of radiotherapy. Like some other pioneers, Lee suffered from the complications of handling radium: he lost two middle fingers from radiation burns, but unlike Kassabian and Grubbé, at least, he did not succumb to malignancy.

References

1. Anonymous. Obituary. BMJ. 1960;2:609.
2. Frame PW. Tales from the atomic age. The legend of Emil H. Grubbé [Internet] Health Physics Historical Instrumentation Collection; 2011 [Cited 2011 Dec 31]. Available from: www.orau.org/ptp/articlesstories/grubbe.htm.
3. Anonymous. Commentary: The Book Forum. J Am Med Assoc. 1965;191:161.
4. Grubbé E. Who was the first to make use of the therapeutic qualities of the X-Ray? Radiological Review. 1933;XXII:184–7.
5. Grubbé E. Priority in the therapeutic use of X-Rays. Radiology. 1933;XXI:156–62.
6. Anonymous. Pioneer in x-ray therapy. Science. 1957;125:18–9.
7. Biography of Emil Grubbé [Internet]. Chicago Radiological Society: Naperville; 2012 [Cited 2012 Oct 30]. Available from: http://www.chirad-soc.org/crs.grubbe_bio.html.
8. Orndorff BH. In Memoriam. Emil Herman Grubbé. Radiology. 1960;75:473–4.
9. Grubbé EH. X-rays in the treatment of cancer and other malignant diseases. Medical Record. 1902;62:692–5.
10. Grubbé E. X-ray treatment: its origin, birth and early history. St. Paul/Minneapolis: Bruce Publishing Company; 1949.
11. Vujosevic B, Bokorov B. Radiotherapy: past and present. Archiv Oncology. 2010;18:140–2.
12. Hodges PC. The life and times of Emil H. Grubbé. Chicago: The University of Chicago Press; 1964.
13. Lowman RM. Review of The Life and Times of Emil H. Grubbé. J History Med. 1965;21:302–3.
14. Brecher R, Brecher F. The rays – a history of radiology in the United States and Canada. Baltimore: Williams and Wilkins Company; 1969.
15. Knight N, Wilson JF. A history of the radiological sciences. In: McLennan B, Gagliardi RA, editors. The early years of radiation therapy, vol. 1. Reston: Radiology Centennial Inc; 1996.
16. Obituary. Frank C. Benson, Jr., MD, ScD, FACS. Professor of Radiology [Internet]. Hahnemann Medical College Yearbook. 1941 [Cited 2012 Aug 1]. Available from: http://archive.org/stream/medic41hahn/medic41hahn_djvu.txt.
17. Federal Writers Project (Pa.). Philadelphia, A Guide to the Nation's Birthplace [Internet]. Philadelphia Historical Commission. Harrisburg: The Telegraph Press; 1937 [Cited 2012 Aug 1].

Available from: http://www.ebooksread.com/authors-eng/federal-writers-project-pa/philadelphia-a-guide-to-the-nations-birthplace-hci/1-philadelphia-a-guide-to-the-nations-birthplace-hci.shtml.

18. Benson FC. Songs of the cricket field and other verses. Philadelphia: James Clark Press; 1932.

19. Sues 4 Women Doctors. Trial begun in physician's action for alleged slander. The New York Times. 1922 Aug 16.

20. Dr. W.H. Dieffenbach dies suddenly at 71. Head of community hospital board of trustees for years – aided other institutions. The New York Times. 1937 Jan 14. p. 21.

21. Dieffenbach WH. Roentgen therapy – its present status and recent developments. J Am Inst Homeopath. 1925;18:13–26.

22. Five cases of cancer cured. Dr. Dieffenbach successfully treats the disease with radium. The Spokane Daily Chronicle. 1905 Oct 13. p. 3.

23. Dieffenbach WH. A new method for the therapeutic application of radium salts. N Am J Homeopath. 1905;LII:769–74.

24. Lockyer, Sir Norman. International Congress on Radiology and Ionization. Nature. 1905;72:611–2.

25. Chapman K. Symposium commemorates Wilder Laboratory's designation as historic site [Internet]. Dartmouth Now. 17 Sept 2012. [Cited 2012 Oct 1]. Available from: www.now.dartmouth.edu/2012/09/symposium-commemorates-wilder-laboratorys-designation-as-historic-site/.

26. Editorial. The radium treatment of cancer. N Am J Homeopathy. 1914;62:236–8.

27. Dieffenbach WH, Helmuth WT. Clinic at Flower Hospital. N Am J Homeopath. 1909;24:419–29.

28. Dieffenbach WH. Report on cancer patients treated with Roentgen or radium rays and remaining clinically cured after more than three years. J Am Inst Homeopath. 1916;IX:430.

29. Steinke CR. Report on cancer patients treated with Roentgen or radium rays and remaining clinically cured after more than three months Int Abst Surg. 1917;XXIV:162.

30. Fisher B. Amazing new jobs for X-rays. Popular Sci. 1928;113:31–2.

31. Cowperthwaite AC. Radium as an internal remedy. Pac Coast J Homeopath. 1916;XXVII:19–23.

32. Dieffenbach WH. Hydrotherapy: a brief summary of the practical value of water in disease for students and practitioners of medicine. New York: Rebman Company; 1909.

33. Book Reviews. Hydrotherapy. Am J Nursing. 1910;X:222–3.

34. Book Reviews. Hydrotherapy: a brief summary of the practical value of water in disease for students and practitioners of medicine. J Adv Ther. 1909;XXVII:396–7.

35. Dieffenbach, radiotherapy specialist dies. Naturopath and Herald of Health. 1937;XXXXI:126.

36. Pope C. Progress in physical therapeutics. Hydrotherapy. J Advanced Therapeutics. 1909;XXVII:37–8.

37. Alderson HE. Heliotherapy in psoriasis. Arch Dermatol Syphilol. 1923;8:79–80.

38. Goeckerman WH. The treatment of psoriasis. Northwest Medicine. 1925;24:229–31.

39. Dieffenbach WH. Practical office applications of the ultra-violet rays. J Am Inst Homeopath. 1925;18:802–5.

40. Lithell H, Bruce A, Gustafsson IB. A fasting and vegetarian diet treatment trial on chronic inflammatory disorders. Acta Dermato-Venereology. 1983;63:397–403.

41. Wolters M. Diet and psoriasis: experimental data and clinical evidence. Br J Dermatol. 2005;153:706–14.

42. Dieffenbach WH. Ultra short wave therapy – a new and important medical discovery. New York: Westerman; 1936.

43. Dickson RJ. The legacy of 179 Lake Avenue: a small private hospital's service to the community. Rochester History. 2008;70:1–21. [Internet]. [Cited 2012 December 29]. Available from: www.rochester.lib.ny.us/rochhist/v70_2007/v7011.pdf.

9

Heartbeat, Heart Failure, and Homeopathy

Homeopathic footprints can be found in cardiovascular medicine. One of medicine's most enduring drugs, nitroglycerin, was introduced by a homeopath in 1847 and was utilized by homeopathy for many years before the regular medical profession applied it for anginal chest pain, for which it has been a mainstay ever since.

Constantine Hering and His Contributions

To make ends meet as an impoverished student, Constantine Hering (1800–1880) agreed in 1820 to write a refutation of the upstart and growing specialty of homeopathy [1] (Fig. 9.1). To the surprise and annoyance of his family and sponsor, Hering was converted as the result of this exercise, becoming a lifelong proponent of homeopathy and, arguably, the most influential person in American homeopathy.

Hering completed his medical training at Leipzig in 1826, but was unable to secure a position that allowed him to practice the way he wanted. As a result, for some years thereafter, Hering was employed in other fields, including mathematics and biology. In 1828, the King of Saxony sent Hering to conduct a botanical and zoological survey in Surinam. In 1835, he settled in the United States, where he established homeopathy as a presence in America with a short-lived medical school in Allentown, Pennsylvania, and then later an enduring school in Philadelphia, where his college became a mecca for homeopathic training. Samuel Hahnemann referred to Hering as the father of homeopathy in America.

Nitroglycerin

Hering remained professionally active up to end of his life. In addition to his far-reaching influence as teacher and mentor, Hering directed many provings of substances that have become part of the homeopathic *pharmacopoeia*. Among these are included *hydrophobinum* for rabies, *Lachesis* (venom from the bushmaster snake), and venom from several other snakes. His claim to fame as a prover of new remedies, however, relates to the original investigations he and his colleagues conducted with nitroglycerine, or to use Hering's term, glonoine/glonoinum, an acronym derived from *Gl*ycyl *O*xyd (glycerin), *N*itrogen, and *O*xygen, with the suffix *-inum* added (Latin: "what is derived"). As noted by Fye, without the unheralded work of Hering and his colleagues, it is quite conceivable that nitroglycerin would never have been introduced into medicine at all, and emergence of the drug as a mainstream treatment for angina pectoris would not have taken place without "the aggressive screening of various compounds by Hahnemann, Hering and their followers" [2].

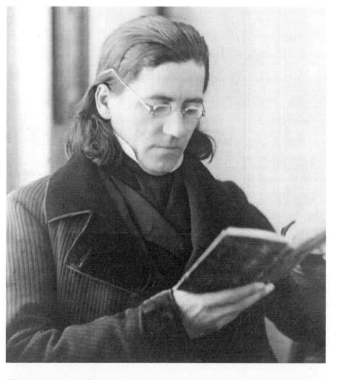

Fig. 9.1 Constantine Hering. Founder of Hahnemann Medical College, Philadelphia, and pioneer in the medical use of nitroglycerin (Image in the public domain)

J. Davidson, *A Century of Homeopaths*,
DOI 10.1007/978-1-4939-0527-0_9, © Springer Science+Business Media New York 2014

The glonoine story has unfolded over nearly 100 years, involving chemists, pharmacologists, homeopaths, allopaths, and Alfred Nobel, the inventor of dynamite. In 1846, the Italian chemist Ascanio Sobrero discovered how to synthesize nitroglycerin from nitric acid, sulfuric acid, and glycerin. In describing the effects of this highly explosive substance, he noted the severe headache following ingestion of even a small quantity. Hering quickly became familiar with Sobrero's report, saw therapeutic potential of the drug, and between 1847 and 1851 conducted provings on 100 homeopaths. He even engaged the assistance of a Philadelphia medical student, Charles Jackson, who took nitroglycerin himself and experienced the same symptoms that provers had reported. Unfortunately, Jackson, who was studying at the Jefferson Medical School, could not persuade any of his colleagues to study this drug because its homeopathic pedigree was a problem and the explosive nature of nitroglycerin made it seem unsafe. It was to be a full decade before orthodox medicine took any further interest, and even then, it was at the instigation of a homeopath in faraway England.

In 1858, a British surgeon, Alfred Field, had been urged by a homeopathic colleague to try nitroglycerin. Although Field approached this experiment with great skepticism, upon placing a minute quantity on the tip of his tongue, he experienced marked headache, fullness in the neck, and nausea. Despite conducting a number of unsuccessful animal experiments with nitroglycerin at a homeopathic pharmacy, Field wrote that "I still thought I had seen and felt enough of the physiological action of the medicine to justify my cautious employment of it in the treatment of disease." Accordingly, he administered the drug to four patients with complaints of pain: a 68-year-old female patient with symptoms suggestive of ischemic chest pain, two with dental pain, and a fourth with headache. All responded well [3]. His report spurred further pharmacological study of the drug by Fuller and Harley at University College Hospital, London, and by others in Germany and the United States. While these investigators replicated the clinical results, they were unable to provide any clear explanation for the effects. In 1879, Murrell was the first to suggest that nitroglycerin was effective for angina pectoris [4]. Because early homeopathic tests clearly indicated that glonoine caused a panoply of symptoms besides headache, such as "oppression of the chest" akin to a feeling of constriction "as if chains were placed about it, and tightened more and more," and a "sensation of numbness, upward in chest and down left arm," it may be asked why homeopaths failed to emphasize glonoine in the treatment of angina. Certainly, it is fair to say that awareness of angina was low among physicians of all schools at the time as it was believed to be a rare condition, but even so, it remains somewhat surprising that the value of the drug for ischemic heart disease was unrecognized for another 30 years. What can be said, though, is that Hering's provings

were a critical first step in the medical use of nitroglycerin. He showed that a powerful explosive could be given as a safe medicine, bringing peace of mind to those who suffer from chest pain due to coronary artery insufficiency.

The nitroglycerin story would be incomplete without mentioning Alfred Nobel. Like Hering, Nobel became acquainted with Sobrero's work soon after its publication and, also like Hering, he recognized considerable potential for the substance. However, Nobel envisaged a totally different use for the compound, wanting to find a method to exploit nitroglycerin's detonative action in a controlled manner. His successful pursuit of this quest is well known, and from the vast fortune he made, funds were set aside to endow the Nobel Prize. Two codas can be added to the nitroglycerin story. Nobel suffered from severe headaches and angina pains in his old age, leading his doctor to recommend none other than nitroglycerin as treatment. Just a few weeks before his death in 1896, Nobel wrote: "…isn't it the irony of fate that I have now been prescribed NGl [nitroglycerine] to be taken internally! They call it Trinitrin, so as not to scare the chemist and the public" [5]. The second coda relates to the much later discovery of NTG's mechanism of action by Murad et al. [6], Furchgott and Zawadski [7], Moncado's group [8], and Ignarro et al. [9] Nitroglycerin releases nitric oxide (NO), which is located in the inner cell lining (endothelium) of arteries and which, when dilated, lowers pressure and relieves angina pain. For their work, many of the above investigators received the Nobel Prize in 1998 [10].

Snake Venoms

Hering should also be remembered for his proving of snake venoms. In 1828, he created the first dilution of snake venom *Lachesis trigonocephalus* (or *Lachesis muta* as it is now known) from the Amazon surucucu snake and published his cases in 1835. It has been said that Hering was the first to take a scientific approach to the study of snake venoms in medicine [11]. Together with rattlesnake and cobra venom, these remedies were incorporated into the homeopathic *materia medica* for treating hemorrhagic conditions [12]. One hundred years later, the same properties were rediscovered, with some acknowledgment of their homeopathic heritage [13] by Peck and colleagues [14]. Peck's work was covered in the popular press, which described how moccasin venom had opposite effects at low and high doses, exactly in accord with homeopathic principles: that is to say that it caused hemorrhage at high dose and staunched bleeding at low dose. Linn Boyd obtained comparable findings for *Lachesis* as an anti-arrhythmic drug (as described elsewhere in this book). Snake venom derivatives are sometimes administered in the treatment of heart disease.

When it comes to the medicinal uses of snake venoms, pride of place goes to homeopathy. Even non-homeopathic sources credit their introduction to the homeopathic school: besides the reference above to Peck, an article by Reed on rattlesnake venom in epilepsy may be cited. This paper appeared in the Lancet-Clinic, a "regular" American medical journal published between 1876 and 1916; it noted that "The first systematic attempt at the use of snake poison in medicine was made … by Constantine Hering … in 1837." The author then went on to say that "Russell and Stokes, in India, later fed the virus [sic] of the cobra to thirteen subjects and noted a large number of symptoms." He further elaborated that these experiments had elicited symptoms suggesting a role in epilepsy, although homeopaths had not exploited this property of the drug – an action which was to be subsequently applied in regular medicine for some time [15, 16]. Reed's mention of Adrian Stokes (1821–1876) and John Rutherford Russell (1816–1867) is important in that both these physicians were homeopaths and were the first to experiment with cobra venom. They published their work in the British homeopathic literature in 1853 and 1859, which was over 10 years before Sir Joseph Fayrer's classic book on Indian snakes appeared [17]. Fayrer was one of the most eminent doctors in the Indian Medical Service and was rewarded for his efforts by a baronetcy [18]. He and Lauder Brunton conducted several studies of cobra and other snake venoms and were aware of Hering's work. For example, in their 1873 report, Brunton and Fayrer compared their results with those of Hering, noting similarities in the rapid onset of action of snake venom [19]. In America, Silas Weir Mitchell wrote an essay on rattlesnake venom two decades after Hering's publications. In the opinion of one expert, Hering's "excellent symptomatic detail" had been "little recked [by Mitchell] … as to either the rattlesnake itself or to the related South American reptile" [20, 21].

Another homeopath who contributed to the cobra venom story was John Hayward, of Birkenhead in England. Hayward was one of the first to administer cobra venom extract in medical practice, recommending low potencies (1X or 2X) by the oral or subcutaneous routes as lifesaving measures for diphtheria, smallpox, and scarlet fever [22]. Homeopaths have thus played an important part in the original study of snake venoms, their effects, and therapeutic applications. Where orthodox medicine went further, however, was the extent to which it investigated the mechanism of action of venom and their effects of specific body organs. As has been noted elsewhere, Hahnemann and most homeopaths showed little interest in mechanisms, preferring to focus on symptoms.

Hering's Law of Cure

In a third capacity, Hering is remembered for what has come to be known as Hering's law. Hering observed that healing often followed a characteristic pattern in which symptoms improved from the head down, from the inside out, from the most important organs to the least, and in reverse order of their first appearance. Thus, it is that sometimes symptom aggravations occur or that new symptoms and the return of old ones in reverse sequence can be seen. While medicine has largely ignored these phenomena, some contemporary physicians acknowledge that they occur (the "rollback" phenomenon) and that they may be therapeutically significant, for example, in psychiatry [23, 24]. It is interesting, by way of linking traditional homeopathy to modern research, that Brien et al. have developed a rating scale to measure Hering's law of cure and have shown that (1) such a scale can be operationally constructed and that (2) the total score predicts outcome [25].

The Cardiovascular Institute (CVI) at Hahnemann Medical College

In the 1930s and 1940s, a talented group of physicians made groundbreaking contributions to cardiology while Hahnemann was still a nominally homeopathic school. In 1948, they formed the Mary Bailey Institute for Cardiovascular Research, often referred to as the Cardiovascular Institute (CVI), named after Charles Bailey's young daughter, who died from hepatitis. Members of the CVI gained worldwide recognition for their work. At the time of its founding, the CVI was the first of its kind in the United States and the second worldwide. While many were involved in the CVI's birth, the cardiologist William Likoff and the cardiac surgeon Charles Bailey provided substantial leadership, raising the funds to obtain dedicated space. The CVI initially employed around a dozen principal investigators, but by the time of Likoff's death in 1987, it had grown to 55 faculty, 15 trainees, and over 100 support staff, making it one of the largest cardiovascular institutes in the United States [26].

The first member of the CVI team to become well known was *George Geckeler* (1894–1989), a 1919 Hahnemann graduate (Fig. 9.2). In 1939, Geckeler produced a series of heart sound recordings which was distributed commercially by Columbia. These long-playing teaching records, or "stethophones" as they were called, were widely used by US medical students and brought national recognition to Geckeler as an educator. He designed the famous "walk-through" heart on exhibit in the Philadelphia Franklin Institute and in 1956 was featured in *Life* magazine for restoring "Harriet," a unique dissection of the human central nervous system that was in the Hahnemann collection, dating back to the nineteenth century (see Chap. 4). Geckeler was the CVI's first director, and in 1950, he received a grant from the newly established National Heart Institute to support his teaching

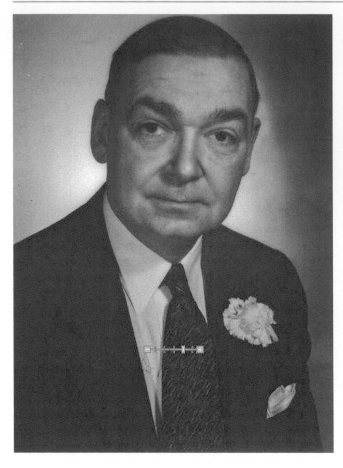

Fig. 9.2 George Geckeler. Hahnemann Medical College cardiologist and first director of Hahnemann Cardiovascular Institute (Image courtesy of National Library of Medicine)

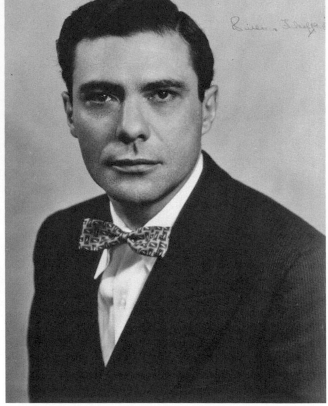

Fig. 9.3 William Likoff. Hahnemann Medical College cardiologist and president. His name was perpetuated through the Likoff Cardiovascular Institute (Image courtesy of National Library of Medicine)

work. Geckeler's career spanned an era that began when Hahnemann was primarily a homeopathic college and concluded after its allopathic refashioning.

One of Geckeler's students, *William Likoff* (1912–1987), a 1938 Hahnemann graduate, joined the CVI group after returning from military duty in World War II (Fig. 9.3). Likoff in turn became a distinguished cardiologist, president of the American College of Cardiology, and executive president of Hahnemann. His legacy endured at the CVI, which was named the William Likoff Cardiovascular Institute.

Charles Bailey was perhaps the most famous member of this group, and, as a surgeon, his story is told in Chap. 4. Likewise, *Kenneth Keown*, the anesthesiologist who was so instrumental in Bailey's triumphs, is discussed in Chap. 5.

Other Contributors to Cardiology

Linn Boyd was a man of many accomplishments and, while known as a cardiologist, merits broader categorization. He is accordingly described elsewhere in Chap. 11. Of the clinical cardiologists, this leaves Milton Raisbeck, whose contributions to medicine will be described here.

Milton Raisbeck

Milton Raisbeck (1888–1988) qualified as an MD at the NYHMC, where he was then appointed to the faculty as instructor in pharmacology and *materia medica*. Raisbeck participated in homeopathic affairs early in his career. He attended a meeting of the Albany County Homeopathic Medical Society on February 10, 1922, where he "gave a stereopticon lecture on electro-cardiographic studies in cardiac pathology." The journal proudly added that "These studies reflected great credit on Dr. Raisbeck," who presented one EKG tracing "that had never before been recorded" and was to "appear in Nelson's loose-leaf set … another assurance that the New York Homeopathic graduates are truly scientific" [27]. (Loose-leaf sets were big business during the first decades of the twentieth century and *Nelson's New Loose-Leaf Medicine* was widely read by those wishing to remain updated about current trends.)

In a lengthy review of a book appraising homeopathy [28], Raisbeck revealed his personal support for scientific testing of homeopathy and the need to move forwards from old-fashioned beliefs [29].

At the 91st annual meeting of the AIH, Raisbeck spoke on the management of chronic congestive heart failure. His recommendations for bed rest, diet, digitalis, and diuretics differed little from what might have been heard from a non-homeopath, and it is striking that he did not include homeopathy in his management plan; his suggested dose of 3 grains (180 mg) digitalis per day was far above the low doses characteristic of homeopathy [30].

Raisbeck conducted a practice in cardiology and held a faculty appointment in the division of cardiology at NYHMC. In 1942, he coauthored a paper with the surgeon Samuel Thompson on surgical treatment of coronary artery disease by creating adhesions of the pericardium (the sac that surrounds the heart) [31]. The authors described a new operative technique in which they used magnesium silicate powder (or "talc") to bring about pericardial adhesion to the heart, which was then followed by a hyperemic reaction producing a collateral arterial circulation to compensate for coronary artery insufficiency. The cases they reported showed encouraging responses.

According to William Beinfield, who trained with Raisbeck at NYMC, Raisbeck was more interested in clinical practice and promoting support for education and research, which may explain his relatively modest output of original research. He was a popular teacher and the residents felt privileged to be associated with the care of his patients. On account of his expertise, he was often the favored cardiologist to care for his professional brethren and their relatives [32].

One of Raisbeck's patients was Miss Ethel Glorney, a wealthy Irish woman. In Miss Glorney's final years, Raisbeck had refused to accept payment for his services but eventually proposed that those monies could be used to fund a foundation, which came into being with Raisbeck as its first president. He remained the foundation's president until 1982, when he was succeeded by Beinfield. In the last year of Raisbeck's long life, he was able to arrange for the Glorney Foundation to endow the New York Academy of Medicine with funds sufficient to support annual training fellowships in cardiology, summer internships for medical students, and an annual lecture and award to honor a distinguished cardiologist. These awards are coveted honors in cardiology, and among the annual lectureship awards are some of America's most famous cardiologists and researchers into heart disease, including a Nobel Prize winner. Through the Glorney-Raisbeck Fellowship program, Milton Raisbeck's name is perpetuated and his contributions remembered. It was appropriate that Raisbeck himself was the first recipient of the Glorney-Raisbeck Award, given posthumously 1 year after his death.

Measuring Cardiovascular Physiology: Nineteenth-Century British Studies

Robert Dudgeon and the Dudgeon Sphygmograph

Robert Ellis Dudgeon (1820–1904) was one of Britain's most influential nineteenth-century homeopaths, serving as editor of the *British Journal of Homoeopathy* for 40 years and president of the British Homoeopathic Society in 1878 and 1890 (Fig. 9.4). Along with Richard Hughes, he was the chief apostle of low-potency homeopathy, adhering to the belief that material drug substance was required for any therapeutic action. Dudgeon was considered to be an independent thinker, unafraid to disagree with Hahnemann.

When Dudgeon died in 1904, the *British Medical Journal* referred to him as "a notable personage, and certainly one of the most distinguished followers of whom the cult of homoeopathy has been able to boast during the past half-century." The obituary noted Dudgeon's creativity and high energy and singled out the Dudgeon sphygmograph as "the handiest and most generally useful of those which have been brought

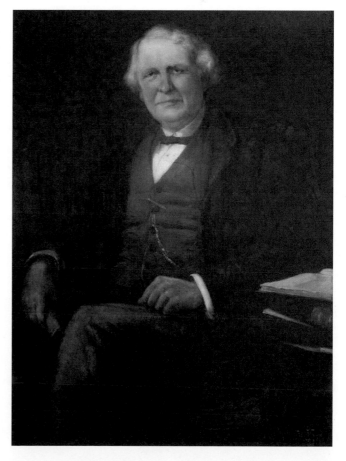

Fig. 9.4 Robert Ellis Dudgeon. British homeopath and inventor of the Dudgeon sphygmograph. Painting by Philip Stretton (By permission, University College London NHS Foundation Trust)

out." It added that this creation "best entitles Dudgeon to a permanent place in the memory of his fellows." The obituary also acknowledged Dudgeon's proficiency in optics; his presentations, papers, and book on the topic; and the design of spectacles which enabled clear vision underwater [33].

The Sphygmograph

In order to noninvasively record variations in the pulse, nineteenth-century physicians and physiologists devised an instrument called the sphygmograph, the first of which was produced in Paris by Marey in 1860, followed by modifications of Fleming in 1877 and Pond in 1879. All of these instruments were cumbersome and little used. The most popular variety of sphygmograph was introduced by Robert Dudgeon in 1881 and enjoyed the advantage of being small and portable (Fig. 9.5). As Lawrence observed, "The Dudgeon soon became the most popular instrument in Britain, rapidly displacing the Marey type," and there are now at least 12 of these in the Wellcome Museum of the History of Medicine [34]. The Dudgeon played an important role in facilitating the growth of experimental physiology and was used by famous experimenters like Lauder Brunton, Sir James Mackenzie, and Thomas Lewis. Mackenzie used the Dudgeon in his pivotal work which laid the foundation of the modern concept of heart failure, calling it "the handiest and most useful" of instruments [35]. The cardiologist, Thomas Lewis, considered the Dudgeon to be "an instrument of considerable delicacy and accuracy" [36]. By 1887, even in Paris, the Dudgeon had supplanted the homegrown Marey apparatus as the sphygmograph of choice among phy-

sicians of that city [37] – a noteworthy achievement wherein performance trumped patriotism.

Writing in 1979, Lawrence attested to the long life of the sphygmograph, which entered British medicine as a tool of experimental physiology, "in which field it still survives." He observed that it never made headway into clinical practice where, as a means of measuring blood pressure, it was replaced by manometry (as in the sphygmomanometer) by the 1880s; by the early twentieth century, the electrocardiogram "usurped almost all its other functions." But in the hands of experienced researchers, the sphygmograph proved its worth in facilitating the triumph of experimental physiology [34, p. 100].

Experimental Physiology at Boston University School of Medicine (BUSM)

Further work in cardiovascular physiology was conducted at BUSM during its homeopathic days.

Arthur Weysse

The department of physiology at BUSM began under the leadership of Professor John Rockwell (1888–1998), who was followed by Frederick Batchelder (1902–1921). Both of these men were BUSM graduates, and they built a respected department. In 1899, the department recruited Arthur Weysse, Ph.D., MD., who was a talented Harvard graduate. Although Weysse was not a homeopath by training, almost 20 years of his tenure at BUSM took place during its era as a homeopathic school, where he held a clinical appointment as lecturer in syphilis and for many years taught 12 h of medical urology and syphilology to third-year medical students. He also taught bacteriology between 1899 and 1903. Weysse is best known however as a physiologist and author of a zoology textbook.

It has been stated that Weysse was the first to introduce the auscultatory method into America for measuring blood pressure. Closer scrutiny of this claim more accurately reveals that he was the first to demonstrate a reliable method of using the technique, but that others had published about auscultation within the year previous to Weysse's 1913 report [38]. He most probably was the first to demonstrate diurnal blood pressure and pulse values [39]. Weysse had a distinguished career as both physiologist and administrator, being dean of the graduate school for 11 years between 1922 and 1933 [40].

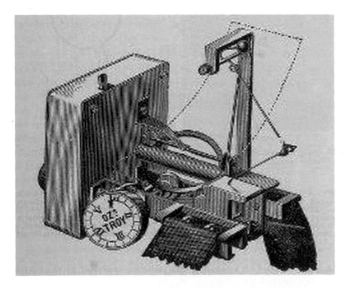

Fig. 9.5 Dudgeon's sphygmograph. Circa 1890 (From Baker et al. [41]. In public domain)

References

1. Stephens LW. German Life. Feb/Mar 1998. p. 42–4.
2. Fye WB. Vasodilator therapy for angina pectoris: the intersection of homeopathy and scientific medicine. J Hist Med Allied Sci. 1990;45:317–30.

3. Field AG. On the toxical and medicinal properties of nitrate of oxyde of glycyl. Medical Times Gazette. 1858;1:291–2.

4. Murrell W. Nitro-glycerine as a remedy for angina pectoris. Lancet. 1879;1:80, 113, 151, 225.

5. Marsh N, Marsh A. A short history of nitroglycerine and nitric oxide in pharmacology and physiology. Clin Exp Pharmacol Physiol. 2000;27:313–9.

6. Murad F, Arnold WP, Mittal CK, Braughler JM. Properties and regulation of guanylate cyclase and some proposed functions of cyclic GMP. Adv Cycl Nucl Prot Phosphoryl Res. 1979;11:175–204.

7. Furchgott RF, Zawadski JV. The obligatory role of endothelial cells in the relaxation of arterial smooth muscle by acetylcholine. Nature. 1980;288:373–6.

8. Palmer RM, Ferrige AG, Moncada S. Nitric oxide release accounts for the biological activity of endothelium-derived relaxing factor. Nature. 1987;327:524–6.

9. Ignarro LJ, Byrns RE, Buga GM, Wood KS. Endothelium-derived relaxing factor from pulmonary artery and vein possesses pharmacological and chemical properties identical to those of nitric oxide radical. Circ Res. 1987;61:866–79.

10. Fye WB. Nitroglycerin: a homeopathic remedy. Circulation. 1986;73:21–9.

11. Leeser O. Actions and medicinal use of snake-venoms. Br Homoeop J. 1958;74:153–71.

12. Besson JH. Snake venoms in therapeutics. Pac Coast J Homeopathy. 1936;47:479–89.

13. Nash EB. Leaders in homeopathic therapeutics. Philadelphia: Boericke & Tafel; 1913. p. 11.

14. Peck SM, Rosenthal N, Erf LA. The value of the prognostic venom reaction in thrombocytopenic purpura. JAMA. 1936;106:1783–91.

15. Reed RC. Rattlesnake venom in epilepsy. The Lancet-Clinic. 1911;106:347–8.

16. Editorial. The rattlesnake venom treatment of epilepsy. JAMA. 1913;60:1001.

17. Fayrer SJ. The thanatophidia of India being a description of the venomous snakes of the Indian Peninsula, with an account of the influence of their poison on life; and a series of experiments. London: J. & A. Churchill; 1872.

18. Fayrer SJ. Recollections of my life. Edinburgh: William Blackwood and Sons; 1900.

19. Brunton TL, Fayrer SJ. On the nature and physiological action of the poison of Naja tripudians and other Indian venomous snakes – Part 1. Proc Roy Soc Lond. 1873;21:358–74.

20. Mitchell SW. Researches upon the venom of the rattlesnake. Smithsonian Contributions to Knowledge. Washington: The Smithsonian Institution; 1860.

21. Morgan JC. The action of serpent poisons upon the blood and upon the nervous system, etc. The Hahnemannian Monthly. 1880;23:349–55.

22. Hayward JW. The absorption of serpent-venom. Br J Homoeopathy. 1882;XL:45–55.

23. Detre TP, Jarecki HG. Modern psychiatric treatment. Philadelphia: Lippincott; 1971.

24. Fava GA, Tomba E. Increasing psychological well-being and resilience by psychotherapeutic methods. J Pers. 2009;77:1–31.

25. Brien SB, Harrison H, Daniels J, Lewith G. Monitoring improvement in health during homeopathic intervention. Development of an assessment tool based on Hering's Law of Cure: the Hering's Law Assessment Tool (HELAT). Homeopathy. 2012;101:28–37.

26. DiPalma J. Profiles in cardiology. In memoriam: William Likoff, 1912–1987. Clin Cardiol. 1987;10:550–1.

27. Anonymous. Miscellany: General News. J Am Inst Homeopathy. 1922;14:878.

28. Dejust LH. Examen Critique de l'Homeopathie. Paris: Vigot Frères; 1922.

29. Raisbeck MJ. A critical examination of homeopathy: a review. J Am Inst Homeopathy. 1923;XV:780–90.

30. Raisbeck MJ. The management of chronic congestive heart failure. J Am Inst Homeopathy. [Internet]. 1935 [Cited 2012 Oct 8]; XXVIII. Paper read at Bureau of Drug Pathogenesis, 91st Annual convention, AIH, New York City, 2–6 June 1935. Available from: www.homeoint.org/hompath/articles/17.html.

31. Thompson SA, Raisbeck MJ. Cardio-pericardiopexy: the surgical treatment of coronary arterial disease by the establishment of adhesive pericarditis. Ann Intern Med. 1942;16:495–518.

32. Beinfield WH. Dr. Milton J. Raisbeck – San Francisco. Bull NY Acad Sci. 1988;64:898–901.

33. Obituary. Dr. Robert Ellis Dudgeon. Br Med J. 1904;2(2284):954.

34. Lawrence C. Physiological apparatus in the wellcome Museum. 2. The dudgeon sphygmograph and its descendents. Med Hist. 1979;23:96–101.

35. Mackenzie J. The study of the pulse. Edinburgh: Young J. Pentland; 1902. p. 8.

36. Lewis T. The interpretation of sphygmograph tracings, and of tracings produced by compressing the brachial artery. Factors which are involved in the production of anacrotism. Practitioner. 1907;78:207–40.

37. Anon. Dr. Dudgeon's sphygmograph in France. The Homoeopathic World. 1887;22:303–4.

38. Weysse AW, Lutz B. A comparison of the auscultatory blood pressure phenomenon in man with the tracing of the Erlanger sphygmomanometer. Am J Physiol. 1913;32:427–37.

39. Weysse AW, Lutz BR. Diurnal variations in arterial blood pressure. Am J Physiol. 1915;37:330–47.

40. Loew ER. Department of Physiology, Boston University School of Medicine (1873–1948). Physiologist. 1984;27:4–12.

41. Baker WM, Harris VD, Kirkes WS. Hand-book of physiology. 13th ed. Philadelphia: P. Blakiston & Sons; 1892. p. 219.

Introduction

The word, allergy, derives from the Greek "allos" (other) and "ergon" (action, energy, or reactivity

The term "allergy" was introduced into medicine in 1906 by Clemens von Pirquet, a pediatrician with an interest in immunity. By introducing a term that denotes the concept of altered biological reactivity, his aim was (1) to draw together a group of conditions that were caused by altered host responsiveness and (2) to describe the nature of the seemingly parallel process of immunity and hypersensitivity [1].

While today allergies and allergic disorders are understood to be common and still on the rise, for a long time, they were regarded as rare and mainly confined to upper socioeconomic groups. For most of the nineteenth and part of the twentieth century, allergy was poorly understood, although this did not in any way stifle vigorous debate about its nature, causes, and treatment.

Many individuals contributed to the growing knowledge base of allergies, and homeopathy can claim two members of this pioneering group: Charles Harrison Blackley and L. Grant Selfridge. Also to be noted briefly is the work of Gregory Shwartzman, a non-homeopathic physician who obtained his medical degree in Brussels and became professor of bacteriology at the New York Homeopathic Medical School between 1923 and 1926, where he began to build his research career before moving to Mount Sinai Medical Center. His initial association with a homeopathic establishment is of some historical interest. Today, Shwartzman is recognized for his pioneering work in anaphylaxis and typhoid vaccination, and his name lives on eponymously in the Shwartzman reaction. At NYHMC, Shwartzman experimented with bacteriophage (a virus that infects bacteria) at dilutions in the range of 10^{-9} (i.e., corresponding to low-potency homeopathic doses) and found them to be capable of producing bacteriolysis under anaerobic conditions [2].

Charles Blackley

Blackley (1820–1900) practiced medicine between 1835 and 1900 and is credited as the first to demonstrate that seasonal hay fever is caused by pollen, along with a number of other important discoveries (Fig. 10.1). Blackley was born in Bolton, England; he received little education and at an early age was apprenticed to a firm of engravers. However, ambition led him to pursue further education through evening classes in chemistry, botany, physics, microscopy, and Greek. From his studies of chemistry, Blackley became intrigued with the fact that a disproportionately small quantity of enzyme was able to catalyze the

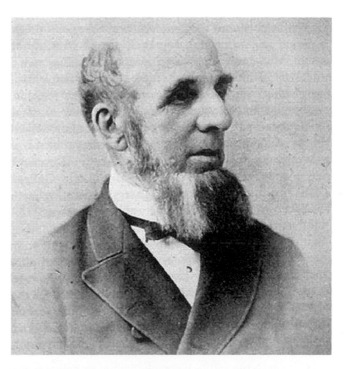

Fig. 10.1 Charles Harrison Blackley. English general practitioner who discovered pollen as the cause of hay fever (Image by courtesy of Stephen Holgate, MD)

J. Davidson, *A Century of Homeopaths*,
DOI 10.1007/978-1-4939-0527-0_10, © Springer Science+Business Media New York 2014

conversion of large amounts of one substance into another, a phenomenon that may have been relevant to his subsequent interest in homeopathy. It is also likely that his personal experience as the patient of a local homeopath gave further impetus to this interest [3]. His fascination with allergies, specifically hay fever, was almost certainly the result of being a hay fever sufferer.

At the age of 35, Blackley changed his career path and enrolled in the Pine Street Medical School in Manchester, graduating as member of the Royal College of Surgeons (MRCS) in 1858. He settled in the nearby town of Holme as a general practitioner. Although trained as an allopathic doctor, Blackley incorporated homeopathy into his practice and later in his career became heavily involved in homeopathic affairs by editing the *Manchester Homoeopathic Observer* and serving as president of the British Homoeopathic Society. In 1874, Blackley made a significant detour and obtained a doctorate of medicine from the University of Brussels. Although his MRCS degree served as a legitimate passport into medical practice, it has been suggested by Taylor and Walker that the Brussels MD degree conferred a greater measure of scholarship, which could have been significant to Blackley because adherents of homeopathy were look at askance by the allopathic medical community. It is believed that on at least one occasion, his homeopathic allegiance resulted in the withdrawal of an offer to collaborate on a hay fever study.

In Blackley's day, debates about hay fever and related allergic conditions focused on their causes, frequency, epidemiology, and treatment. There were different notions as to what caused hay fever, which was initially termed *catarrhus aestivus* (summer catarrh) by Bostock in 1827 and then "hay asthma" by the poet Robert Southey, who suffered from the condition. The term "hay fever" was introduced in 1828 [4]. Simultaneously, hay fever came to the attention of a famous London consultant physician, John Elliotson (1786–1868), who in 1831 affirmed his belief that the condition was caused by grass flowers, most likely the pollen. However, Elliotson never demonstrated this was so and encountered serious problems of credibility with his colleagues when he advocated hypnosis as a form of anesthesia. Thus, for their beliefs, Blackley and Elliotson were marginalized by the medical community and their insights about hay fever failed to receive due attention, with the result that knowledge of its cause was retarded by almost 50 years [5].

In order to pursue the possible cause of hay fever, Blackley commenced a series of painstaking and systematic experiments in 1859, which continued over at least the next 15 years. As he lamented in his book, their slow progress was

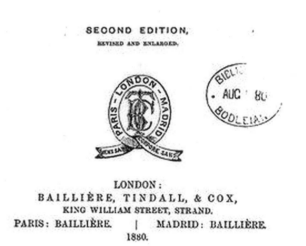

Fig. 10.2 Title page of Hay Fever: Its Causes, Treatment and Experimental Researches. 2nd Edition. 1880 (Image in the public domain)

due to difficulty taking time off from his practice in the summer months. He described the results of many of his experiments in his 1873 book *Experimental Researches on the Cause and Nature of Catarrhus Aestivus (Hay-Fever or Hay-Asthma)* [6], as well as in a second book in 1880 (Fig. 10.2). Blackley experimented on himself since he was unable to find a patient willing to devote the time. He administered pollen from over 100 species of grass and flowers by different routes to the nasal mucosa, larynx and throat, conjunctiva, tongue and lips, and upper and lower limbs. He took the precaution of including an inactive control substance for comparison. Blackley observed reactions of different intensities but they all pointed to grass pollen as the cause of his symptoms, which included itching, nasal discharge, swelling, and even asthma. After challenge with higher doses, more severe symptoms emerged, including rapid heartbeat, fever, and sweating up to 48 h in duration. Some reactions were extraordinarily severe, as shown by the appearance of a wheal ½″ high and over 2″ round following injection of pollen into the skin of his arm. As pointed out by Hurwitz, by using the diagnostic scratch and mucous membrane tests, Blackley may be credited for anticipating by 25 years their more widespread use in medicine. From his experiments, Blackley concluded that pollen was the cause of seasonal hay fever.

Blackley's next goal was to ascertain whether a relationship existed between atmospheric pollen content and symptom severity. To answer this question, in the summer months of 1866, he devised some intricate experiments in which he attached a glass-slide apparatus to kites flown at different altitudes between 500 and 2,000 ft, from which he collected pollen samples. Symptom intensity was found to correlate with pollen count. He also found that rainy and cool weather brought about a reduction in the pollen count and in his symptoms.

The results from all of these experiments were published in his 1873 book on the causes and nature of hay fever, which drew favorable attention from the press and from certain prominent people, including Charles Darwin, with whom Blackley engaged in correspondence. Darwin found Blackley's work to be "ingenious and profoundly interesting" [7]. The *Lancet* gave a favorable review to Blackley's book as being "one of the most interesting that it has been our fortune to read" [8], but the reviewer quite reasonably concluded that since the findings were based on one subject, it would be necessary to replicate them (Fig. 10.3). In 1929, Bosden Leach, writing in the *British Medical Journal*, characterized Blackley as "the first who brought extensive experimental evidence to show that pollen is the one cause of hay fever … (that he was) looked upon as somewhat of a faddist – a man who played with grass – … (that he was) certainly not sufficiently recognized in England." Leach observed that more enquiries were received from America about Blackley than from Britain at that time [9].

Blackley made other observations relevant to hay fever. He conjectured that the low rate of hay fever in farmers, who were in frequent contact with grass, could reflect the buildup of immunity ("insusceptibility"). He also asserted that a "nervous temperament" was one predisposing factor for hay fever and that hay fever increased in incidence as population patterns shifted from rural to urban and as life became increasingly competitive [6, p. 159]. He created what is perhaps the first pollen counter to measure the quantity of pollen in relation to symptoms of hay fever (Fig. 10.4). In affirming the

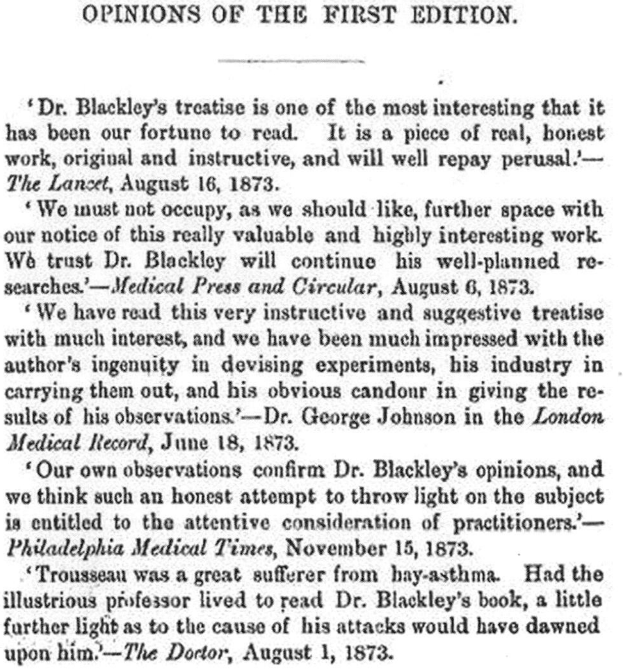

OPINIONS OF THE FIRST EDITION.

'Dr. Blackley's treatise is one of the most interesting that it has been our fortune to read. It is a piece of real, honest work, original and instructive, and will well repay perusal.'— *The Lancet*, August 16, 1873.

'We must not occupy, as we should like, further space with our notice of this really valuable and highly interesting work. We trust Dr. Blackley will continue his well-planned researches.'— *Medical Press and Circular*, August 6, 1873.

'We have read this very instructive and suggestive treatise with much interest, and we have been much impressed with the author's ingenuity in devising experiments, his industry in carrying them out, and his obvious candour in giving the results of his observations.'— Dr. George Johnson in the *London Medical Record*, June 18, 1873.

'Our own observations confirm Dr. Blackley's opinions, and we think such an honest attempt to throw light on the subject is entitled to the attentive consideration of practitioners.'— *Philadelphia Medical Times*, November 15, 1873.

'Trousseau was a great sufferer from hay-asthma. Had the illustrious professor lived to read Dr. Blackley's book, a little further light as to the cause of his attacks would have dawned upon him.'— *The Doctor*, August 1, 1873.

Fig. 10.3 Book reviews of Blackley first book, *Experimental Researches on the Causes and Nature of Catarrhus Aestivus*. 1873 (Image in the public domain)

causative role of pollen, Blackley had ruled out other possible candidates, such as ozone, coumarin, dust, light, and heat.

In addition to these discoveries, Blackley explored the relationship between symptoms and dose. While his work seems quite clearly supportive of pollen effects at homeopathic dose, this aspect of his work was not so well recognized. In a paper published in 1882 [10], Blackley assembled evidence that extremely low doses could, in general, be biologically active and that this applied to pollen sensitivity. He initially referred back to work with the enzyme diastase which, it was found, could convert 40,000 times its weight of starch into sugar. He then reviewed Darwin's work with insectivorous plants, such as *Drosera rotundifolia*, in which quantities of ammonia phosphate as low as 1/20,000,000th of a grain (one grain, often abbreviated as "gr."=60 mg) could exert physiological action in the leaf glands of this plant. Darwin admitted incredulity to himself at this finding, likening it to the application of one drop of the salt to a 31 gallon cask of water and still finding biological activity. A dilution this great is definitely in the homeopathic range, that is, 10^7 or 7X. In his paper, Blackley derived a calculation that showed that 1/2,000,000th gr. of pollen could bring on hay fever symptoms, a dilution that represents a homeopathic quantity of around 6X.

Fig. 10.4 Blackley's pollen counter – the first of its kind (Image in the public domain)

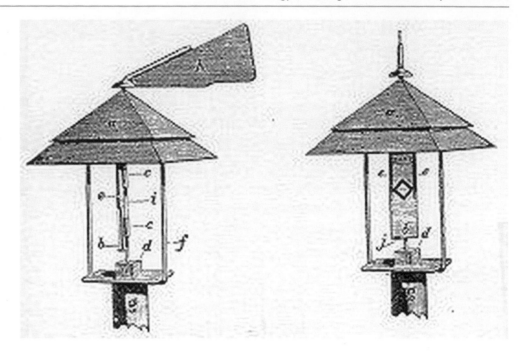

In attempting to explain how such infinitesimal doses could produce clinically evident effects, Blackley (1882) understood that it was not the result of "ordinary chemical affinity" and that "it does not derive its marvelous endowments from its material substance." He believed that the stimulating granular matter contained potential energy that became charged at the moment the stimulus was brought into contact with the responding tissue. In his speculations, Blackley anticipated the direction taken by more recent theoreticians in trying to explain the mechanisms of action of homeopathy.

One might be tempted to dismiss Blackley's findings on the infinitesimal dose were it not for later work by Noon and Freeman [11, 12]. In 1911, these consultant physicians reported on the use of hypodermic pollen desensitization, or pollen vaccination as they sometimes named it, to treat hay fever. In their clinic at St. Mary's Hospital in London, Noon and Freeman used initial doses of Timothy grass (*Phleum pratense*) as low as 1/1,000,000 dilution, that is, in the amount of 1/1,000,000 g, or 1 microgram (μg). Half a century later in the practice of sublingual immunotherapy [13, 14], nanogram (ng) doses of house dust mite allergen were found to produce an effect, which are again within the "infinitesimal" dose range described by Blackley, corresponding to homeopathic dilutions of 6–9X.

Grant L. Selfridge

While Blackley's major contribution to allergy lays in the careful experiments that helped him to identify the cause of hay fever, another homeopath from a later generation contributed in different ways, less through science (although

that was not altogether neglected) and more by shaping the new medical specialty of allergic diseases. Grant Selfridge (1863–1951) received his medical training at Hahnemann Medical College in San Francisco and joined the California State Homeopathic Medical Society. Although on record as attending its meetings, it is not clear how much he used homeopathy in his own clinical practice. He first became aware of pollen as a factor in hay fever through friendship with Dr. Joseph Goodale of Boston, a pioneering allergy researcher. Selfridge later specialized in otolaryngology, allergy, and nutritional medicine; he is reputed to have been the first surgeon in San Francisco to perform a tonsillectomy [15, p. 126]. Known for using salty language and frequent swear words when he encountered difficult cases of deafness, he earned the moniker of "the little Goddamn," so named as there was another San Francisco surgeon who had already secured a reputation as "the big Goddamn." Selfridge ultimately went on to achieve national fame, being cited in *Time* magazine in 1939 for his use of vitamin B to treat deafness [16].

Similar to anesthesiology and other nascent branches of medicine, allergy had not yet evolved into a recognized specialty during the 1920s, and Grant Selfridge was one of the first to change that. Along with two colleagues, Albert Rowe and George Piness, he established the Western Society for the Study of Hay Fever, Asthma, and Allergic Diseases in 1923 and was elected its first president. As this regional society increasingly drew members from a wider catchment area, it metamorphosed into the American Association for the Study of Allergy (AASA). In turn, the AASA amalgamated with its Eastern counterpart, the Society for the Study of Asthma and Allied Disorders, to form the American Academy of Allergy. These associations all played a pivotal role in establishing allergy as a scientifically and medically credible specialty.

Selfridge's role has been described by Cohen [17], who saw Selfridge as the senior and most forceful personality of the three founders. His impact was clearly visible during his terms as the first and second president of the Western society between 1923 and 1925 and then for the ensuing 5 years as a director of the organization. Perhaps because Selfridge resigned his membership in 1932 due to other interests related to the use of vitamin B, Cohen believes that later generations of allergy specialists never sufficiently recognized his achievements in establishing allergy as a medical specialty. Another initiative taken by Selfridge was his attempt to set up a governmental institute of nutrition in San Francisco; although this was not immediately successful, ultimately, such an institute came about and evolved into a component part of the National Institutes of Health in Bethesda.

Selfridge commissioned a comprehensive botanical survey of the western US states. The background to this survey was related to disability from seasonal allergy in a Southern Pacific Railroad Company employee who consulted with Dr. Selfridge. Selfridge quickly realized the possible economic implications for the employer if many of its employees were losing time from work because of seasonal allergies. Following the encounter with his patient, Selfridge conducted a survey to determine the number of hay fever cases in the company who reported sick each year. He learned that the number was about 500, far more than the authorities had believed. This review was succeeded by two surveys of grass, shrub, and tree pollen, the largest of which was supervised by Henry Hall, professor of botany at Stanford University, who organized the collection of pollen samples along the rail path. Hall identified those most likely to cause hay fever, and Selfridge then experimented on many of them to identify allergens and for desensitization. In his 1918 report, Selfridge described a method of testing for pollen allergy and then noted very positive results in 90 % of patients who were desensitized. His paper concluded by noting the value of (1) a careful botanical survey of local flora, (2) testing pollen extracts, (3) removing focal infections, (4) cross-disciplinary teamwork, (5) pollen therapy as the most beneficial therapy, and (6) starting treatment at least 60 days before the hay fever season begins. He also made a cogent plea for pharmaceutical companies to put patient interests ahead of commercial interests in the content of pollen preparations, many of which he found to be useless, although they were accompanied by extravagant claims [18].

Beyond his concern with allergic diseases, Selfridge was convinced that vitamin B was a contributing factor in hearing loss. In 1934, Selfridge observed that most of his deaf patients were consuming very small amounts of food that contained vitamin B, which led him to add vitamin B tablets, rice bran, or injections in over 100 patients with nerve deafness. After as few as six injections, some patients noted substantial improvement; for older patients, a longer course of treatment was necessary and recovery was rarely as good as in younger cases. While it is hard to discern the long-term effect of Selfridge's insights about vitamin B in relation to deafness, he may well have identified a true phenomenon [19]. As a result of his clinical work, he suggested to the young otolaryngologist W.P. Covell that it would be worthwhile investigating the matter further. This resulted in a publication that is still cited in today's literature, demonstrating a relationship between low levels of the vitamin B complex (B_6 and B_{12}) and other vitamins and damage to the auditory nerve in animal experiments [20]. Recent work has to some extent confirmed Selfridge's views about the relationship between vitamin B and deafness [21], and one study has found that hearing was improved by administration of vitamin B_{12} [22]. However, not all studies have supported the claims of Selfridge and Covell [23]. Among the various recommendations that have been made to preserve optimal hearing function in older adults, Johnson et al. write that "nutrients of particular importance include vitamin B_{12}, folacin, vitamin D and calcium" and that generous dietary intakes are encouraged in the elderly [24].

Homeopathy, Immunology, and Allergy: Other Considerations

While Blackley and Selfridge have been singled out, they were not the only homeopaths to carve out a place in the history of allergy and immunology.

In A History of Medicine, Inglis states that homeopathy can lay some claim to the paternity of immunization [25]. He quotes Emil von Behring, winner of the first Nobel Prize in medicine for his discovery of diphtheria antitoxin and renowned for demonstrating that immunization was a practical therapeutic procedure. Von Bering said that "Pasteur traced the origin of (Jenner's discovery of smallpox vaccination) to a homeopathic principle.... And by what technical term could we more appropriately speak of this influence, exerted by a similar virus, than by Hahnemann's word 'Homeopathy'? I am touching here upon a subject anathematized till very recently by medical pedantry: but if I am to present these problems in historical illumination, dogmatic imprecations must not deter me."

Coulter [26] also quotes trenchantly from a speech given by von Behring to the Berlin Physiological Society in 1905, in which von Behring described having demonstrated in 1892 the immunizing property of homeopathic ("infinitesimal") doses of tetanus antitoxin and that he found the lower the dose, the better the effect. Not surprisingly, a colleague then reproved von Behring for such a comment, as it was "grist for the mill of homoeopathy" [27]. Reportedly, von Behring had been advised to suppress these 1892 experiments on account of their propaganda value for homeopathy, and not until 13 years later, after gaining the Nobel Prize, was he to disclose this work [15, p. 117].

Charles Frederick Millspaugh

As far as hay fever and other allergies are concerned, there is evidence that a homeopath was the first to use pollen to protect against seasonal allergy. In the 1880s, Millspaugh successfully applied ragweed pollen (*Ambrosia artemisiifolia*) in the third centesimal (3C) dose to several patients with hay fever [28], antedating by over 20 years the work of Noon and Freeman. Millspaugh (1854–1923) was trained in homeopathy at the New York College, graduated in 1881, and practiced medicine for 9 years (Fig. 10.5). The first two cases were treated in 1884, when Millspaugh was working

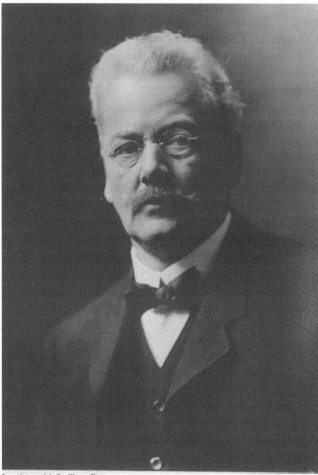

CHARLES FREDERICK MILLSPAUGH

Fig. 10.5 Charles Millspaugh. Possibly the first to use low-dose treatment for pollen allergy. Source: Eve Watson Schutze (Image by permission. Author E.F. Sherr. By permission University of Chicago Press)

on *Millspaugh's Medical Plants*. Four more patients were reported in the *Homeopathic Recorder* (a journal of which Millspaugh was an editor) in 1889. The cures were remarkable and long-lasting. Thus, as noted by Dewey, "The first suggestion that ambrosia artemesiafolia [sic] might prove a remedy of value for in hay fever comes from a homeopathic physician" [29]. Around 1890, Millspaugh gave up medical practice for a career in botany and became one of the country's most distinguished botanists. His 1887 publication, *American Medicinal Plants*, has been referred to as "one of the monumental works in its line" [30]. Millspaugh spent a brief 3 years as professor of botany at the University of West Virginia, yet bequeathed an enduring legacy with its herbarium and his botanical survey of that state. From 1894 until his death, he was the Curator of Botany the Field Museum of Natural History in Chicago, where he assembled a large collection of valuable materials that would eventually make the field a foremost center of taxonomic research. Many honors were bestowed upon Millspaugh, including the naming of some plants (the *Millspaughia* and *Neomillspaughia* genera), fellowship of the American Association for the Advancement of Sciences, and honorary fellowship of the Mexican and Brazilian colleges of medicine.

Of further importance is the more recent work by Reilly and colleagues at the Glasgow Homoeopathic Hospital. In a series of small, well-designed, and carefully conducted studies, they have affirmed the benefit of homeopathic pollen treatment or, more accurately, "isopathic" treatment, since the exact same substance that causes the disease is given to treat it. In summary, over the course of a 15-year period, Reilly's group has conducted four placebo-controlled double-blind trials of homeopathically prepared allergen at 30C vs. placebo for atopic disorders. In other words, the 30C potency ensured that no material trace of the original allergen was believed to be present. The 253 subjects in the four studies suffered, respectively, from hay fever (studies 1 and 2), asthma (study 3), and allergic rhinitis (study 4). Homeopathy proved superior to placebo in every study on some (but not all) outcome measures. Two conclusions can be drawn from this work, even conceding that the studies, as with all clinical trials, had their flaws. Firstly, they provide evidence of benefit for one type of homeopathy, isopathy (i.e., use of the toxin or "cause" of the illness), in the treatment of certain allergic states. Secondly, it is important that Reilly's group replicated their findings in several studies. Replication is a basic requirement of experimental therapeutics, and medical research does not always do well in reproducing positive findings [31]. In 2009, the reported success rate for promising new drugs in phase II (i.e., drugs that initially yielded positive results) was a low 18 % [32]. Although not all trials attempting to replicate Reilly's work have yielded positive results [33], we may still be inclined to agree with Reilly's appraisal that his repeated positive findings are incompatible with the belief that ultramolecular isopathy is a placebo [34].

While the Reilly studies clearly provide no final answers, they keep the flame burning and pose intriguing questions concerning efficacy and mechanism of action of high-potency homeopathy, especially in relation to allergic disorders.

References

1. Jackson M. Allergy: the history of a modern malady. London: Reaktion Books; 2007. p. 33.
2. Shwartzman G. Studies on regeneration of bacteriophage. I. The influence of partial anaerobiosis upon regeneration of a highly diluted lytic principle. J Exp Med. 1925;42:507–16.
3. Taylor G, Walker J. Charles Harrison Blackley, 1820–1900. Clin Allergy. 1973;3:103–8.
4. Waite KJ. Blackley and the development of hay fever as a disease of civilization in the nineteenth century. Med Hist. 1995;39:186–96.
5. Hurwitz SH. The development of specialization in allergy. A historical review and a view ahead. Calif Med. 1953;78:216–21.
6. Blackley CH. Experimental researches on the causes and nature of catarrhus aestivus (Hay-Fever or Hay-Asthma). 1873. Abingdon. Re-published by Oxford Historical Books. 1988.
7. Young S. Sue Young Histories. Biographies of Homeopaths. 21 Nov 2008 [Internet]. The Blackley Family and homeopathy. [Cited 2011 Sep 29]. Available from: http://sueyounghistories.com/archives/2008/11/21/the-blackley-surname-and-homeopathy/.
8. Anon. Opinions of the first edition Lancet. 1873;ii:231–2.
9. Bosden Leach F. Charles Harrison Blackley of Manchester and hay fever. BMJ. 1929;1:1171–2.
10. Blackley CH. On the influence of infinitesimal quantities in inducing physiological action. Monthly Homoeopathic Review. 1882;26:604–18.
11. Noon L. Prophylactic inoculation against hay fever. Lancet. 1911;i:1572–3.
12. Freeman J. Further observations on the treatment of hay fever by hypodermic inoculations of pollen vaccine. Lancet. 1911;ii:814–7.
13. Scadding G, Brostoff J. Low dose sublingual therapy in patients with allergic rhinitis due to house dust mite. Clin Allergy. 1986;16:483–91.
14. Platts-Mills TAE. Oral immunotherapy: a way forward? J Allergy Clin Immunol. 1987;80:129–32.
15. Ullman D. The homeopathic revolution. Berkeley: North Atlantic Books; 2007.
16. Medicine: B for Ears. Time. 19 Jul 1939. [Cited 2011 Sep 2]. Available from: www.time.com/time/magazine/article/0,9171,761531,00.html?artid=761531?contType=article?chn=us.
17. Cohen SG. The American Academy of Allergy: an historical review. J Allergy Clin Immunol. 1979;64:332–466.
18. Selfridge G. Spasmodic vaso-motor disturbances of the respiratory tract, with special reference to hay fever. Cal State J Med. 1918;16:164–7.
19. Selfridge G. Menière's symptom complex in relation to chemistry: an etiologic study. Arch Otolaryngol. 1949;49:1–15.
20. Covell WP. Pathological changes in the peripheral auditory mechanism due to avitaminosis. Laryngoscope. 1941;50:632–47.
21. Shemesh Z, Attias J, Ornan M, Shapira N, Shahar A. Vitamin B12 deficiency in patients with chronic-tinnitus and noise-induced hearing loss. Am J Otolaryngol. 1993;14:94–9.
22. Durga J, Anteunis LJC, Schouter EG, Bots ML, Kok FJ, Verhoef P. Association of folate with hearing loss is dependent on the 5,10-methylenetetrahydrofolate reductase $677C \rightarrow T$ mutation. Neurobiol Aging. 2006;27:482–9.
23. Houston DK, Johnson HA, Nozza RJ, Gunter EW, Shea KJ, Cutler GM. Age-related hearing loss, vitamin B-12, and folate in elderly women. Am J Clin Nutr. 1999;69:564–71.
24. Johnson MA, DeChiccis AP, Willott JF, Shea-Miller KJ. Hearing loss and nutrition in older adults. In: Bales CW, Ritchie CS, editors. Handbook of clinical nutrition and aging. Totowa: Humana Press; 2004. p. 291–307.
25. Inglis B. A history of medicine. London: Weidenfeld & Nicholson; 1965. p. 125.
26. Coulter HL. The divided legacy, vol. IV. Berkeley: North Atlantic Books; 1994. p. 98.
27. von Behring E. Moderne phthisiogenetische und phthisiotherapeutische Probleme in historischer Beleuchtung. Marburg: Selbsteverlag des Verfassers; 1905. p. xxvii. German.
28. Millspaugh CF. Ambrosia artemisiaefolia. Homeopathic Recorder 1889;IV: 256. Reported in Anschutz EP. New, old and forgotten remedies. 2nd ed. Philadelphia: Boericke & Tafel; 1917, p. 16–17.
29. Dewey WA. Ambrosia artemisiifolia in hay fever. Am Physician. 1903;XXIX:208–9.
30. Sherff EE. Charles Frederick Millspaugh. The Botanical Gazette. 1924;77:228–30.
31. Naik G. Scientists' elusive goal: reproducing study results. The Wall Street J. 2011.
32. Arrowsmith J. Phase II, failures: 2008–2010. Nat Rev Drug Discov. 2011;10:1.
33. Lewith GT, Watkins AD, Hyland ME, Shaw S, Broomfield J, Dolan G, et al. A double-blind, randomized, controlled clinical trial of ultramolecular potencies of house dust mite in asthmatic patients. BMJ. 2002;324:520–3.
34. Taylor M, Reilly D, Llewellyn-Jones RH, McSharry C, Aitchison TA. Randomized controlled trial of homoeopathy versus placebo in perennial allergic rhinitis with overview of four trial series. BMJ. 2000;321:471–6.

At the beginning of the twentieth century, the three top-tier homeopathic medical schools were Hahnemann Medical College in Philadelphia, the New York Medical College, and Boston University School of Medicine. Second-tier schools existed at Michigan, San Francisco, and Ohio State. Together, these six institutions developed scholarly research programs and graduated a number of talented doctors who kept homeopathy on the national map.

Once American homeopathy began to fade after World War I, and its professional societies withered, homeopaths at the universities had little choice but to adapt to the new world of American medicine if they aspired to an academic career. Thus, in the 1920s and 1930s, some prominent homeopaths began to make their mark in regular medicine. This chapter focuses on Roy Upham, Conrad Wesselhoeft, Lynn Boyd, and Thomas McGavack. It could be argued that others (e.g., surgeons, anesthesiologists, cardiologists, psychiatrists, etc.) warrant inclusion here, but these individuals can more easily be categorized according to their specialty and are better addressed in the appropriate sections.

Roy Upham: Promoter of International Homeopathy

Roy Upham (1879–1956) received his medical degree from the New York Homeopathic Medical College in 1901. He remained on the NYHMC faculty, first as an assistant professor and then later as professor of gastroenterology, directing that department for many years. He was a staunch advocate of homeopathy, being heavily involved in the American Institute, serving as its president in 1921. Additionally, he was one of the founders and first president of the *Liga Medicorum Homeopathica Internationalis* (LMHI) in 1925 – an organization that remains the premier international homeopathic organization today. An illustration of Upham's commitment to homeopathy is evident in a 1921 publication, where he wrote "Our school of scientific medicine has made a record of which we can well be proud and our flag should fly not in

arrogant flapping but with a conscious satisfaction that the world may take notice of its standards," and he urged his colleagues to "let your light shine and you will give courage to every man who sees it" [1].

As homeopathy declined, Upham adjusted to the new order and earned a fine reputation in allopathic medicine, publishing, mentoring, and practicing at his alma mater. Upham's greatest legacy to his institution, and more widely to medicine, was endowing the gastroenterology clinic (later division of gastroenterology) at NYHMC in his mother's name. Thus was born the Sarah C. Upham Division of Gastroenterology at New York Medical College, as well as an endowed chair of gastroenterology and liver diseases in her name. As of 2011, the trust provided between $250,000 and $400,000 in support of the program [2]. Upham's philanthropy not only attested to his institutional loyalty, even after the school's abandonment of homeopathy, but also planted the seeds for future medical breakthroughs. As noted on the school's website, the division has nurtured some excellent science, for example, the work of Jerzy Glass on gastrointestinal hormones, Slomiany's discoveries in relation to gastric mucus, Rigas' breakthroughs in chemoprevention of colon cancer, and the role of a new hepatitis virus [3].

Even as Upham embraced regular medicine, he did not forsake homeopathy and was presenting talks as late as 1937, when he spoke at the LMHI meeting in Berlin on snake venoms and their application in treatment, including in seasickness. One minor measure of his recognition in public can be gained from an announcement in the *Montreal Gazette*, which singled him out from over 1,000 passengers who were arriving in New York on the steamship *New York*, referring to his participation at the Liga meeting in Europe [4].

Conrad Wesselhoeft: Physician in Search of an Identity

The Wesselhoeft family arguably represents one of medicine's longest dynasties, stretching unbroken for more than 200 years from the time of Goethe up to the present day.

J. Davidson, *A Century of Homeopaths*,
DOI 10.1007/978-1-4939-0527-0_11, © Springer Science+Business Media New York 2014

Its most recent scions are Conrad W. Wesselhoeft (born 1933), pediatric surgeon and clinical professor at Brown University [5], Robert Wesselhoeft III (1944–2007) of Tufts University, and Hadwig Wesselhoeft (born 1926), a pediatric cardiologist on the German side of the family. All have made enduring contributions to modern medicine. Conrad published several important articles on thoracic surgery in children [6], while Robert played a significant role in developing family medicine as an academic discipline, emphasizing patient-centered care and humanistic values. He became the first chief of family medicine at Tufts University Medical School, and his influence was felt by his many students who chose family medicine as a career. He also established training opportunities in Europe and Africa and a family clinic in New Zealand [7]. Hadwig Wesselhoeft spent some years in the United States before returning to Germany, and she has contributed a number of publications in leading journals of cardiology [8, 9].

These modern-day Wesselhoefts were preceded by at least four generations of Wesselhoeft physicians, of whom Conrad Wesselhoeft 2nd (1884–1962) is the focus here. He was the ninth physician in his family and, like all previous Wesselhoefts, practiced homeopathy. When Boston University School of Medicine (BUSM) opened its doors in 1873, 3 of the 17 founding faculty were Wesselhoefts. As far as this author is aware, no Wesselhoefts are currently practicing medicine, although two are now living in retirement [10, 11].

The dynasty began with the sons of Karl Wesselhoeft, a successful publisher in the city of Jena, Germany, in the late eighteenth century. The Wesselhoeft family was on friendly terms with Goethe, who often visited them at home and took a kindly interest in Karl's young son, William, born in 1794. After completing his medical studies in Europe, William Wesselhoeft (1794–1858) came to the United States, followed later by his younger brother Robert (1795–1852), where they embraced homeopathy. William was instrumental in establishing the first homeopathic teaching academy in Allentown, PA, and shortly afterwards moved to Boston, where he established a homeopathic practice. Robert also settled in the same town.

In 1842, the two brothers earned a measure of fame when Oliver Wendell Holmes attacked the popular Dr. Robert Wesselhoeft in his vilification of homeopathy as a form of quackery. Following this attack, Robert moved to Brattleboro, Vermont, where he and his brother opened the Wesselhoeft Water Cure, a hydropathic establishment, which grew into a most successful enterprise, although a leading Boston medical journal castigated hydropathy as "one of the last of the great medical farces being played for the diseased imaginations of semivaletudinarians" [12]. Nathaniel Hawthorne was to base his novel, *The Blithedale Romance*, on these events. In another story, *Rappaccini's Daughter*, he also immortalized Robert Wesselhoeft, about whom he had

negative feelings due to Wesselhoeft's use of hypnosis on Hawthorne's wife without permission.

Robert Wesselhoeft had three sons, Conrad Wesselhoeft 1st (1834–1904), Reinhold, and Walter. Conrad practiced, published, and taught at BUSM, and among his patients were Ralph Waldo Emerson, Henry Wadsworth Longfellow, Harriet Beecher Stowe, Emily Dickinson, and Louisa May Alcott. Conrad too earned his day of literary fame as the dedicatee of Louisa May Alcott's novel, *Jo's Boys*. Reinhold was strongly attracted to a medical career, but was denied the opportunity. While serving in the Union Army at Ball's Bluff, his regiment was trapped on the southern side of the Potomac River. Attempting to escape capture, he drowned while trying to save a colleague who had been shot by Confederate troops. Walter's third son, Conrad Wesselhoeft 2nd (1884–1962), entered medicine and became one of the few Americans of his time to explore the scientific foundation of homeopathy [13] (Fig. 11.1). Later in his career, he acquired fame as an infectious disease specialist [14].

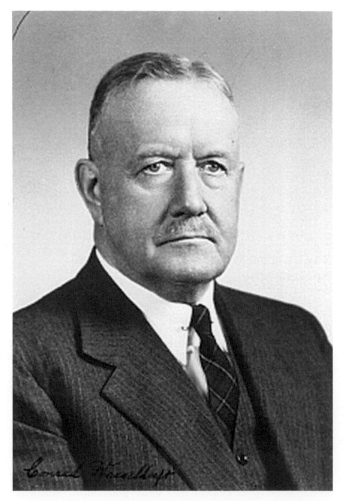

Fig. 11.1 Conrad Wesselhoeft. Expert in infectious disease (Image from the National Library of Medicine, in the public domain)

Conrad Wesselhoeft occupies a central place in any historical account of the intersection between homeopathy and conventional medicine. He began his career as a homeopath and later became a distinguished researcher and clinician in both schools. In his approach to medicine, he demonstrated exemplary objectivity and conducted some of the earliest, largest, and best (for the time) controlled studies of homeopathic remedies. Wesselhoeft provides a lens through which we can observe an individual who successfully practiced homeopathy and orthodox medicine at the highest academic level. Conrad Wesselhoeft journeyed from being an important contributor to homeopathy to a Harvard-based authority on infectious disease. After his death, he was saluted with obituaries in the *New England Journal of Medicine (NEJM)* and *Journal of the American Medical Association (JAMA)* [15]. The obituary in *NEJM* is quite comprehensive and speaks to Wesselhoeft's entire career, whereas *JAMA* restricts its tribute to Wesselhoeft the allopath, avoiding mention of his homeopathic affiliations.

Mary Kraft [16] has summarized the fascinating story of the Wesselhoeft family, remarking (as noted above) that Conrad was preceded by eight other Wesselhoeft doctors. Although Conrad's father, Walter, was a homeopathic professor of anatomy at BUSM, he was unconvinced about homeopathy's superiority, referring to himself as a mugwump in this respect (i.e., sitting on the fence). Reflecting on his life, Walter Wesselhoeft wrote in his memoirs: "I am glad and thankful to retire. My disapproval of the school and hospital (Boston University) were deep within me … On all my inward conflicts, on all my suffering and sacrifices on behalf of the cause I really had at heart … I now look without the heartfelt joy a long life of hard work … should bring" [17].

Notwithstanding his ambivalence about homeopathy, Walter Wesselhoeft overcame initial skepticism by his community and colleagues and built up a successful homeopathic practice, firstly in Halifax, Nova Scotia, and later in Boston. Moreover, and despite their professional differences, father and son shared coverage of each other's patients when one of them was away.

Walter Wesselhoeft bequeathed his inner struggle for his son Conrad "to bring together allopathy and homeopathy" – a burden to place on anyone's shoulders, but Conrad Wesselhoeft was ideally prepared to meet the challenge. His personal voyage in this regard will be described.

Wesselhoeft completed 3 years of undergraduate study at Harvard University, but before graduating, he entered BUSM. After a year there, he transferred back to Harvard in order to fulfill his father's charge that Harvard would expose him to the best allopathic training. He graduated in 1911 and then accepted an internship at the Massachusetts Homeopathic Hospital, where he studied homeopathy for treating diphtheria. For much of the next 15 years, Wesselhoeft continued his homeopathic research and for many years was a prominent figure in the homeopathic community.

Homeopathic Career

Wesselhoeft belonged to the American Institute of Homeopathy and in 1913 was appointed an assistant editor of the *New England Medical Gazette*, being promoted to full editor in 1917. He conducted substantial clinical research into homeopathy and it may well be asked how this was made possible. Such research was supported by the Evans Memorial Research Center, endowed through a bequest from Mrs. Maria Antoinette Evans, widow of a wealthy Boston businessman, Robert Dawson Evans. As briefly outlined in Chap. 6, Mr. Evans was fatally injured when thrown from his horse in 1909 and received terminal care at the Massachusetts Homeopathic Hospital. Mrs. Evans was so impressed with the care given that she made the bequest to establish a research program; the endowment was created in 1910 and research began in 1912. Wesselhoeft worked in the department of pharmacology at the Evans Memorial. Other research occurred at Evans, both homeopathic and allopathic, and there are two interesting accounts of the Evans program at the time. One of these accounts was provided by the neurologist James Putnam, who referred to plans for research into psychoanalysis, and another account by Elmer Southard reported on the significance of a homeopathic foundation for clinical research and preventive medicine [18, 19]. For several years, the Evans Building provided a base for Conrad's work, and it still stands today, home of the BU Department of Medicine, although the time has long since passed since any homeopathic research has been performed there (Fig. 11.2). In 2012, the Evans Memorial celebrated its first 100 years with a commemorative conference.

Wesselhoeft's reports on the treatment of constipation, malaria, scarlet fever, diphtheria, and digitalis will be described. In these papers, Wesselhoeft was candid about the problems bedeviling homeopathic practice and the profession's reluctance to deal with them. Because these issues are as relevant today as they were a century ago, they will be discussed in the following paragraphs, along with a review of Wesselhoeft's clinical career at Boston and Harvard Universities.

Constipation

One of Wesselhoeft's earliest trials was a placebo-controlled comparison of individualized homeopathy in 166 patients with constipation. Potencies ranged from the third to sixth, that is, these were low dilutions that would have been pharmacologically active. Recovery rates were the same in both groups: 78 and 66 % for homeopathy and placebo, respectively. He emphasized the power of suggestion in his series. Despite finding no difference, Wesselhoeft wrote, "This small experience with cases of constipation has far from led me to a state of therapeutic nihilism … I shall still console myself with the idea that the patients do better in other

Fig. 11.2 Evans Memorial
Institution. One of the earliest
endowed university medical
research units. Centennial
celebrated in 2012 (Image by
permission of Boston University
School of Medicine)

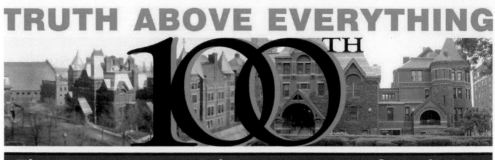

respects under Homoeopathy until this is proved to the contrary, even if the constipation effectively takes care of itself" [20]. He believed that homeopathy had more widespread effects than simply the easing of constipation, but as he noted in his report, the absence of any other measures made it impossible to demonstrate.

Quinine for Malaria

In 1913, Wesselhoeft published a study of quinine's mechanism of action in malaria, one form of which is transmitted by the parasite, *Plasmodium vivax*. Wesselhoeft wished to ascertain whether the drug acted indirectly by stimulating host defense mechanisms or directly via action on the parasite. In so doing, he could potentially show if the mechanism of action was compatible with homeopathic teaching, which held that quinine worked indirectly through stimulation of host resistance, or "vital force," which is what his study did in fact show [21].

Scarlet Fever

In 1917, Wesselhoeft published an article on the effect of homeopathic belladonna to prevent and treat scarlet fever [22]. The paper began with some pertinent observations about two disturbing trends in homeopathy at that time. Firstly, he noted there was a drift away from careful experimentation into either formulaic uses of remedies without trouble being taken to individualize treatment – a state of clinical laziness or "cut and dried homeopathy" as he put it. Secondly, many homeopaths had turned their attention to the more remunerative practice of surgery (albeit with some considerable success as described in Chap. 4). Additionally, Wesselhoeft made a fundamental point that applies to all clinical research. He emphasized that clinical researchers need to be well versed in the nature and course of the disease under study, as well as being familiar with its relevant literature. He further stated that clinical research is the "final criterion of the efficacy of all therapeutic measures and is attended by many snares and pitfalls."

His scarlet fever paper assessed a time-honored homeopathic remedy, belladonna, given as open-label (i.e., not blinded) treatment for nurses about to be exposed to cases of scarlet fever on the wards. Ten of 26 (38 %) who received triturated belladonna 3X, two tablets twice a day, developed scarlet fever. The next year, another sample of 26 nurses received atropine 3X, with the same number (38 %) acquiring the disease. The third winter saw another sample of 28 nurses who received no treatment, of whom 10 (36 %) developed scarlet fever. Wesselhoeft concluded there was no evidence that the remedies prevented scarlet fever.

In the second part of his report, the author compared belladonna to no treatment in 227 established cases of scarlet fever. No differences were found between groups in the length of hospital stay or rates of complications. Wesselhoeft opined that belladonna may not be the best remedy for some cases and that he had good experience with *Mercurius corrosivus* 6X and *Lachesis* 6X. Despite his negative findings, Wesselhoeft concluded that he still preferred homeopathy, mainly because the alternative measures were quite toxic. He exhorted his colleagues to take these results as a challenge and pursue systematic evaluation of homeopathic remedies themselves.

A note of pessimism can be detected in some of these reports, primarily Wesselhoeft's remarks on the difficulty in assigning sufficient time to individualize the choice of remedy. Although he did not explicitly say so, he implied that a major limitation to the homeopathic method lies in its time-intensive history gathering for busy practitioners. He also alluded to unresolved matters of doctrine around high vs. low potencies and how remedies should be given (e.g., alternating the remedy each day or staying with one remedy) for which there was virtually no data but strong opinions. Regrettably, there was almost no response to these challenges by the homeopathic or allopathic communities.

Whooping Cough

Wesselhoeft wrote a thoughtful account of the homeopathic treatment of whooping cough in 1917 [23], in which he expressed vexation with homeopathic colleagues who had no interest in testing fundamental theories. One is struck by his comment that "… no comparative statistics of any moment have been produced to show the relative efficacy of low potencies over high potencies, of the value of a particular repertory over another, of the value of alternating or combining over the single remedy." Remarkably, almost 100 years have passed since he wrote these words, yet there has been extraordinarily little progress on these still relevant questions. Wesselhoeft also drew attention to the unresolved matter of selecting the remedy based on the entire individual profile vs. choosing the remedy according to the peculiar disease features in that individual: a subtle but important difference. He also made the point that individualized homeopathy was simply impractical during epidemics. In his report, Wesselhoeft deplored Hahnemann's tendency to dismiss enquiry into the mechanism of action for remedies in favor of dogmatic assertion of natural laws – Hahnemann had little interest in how drugs worked.

In his whooping cough review, Wesselhoeft stated that he had been unable to make significant inroads when treating the disease, no matter what approach he used, but that he preferred homeopathy for its gentleness. He summarized and critiqued the main homeopathic sources of guidance for whooping cough and concluded that there were five principal remedies whose proving symptoms matched those of the disease: aconite, ipecacuanha, belladonna, cuprum, and magnesia. He tended to attribute his negative results to a lack of prescribing expertise. While this might have been a factor, one is tempted to think that his modesty was misplaced and that homeopathy was simply ineffective.

Mumps Orchitis

By the early 1920s, Wesselhoeft was moving away from homeopathy and began to publish in journals such as the *Boston Medical and Surgical Journal*, which was soon to become the *New England Journal of Medicine*. One such example was his account of mumps orchitis, in which he described the main forms of treatment, referring to homeopathy as one historical option of limited value. Specifically, he singled out pulsatilla, lead, and mercury as homeopathic approaches that had been used and referred to two different case series, one of which originated from his own hospital, showing no benefit for pulsatilla. All in all, the evidence favoring these three remedies was "meager" [24].

Digitalis for Heart Disease

Wesselhoeft obtained experience with digitalis in heart disease at both homeopathic and regular doses and expressed his view that the drug was generally more effective at material doses rather than high dilutions such as 30C. He did not, however, think it was necessary to push the dose so high as to produce side effects like nausea and vomiting. He recommended digitalis for heart disease caused by rheumatic

fever but felt that it was contraindicated in heart disease caused by diphtheria, where it could make things worse: he described the different etiologies of heart failure as being responsible for the difference. In this scholarly review, Wesselhoeft describes the history of digitalis and its use in homeopathy; he reveals that the German homeopath Bernard Baehr was the first to recognize the peculiar affinity of digitalis for treating rheumatic heart problems in his 1859 essay *Digitalis Purpurea: Its Physiological and Therapeutic Action* [25] and that if conventional medicine had heeded Baehr's report, many years of delay could have been avoided in determining optimal use of the drug [26]. Wesselhoeft referred to Baehr's essay as "the second classic on digitalis, as Withering's was the first." (William Withering (1741–1799) had discovered that digitalis was the active ingredient in foxglove, a plant traditionally used by herbalists for heart failure.)

Appraisal of Hahnemann

In 1921, Wesselhoeft wrote an editorial arguing that Hahnemann's contributions had been grossly underestimated. Some of the reasons why this was so have been alluded to in Chap. 2. It was Wesselhoeft's opinion that many of the accepted therapeutic principles in contemporary medicine originated in Hahnemann's writings. Among these ideas, Wesselhoeft counted Hahnemann's clinical experimentation with quinine, the concept of small dose effects, vaccination, and use of the single remedy. Rather than seeing homeopathy as merely bringing about the disappearance of barbarous treatment practices, Wesselhoeft concluded: "The negative value of homeopathy to modern medicine … is only equaled by the enlightenment of medical thought through the principles of pharmaco-therapeutics propounded by Samuel Hahnemann" [27].

Some years after being branded as a homeopathic heretic, Wesselhoeft still acknowledged a role for homeopathy in diphtheria. In a 1924 address to the Bureau of Pedology (i.e., pediatrics) at the American Institute of Homeopathy, for example, he claimed that, in mild diphtheria, homeopathy was as effective as antitoxin, but that in severe cases, antitoxin was the treatment of first choice. Wesselhoeft qualified his opinion by saying that it was not on account of homeopathy's ineffectiveness: it was more a limitation due to the high level of homeopathic expertise necessary for this treatment to work and that, without such skill, the risk of failure was too great. With antitoxin, on the other hand, all that was required was competence in making the diagnosis [28]. From this standpoint, homeopathy suffered from the considerable drawback of not being a "user-friendly" treatment, and, as Wesselhoeft had pointed out elsewhere, homeopathy did not lend itself as a form of treatment during epidemics as it required the practitioner to spend time for thorough individual assessment of the patient.

Career in Regular Medicine

In 1920, Wesselhoeft resigned his membership of the American Institute of Homeopathy after being branded by some homeopathic colleagues as a heretic for advocating diphtheria antitoxin therapy over homeopathy. Shortly afterwards, he joined the Massachusetts Medical Society (in which he eventually served as president). Wesselhoeft repeatedly urged his colleagues to discard the old-fashioned language and concepts of homeopathy in favor of current medical concepts. Wesselhoeft practiced what he preached as he turned towards allopathy and became an authority on infectious disease. Among his later publications are papers on sulfonamides in scarlet fever [29], cardiovascular disease in diphtheria [30], the course of otitis media in scarlet fever [31], the treatment of scarlet fever and diphtheria [32], fatal equine encephalitis in humans [33], and nephritis in scarlet fever [34]. Some of his publications on immunity and infectious disease continue to be cited in the literature decades after his death [35, 36]. His report on sulfonamides for scarlet fever is instructive, since sulfa drugs had just been introduced into medicine and high hopes were attached to their role in treating infectious diseases like scarlet fever. Wesselhoeft and Smith's measured assessment found that the sulfa drugs were unhelpful for many aspects of the disease, but that sulfanilamide was indicated for septicemia and meningitis associated with the condition. In their report, the authors invoked the old concept of the host defense reaction in explaining the drug's action, similar to Wesselhoeft's earlier paper on quinine, tipping his hat to homeopathic thinking.

As a teacher, Wesselhoeft was well liked and well respected. One former Harvard student still vividly recalls Wesselhoeft's lecture on measles, in which the illness came alive as Wesselhoeft imitated the measles cough with his high, shrill voice [37].

A more practical side of Wesselhoeft is evident in a publication describing the design of a weighted retractor to facilitate smoother tracheotomy operation [38]. In a second paper, he described how a nephew had developed a hydraulic lift to assist daily function in patients coping with polio. Wesselhoeft adapted this device for wider use in his hospital, where it proved valuable in rehabilitating polio patients [39].

Homeopathy is barely mentioned in Wesselhoeft's later publications on contagious disease and this may be because ultimately he found it to be largely ineffective in this context. Another possibility is that he (or the journal editors) knew there would be little interest among readers, unless it was to berate homeopathy. Yet further, it is possible that Wesselhoeft desired to keep his hands clean of homeopathic associations, at least in public. Whatever the reason, one is left to guess about Wesselhoeft's true feelings towards homeopathy as he matured professionally. However, there is good evidence of

continuing allegiance, since Wesselhoeft remained a consultant to the Brighton Homeopathic Hospital, where he was ultimately treated for his terminal illness in 1962. After his death, the hospital paid the following tribute: "It is with a sense of deepest loss and sorrow that the staff of the Hahnemann Hospital records the death on December 2, 1962 at this hospital of Doctor Conrad Wesselhoeft, a member of the Associate Staff…. The Hahnemann Hospital, while being one of his less[er] interests, was honored in having him on its staff and at all times he was a willing and dependable consultant. This hospital and staff have received much more than we gave from our association with Doctor Wesselhoeft" [40]. Thus, while the ink on his prescriptions reflected Wesselhoeft's practice of conventional medicine, a permanent place was reserved in his heart for homeopathy.

Was Wesselhoeft able to fulfill his father's almost impossible charge to bring together allopathy and homeopathy? Significantly, the Hahnemann memoriam quotes from a eulogy given by Paul Dudley White, former Harvard classmate, lifelong friend, and world-famous cardiologist. Such affection between the two who were so prominent in medicine, one exclusively in allopathy and the other in allopathy and homeopathy, was a rarity. Wesselhoeft united the two streams in another more personal way, as illustrated in a letter to his sister, Gertrude, dated July 12, 1940 [41]. In this letter, written to acknowledge birthday greetings from Gertrude, Wesselhoeft has this to say: "My big birthday present was to be appointed professor of communicable diseases at the Harvard School of Public Health." In the fall of that year, he would be given a similar appointment in the Harvard Medical School. Mindful of family tradition and expectations, he went on to write: "Can't you imagine what this means to the family after 100 years. Grandfather, Father and Uncle Conrad redeemed. I went out to the cemetery and stood before Mama's and Father's graves. I felt that I had to express my gratitude for what they had given me, for it was an inheritance that has enabled me to get up to this position – and I never aspired to it." He then expressed his disbelief that "I am a Harvard Professor – and the first one to have this title (i.e., in his specialty). My predecessors were assistant or associate professor." Wesselhoeft's father could rest content that his son Conrad had succeeded in "bringing together" the two worlds of homeopathy and allopathy.

Conrad Wesselhoeft was conspicuous in his bravery, as exemplified by multiple decorations in World War I: two Distinguished Service Cross (DSC) awards, the Silver Star with Oak Leaf Cluster, the Purple Heart, and *Croix de Guerre* (Fig. 11.3). (The DSC is the US army's second highest award; in Wesselhoeft's case, they were given for exceptional bravery in tending to the wounded close the front line during the Aisne-Marne and Verdun offensives in 1918.) His grandson, Conrad Wesselhoeft, epitomized his grandfather as follows: "Courage – both physical and intellectual –is at the heart of

Fig. 11.3 Conrad Wesselhoeft caricature (Image by courtesy of Conrad Wesselhoeft (grandson))

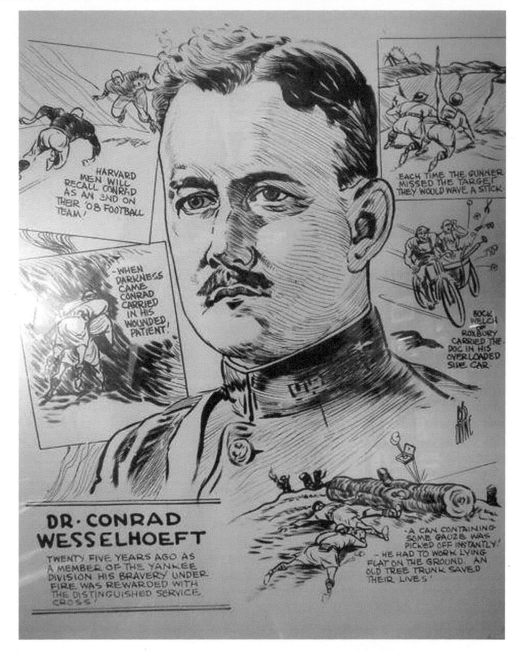

who he was" [42]. As a physician, few have come closer to the ideal image of a doctor than Conrad Wesselhoeft, "the great white-haired father who knew how the patient felt," according to Tenley Albright, a former patient of his, Olympic gold medalist, and famous surgeon [43]. Wesselhoeft's obituary in the *New England Journal of Medicine* described him as "deeply devoted to the truth as he saw it, and intolerant of anything resembling subterfuge or dishonesty…. His standards were high, whether in the accuracy of the statistics in his papers or in the wise, sympathetic and devoted care he gave his patients." One of his patients, Anne A. Ramsey, felt so positively about the care he gave her that she left an endowment to support a chair in medicine at Boston City Hospital in

his honor. This endowed chair has been filled by some very distinguished doctors, including Franz Ingelfinger and Arnold Relman, editors of the *New England Journal of Medicine*. Conrad Wesselhoeft's life coincided with a biramous juncture in American homeopathy, which was poised to advance as a scientific discipline in American medical schools or to remain bogged down in old dogmas – unfortunately, the latter outcome prevailed. Homeopaths did not follow his pleas for controlled trials: resistance to science remained strong and many homeopaths were lulled into complacency by their lucrative practices including, as noted, the practice of surgery. While the factors behind homeopathy's disintegration are complex [44], after the end of World War I, the potential existed for homeopathy to retain a presence in US medical schools, as Wesselhoeft himself noted in 1921. His drift away from homeopathy was inevitable in retrospect, for there was no longer a critical mass to support its best academicians.

Linn J. Boyd: From Homeopathic Philosophy to Cardiology

Linn Boyd (1895–1981) trained in homeopathy at the University of Michigan, graduating in 1918, and was then appointed an assistant professor of homeopathic medicine (Fig. 11.4). Thus, he began a productive and lengthy academic career, initially at Michigan until 1926 and then for the remainder of his life at the New York Homeopathic Medical College and Flower Hospital, which recruited Boyd to improve its clinical clerkship [45]. The reason for Boyd's departure from Michigan was allegedly due to hostility on the part of ultraorthodox homeopathic colleagues who objected to his use of animals in research [46]. Furthermore,

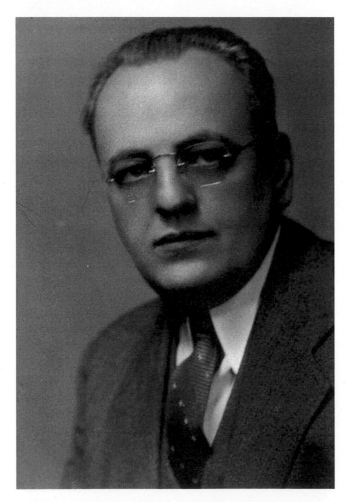

Fig. 11.4 Linn Boyd. Cardiologist, homeopathic scholar, and editor of the *Journal of American Institute of Homeopathy* (Image courtesy of National Library of Medicine, in the public domain)

it is probably relevant that Michigan was in the process of dissolving its homeopathic program, and the future for its young and ambitious faculty was bleak. At New York, between 1926 and 1959, he variously held appointments as professor of medicine and head of the department of medicine, pharmacology, and homeopathic therapeutics, director of the department of medicine, and director of the division of graduate studies.

While homeopathy still remained a force in American medicine, Boyd made many important contributions. In the mid-1920s, the New York Medical College devoted 140 h to the teaching of homeopathy in years 1 and 2. Year 1 consisted of lectures by Drs. Atkins and Wilson on essential and characteristic actions of drugs based on provings in healthy subjects, on the sick, and in toxic poisoning. In year 2, Professor J.W. Krischbaum and Dr. C.E. Krischbaum taught pathogenesis and symptomatology of the various drugs [47]. Ten years later, these 140 h had been whittled down to a mere 32 h [45] as homeopathy was pushed aside at the college, which eventually dropped the word "homeopathic" from its name in 1936. (Of note, it took until 1985 for NYMC to sever its last formal contact with homeopathy, when the board of trustees voted to remove the image of Samuel Hahnemann from the school's official seal.) [48] Not surprisingly, Boyd's homeopathic output declined, but his productivity grew in other ways. During the years he was a card-carrying homeopath, he served capably as editor of the *Journal of the American Institute of Homeopathy* (*JAIH*), putting it on a self-sustaining footing and attracting submissions from the leading homeopathic researchers, as well as advertising from major pharmaceutical and homeopathic companies. He was a prolific publisher in the homeopathic literature and authored a book that is still regarded as a homeopathic classic [49], *A Study of the Simile in Medicine*, which Guttentag referred to as "one of the most important books concerning the history and the concepts of homeopathy." Boyd wrote this book as part of the terms by which the University of Michigan dissolved the homeopathic medical school, and he dedicated it to the Board of Regents of the University of Michigan. It seems unlikely that many of the university trustees would have taken the time to read Boyd's book, which must have surely constituted a poor trade-off for homeopathy in exchange for giving up a medical school.

Boyd was partly responsible for bringing Otto Guttentag to the United States and also for providing Karl Koetschau the opportunity to spend sabbaticals in his laboratory at NYHMC. Among Boyd's homeopathic publications are an introduction to Koetschau's scientific basis of homeopathy [50], a review of factors responsible for the recent progress in homeopathy [51], a study of *Chelidonium* as an anti-infective [52], a review on the place of *Cocculus indicus* in medicine [53], and an essay on homeopathy in liver cirrhosis and the difficulty in finding effective remedies for that condition [54]. In 1922, at an early point in his career, Boyd published two articles on venom as a homeopathic remedy. The first paper provided an account of the action of lizard and snake venoms [55] and the second comprised a review on the effects of black widow spider venom, *Latrodectus mactans* [56]. His obituary makes reference to the fact that Boyd pioneered the therapeutic use of snake and spider venom for treating angina [57] and Boyd himself accepts credit for "human experiments ... which lead medical science to the discovery that poison from the black widow spider, given intradermally at a dilution of 1:10,000 in saline, was a successful treatment for angina pectoris" [58, 59]. He was reported to have remarked that his discovery of this property was the result of over 10 years' research, that many doctors began to use *Latrodectus* for angina, and that black widow spider "farms" were proliferating in South America [60]. In making this statement, it is likely that Boyd was referring to homeopathic physicians since black widow venom has not been widely used in conventional medicine. Although Boyd claimed that he was inspired by Noguchi's work with cobra venom for malaria, it should not escape notice that in 1889 a homeopath by the name of Samuel Jones had proposed the poison might benefit angina pectoris [61], and Boyd was well aware of this literature, as well as allusions to venom in the regular literature.

Further studies were undertaken with bushmaster snake venom (*Lachesis lanceolatus*). *Lachesis* had earlier been proved in considerable detail by Hering, who was first to conduct meaningful medical research on snake venoms [62, 63], and he described the cardiac symptoms it produced. Boyd was among the first person to demonstrate that *Lachesis* had anti-arrhythmic properties, after having previously shown that it induced arrhythmia in cats with a normal heart beat [64]. Later, when given at a dose of 0.025 mg per kilogram to cats in which arrhythmia had been induced experimentally, the drug quickly and lastingly corrected this irregularity [65]. Boyd was at the forefront of research into snake and spider venoms for over a decade. Among his studies was the large proving he conducted on NYHMC medical students in 1927, in which he administered venoms and lactose control to 50 medical students. Although it is unclear whether this study was ever published, it received attention in the national press [66]. According to Swiderski [67], this proving study "left many of the participants in physical distress and mental depression." Boyd continued his proving experiments in readily accessible medical student samples and in 1935 conducted a study of lead, aluminum, and sulfur in 72 subjects [68]. Boyd was one of the first to publically call for human testing of all drugs that were to be developed for the market, saying that such studies would provide information that was unavailable from animal studies: he correctly predicted a time in the future when such testing would be made obligatory.

At the same time, others were exploring the effects of venom on pain, bleeding, cancer, and arthritis, but there seems to have been little interest in their cardiological applications until more recently [69]. Since Boyd was well known, particularly as a cardiologist, it is hard to believe that his peers would not have known of his work. In more recent years, a number of venom-derived drugs, such as tirofiban (Aggrastat) and eptifibatide (Integrilin), were developed in the pharmaceutical industry for treating acute coronary syndrome; Boyd may have been one of the earliest to recognize their potential for this condition, although by building on established homeopathic knowledge [70, 71] and following a somewhat different path.

Boyd's name appears many times in the allopathic literature over a 35-year period and his publications reflect broad expertise and productive collaboration with peers from different disciplines, including psychiatry, surgery, gastroenterology, trauma, and infectious disease. That he was not simply a "jack-of-all-trades-and-master-of-none" is clear by the fact that he received Fellowships of the American Colleges of Physicians, Cardiologists, and Gastroenterologists, the last of which was an honorary award. In 1924, while still an assistant professor of homeopathy, he published a study of 4,000 cases of aortic aneurysm [72], and in 1959, he was a coauthor of a publication from the NYMC obesity clinic on a double-blind trial of T_3 (a thyroid hormone) with an amphetamine and barbiturate combination in comparison to amphetamine and barbiturate alone [73]. He also published a double-blind trial of the antianxiety sedative meprobamate vs. placebo in older patients, to evaluate the potential of that drug for producing dependency and withdrawal [74]. His meprobamate study not only revealed his interest in the problem of addiction but also indicated a solid reputation as an addiction specialist. In response to a request from the US Congress, he was invited to serve on the Committee on Public Health of the New York Academy of Medicine with other distinguished colleagues to address the growing national problem of narcotic addiction and was a coauthor of the ensuing report [75]. He coauthored publications on the early use of cycloserine for tuberculosis [76], gastric secretions after gastric surgery [77], and a hematology report on vitamin B_{12} and gastric hematopoietic factor [78]. Other publications between 1948 and 1958 in the *New York State Journal of Medicine* covered topics such as coma and unconsciousness, sleep induction with salicylamide and acetophenetidin, serological tests for cancer, and, in collaboration with Thomas McGavack, tolerance studies of the antihistamine drug Thephorin.

Boyd was interested in peripheral circulatory problems and worked together with a surgical colleague in the study of frostbite and gangrene. He coauthored a report with Kurt Lange on the intravenous use of fluorescein sodium as a diagnostic test to help detect which patients needed immediate surgery for gangrene or strangulated hernia, this being the first publication of its type. If the red fluorescein dye circulated round the body in 20 s, including through the gut or foot, then blood circulation was still present in the diseased area. If, on the other hand, there was absence of a green-yellow glow in the diseased region, this indicated that the blood supply had been shut off and that amputation of the foot or removal of the gut was indicated. The test, which was described by Lange and Boyd in 1942 [79], attracted much attention in the popular press [80] and was referred to 40 years later in the literature on predicting leg viability [81], which described the subsequent evolution of technical refinements to the Lange and Boyd procedure. In 1945, the authors wrote further on the prevention of gangrene from frostbite [82].

Perhaps it was as a cardiologist that Boyd was best known outside of his homeopathic work. Among his publications was a jointly edited textbook on clinical electrocardiography, which ran into several editions [83]. His journal publications included a double-blind placebo-controlled trial demonstrating antihypertensive effects for meprobamate in elderly hypertensives [84].

Boyd was a prolific translator who made contemporary German medical and homeopathic literature accessible to the English-speaking world. His output included translations of homeopathic works by Karl Koetschau (on dose effects), August Bier (on circulation), and Hans Wapler (on homeopathic philosophy), Otto Leeser's textbook of homeopathic *materia medica*, a pharmacological study of the biphasic effects of cocaine by Edward Rentz, a cardiology book on Roentgen diagnosis of the heart by Erich Zdansky, and a book by Max Neuberger on the historical study of the doctrine of the healing power of nature, which received a very positive review [85].

Boyd's name rarely appears in the homeopathic literature today – in fact, it is the name of William Boyd of the mustard-gas experiments and emanometer fame that receives greater mention, although his achievements fall well short of Linn Boyd's. With such productivity and scholarship, how could Linn Boyd have been "lost" to homeopathy? The truth appears to have been that, as in the case of Conrad Wesselhoeft, homeopathy may not have been ready for what Boyd had to offer. More specifically, Boyd fell casualty to the doctrinal infighting that took place in homeopathic circles, coupled with the old guard's reluctance to leave the safe bield of comforting dogma in favor of scientific questioning. There was also objection to Boyd's use of animals in experimentation. These factors reportedly caused Boyd to resign from the American Institute of Homeopathy, according to Otto Guttentag [86]. It was Guttentag's opinion that Boyd's loss was most unfortunate for the cause of American homeopathy. At least one of Boyd's promising students, Thomas H. McGavack, joined him in resigning and then, like

Boyd, went on to a stellar academic career. Boyd therefore remains a somewhat neglected figure in the twentieth-century medicine. Like Wesselhoeft, he was one of the few who could move freely between homeopathy and allopathy. With the demise of homeopathy, Boyd and Wesselhoeft made impressive transitions. Indeed, had they been unable to do so, they would have been eased out of their faculty posts, as happened in New York to the traditional homeopathic clinicians, who were no longer wanted on faculty in the 1930s and 1940s [87].

Thomas H. McGavack: Embracing Homeopathy, Endocrinology, and Gerontology

Thomas McGavack (1898–1973) obtained a homeopathic MD degree from Hahnemann Medical College, Philadelphia (Fig. 11.5). In 1923, he was appointed to the faculty at the University of California, where he later headed the department of homeopathy. In 1936, he was appointed professor of clinical medicine at the New York Homeopathic Medical College, where he remained until 1957. He was then appointed associate chief of staff at the Martinsburg Veterans

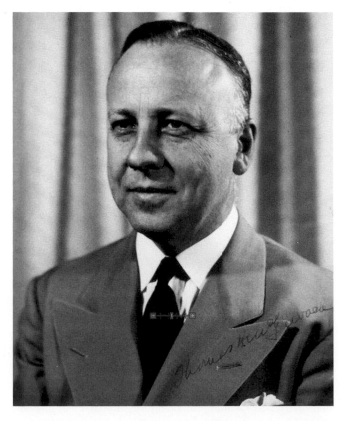

Fig. 11.5 Thomas McGavack. Gerontologist (Image courtesy of National Library of Medicine, in the public domain)

Administration Hospital, West Virginia, where he practiced until retiring.

McGavack practiced and conducted research in homeopathy for the first two decades of his career. Boyd referred to him as one of those engaged in the modern scientific movement [49, p. 152]. In 1932, he authored a book entitled *The Homeopathic Principles in Therapeutics* [88] and was an active member of the American Institute of Homeopathy, serving as its president. Even after resigning, he continued to attend annual meetings of the institute and made an interesting comment at the 1937 conference when he warned the assembled group about the workplace risks of exposure to cadmium [89], which he had found to cause kidney and liver damage in rabbits [90, 91]. In 1941, the government announced federal standards concerning safe limits, and while there is nothing to suggest that this was connected to McGavack, it is evident that he showed an early concern about occupational safety.

McGavack turned his attention to other areas of medicine and became a well-known endocrinologist and gerontologist. His other publications concerned the detection of silica in the body, sickle cell anemia, clinical studies with diphenhydramine (Benadryl™) and other antihistamines, and books on obesity and cerebral ischemia. A literature search yields more than 30 peer-reviewed papers over a 35-year period. Many of his publications concerned the thyroid gland, including his textbook *The Thyroid* [92], which appeared in 1951 and was favorably reviewed by the *Journal of American Medical Association* and *British Journal of Surgery* [93, 94].

As a gerontologist, McGavack was considered to have "made major contributions toward the growth of the science of gerontology and particularly in interesting the medical profession in this major phase of health care" [95]. He received recognition from the American Geriatrics Society by an award of Fellowship, election to its presidency and board membership. In 1962, he was honored as the first recipient of the society's Edward Henderson Award for Research. He also served as council member of the International Association of Gerontology and was awarded Fellowship of the Gerontological Society. Many of his publications concerned geriatrics, including a paper in which he described an innovative program he had developed and implemented at the Martinsburg VA Hospital, for which he coined a new word: remocreaction [96], an acronym for remotivation, reassurance, recreation, rehabilitation, creativity, action, reintegration, and restoration. McGavack thought that it was important to strive for a wider understanding of rehabilitation than simply trying to return people to purposeful employment or activity in the community and that the creation of a different name would help promote his newer concept. McGavack's remocreaction program demonstrated that the hopelessness and passivity that often characterized the chronically ill could be reversed, even when the outlook appeared dismal. To implement his program, McGavack created a special inpatient unit where the emphasis was placed on multidisciplinary teamwork.

McGavack was a successful clinician, who included among his patients Ronald Reagan (before he became president), Jane Wyman, Danny Kaye, and Edgar Bergen. An endowment that he left to his undergraduate college, Hampden-Sidney, currently supports a chair in biochemistry [97].

Thomas McGavack had much experience in treating obesity and served as expert witness in a lawsuit by the US government against Republic Drug Company for illegal interstate shipment and false claims over their product, Unitrol, which they claimed was an effective appetite suppressant. The court found in favor of the libellant, for whom McGavack had served as an expert [98]. He treated over 5,000 patients with obesity and conducted several studies to assess drug efficacy. In the course of his career, he published over 300 articles and several books and served on editorial boards of numerous journals. He was the director of the New York Medical School Metropolitan Hospital Research Unit, where he worked mostly in endocrine and metabolic diseases, and later became the director of the Geriatric Research Laboratories at the Martinsburg VA Medical Center.

Harold Griffith, who never lost his belief in homeopathy as an effective method of treatment, wrote in 1930 that "today there is genuine curiosity and interest in some 'old school circles' about homeopathy." He enumerated the names of Bier, Boyd, Hinsdale, Boericke, Wesselhoeft, Koetschau, and others as "making it easier for us to talk about homeopathy in terms of modern science, and to offer some objective laboratory proof of our theories." He further commented that "of equal importance is the need for convincing clinical statistics of the effect of homeopathic treatment … and very few that are of value have been published." As he wrote these lines [99], homeopathy's trail in academic medicine was about to disappear, not to resurface for another 50 years, when a new homeopathic spring arrived, mainly in Europe and to a lesser extent, in the United States.

References

1. Upham R. National homeopathic clinic day: Tuesday, October 18, 1921. J Am Inst Homeopath. 1921;14:360–1.
2. New York Medical College Annual Report 2010–2011. [Internet]. p. 9 [Cited 2012 Oct 21]. Available from: http://www.nymc.edu/AboutNYMC/AnnualReport/DownloadTheAnnualReport.pdf.
3. New York Medical College Sarah C. Upham Division of Gastroenterology and Hepatobiliary Diseases [Internet] [Cited 2012 Oct 21]. Available from: http://www.nymc.edu/depthome/academic/medicine/gastro_fellowship.pdf.
4. New York Due Today. The Montreal Gazette. 1937 Oct 1. p. 19.
5. Pediatric Surgery @ Brown [Internet] [Cited 2012 Apr 6]. Available from: http://med.brown.edu/pedisurg/Brown/Wesselhoeft.html.

6. Wesselhoeft Jr CW, DeLuca FG. A simplified approach to repair of pediatric pectus deformities. Ann Thorac Surg. 1982;34:640–6.

7. Tufts Alumni: who we are [Internet]. Boston; 2012 [Cited 2012 Mar 25]. Available from: http://tuftsalumni.org/who-we-are/alumni-recognition/tufts-notables/tufts-service-3/#wesselhoeft.

8. Wesselhoeft H, Salomon F, Grimm T. The spectrum of supravalvular aortic stenosis: clinical findings of 150 patients with Williams-Beuren syndrome and the isolated lesion. Z Kardiol. 1980;69:131–40.

9. Wesselhoeft H, Hurley PG, Wagner HW, Rowe RD. Nuclear angiography in the diagnosis of congenital heart disease in infants. Circulation. 1972;45:77–91.

10. William Johannes Wesselhoeft. Personal communication. 26 Mar 2012.

11. Dianne Wesselhoeft. Personal communication. 7 Apr 2012.

12. St. John T. Dr. Wesselhoeft in "Rappaccini's Daughter." [Internet]. Brattleboro History, Brattleboro [Cited 2012 Mar 25]. Available from: http://hawthornessevengables.com/chapters/dr-wesselhoeft-in-rappaccinis-daughter.html.

13. Wapler H. The incorporation of homeopathy into scientific medicine. J Am Inst Homeopath. 1932;25:3–11.

14. Conrad Wesselhoeft, M.D. 1884–1962. N Engl J Med. 1962;267:1373

15. Deaths: Wesselhoeft, Conrad. J Am Med Assoc. 1963;184:511–12.

16. Kraft M. The Doctors Wesselhoeft. Centerscope, Boston University School of Medicine. 1973. p. 18–9.

17. Hoffmann WW. The Wesselhoeft family: from Buxtehude to Boston and beyond. 1969. p. 53. Unpublished manuscript. Courtesy of Caroline Williams

18. Putnam JJ. The significance to neurology of the Robert Dawson Evans Memorial. Boston Med Surg J. 1912;166:584–5.

19. Southard EE. The significance of a homeopathic foundation for clinical research and preventive medicine. Boston Med Surg J. 1912;166:585–7.

20. Wesselhoeft 2nd C. The relative value of homoeopathy in a series of 166 hospital cases exhibiting constipation. N Engl Med Gazette. 1913;48:399–409.

21. Wesselhoeft 2nd C. Studies in regard to the action of quinine on the malarial plasmodia. II. N Engl Med Gazette. 1913;48:637–53.

22. Wesselhoeft C. Homoeopathy in the prophylaxis and treatment of scarlet fever. N Engl Med Gazette. 1917;LII:461–75.

23. Wesselhoeft C. The homeopathic treatment of whooping cough. N Engl Med Gazette. 1917;52:297–319.

24. Wesselhoeft C. Orchitis in mumps. Boston Med Surg J. 1920;183:520–4.

25. Baehr B. Digitalis Purpurea in ihren physiologischen und therapeutischen Wirkungen, Gekroente Preiseschrift, Leipsig; 1859. German. (Cited in Wesselhoeft C. Digitalis as a homeopathic remedy in disorders of the heart. J Am Inst Homeopath. 1922/1923;15:412–34).

26. Wesselhoeft C. Digitalis as a homeopathic remedy in disorders of the heart. J Am Inst Homeopath. 1922/1923;15:412–34.

27. Wesselhoeft 2nd C. Hahnemann's place in "the dawn of modern medicine. J Am Inst Homeopath. 1921;13:712–6.

28. Wesselhoeft C. The scope and limitations of homeopathy in the treatment of the common contagious infections. J Am Inst Homeopath. 1924;16:488–501.

29. Wesselhoeft C, Smith EC. The use of sulfanilamide in scarlet fever. N Engl J Med. 1938;209:947–53.

30. Wesselhoeft C. Communicable diseases: cardiovascular disease in diphtheria. N Engl J Med. 1940;223:57–66.

31. Wesselhoeft C. Factors influencing the incidence and course of otitis media in scarlet fever. Ann Intern Med. 1939;12:1473–85.

32. Wesselhoeft C. Treatment of scarlet fever and diphtheria. Med Clin North Am. 1936;19:1389–407.

33. Wesselhoeft C, Smith EC, Branch CF. Human encephalitis: eight fatal cases, with four due to the virus of equine encephalomyelitis. J Am Med Assoc. 1938;111:1735–41.

34. Wesselhoeft C. Nephritis in scarlet fever and its treatment. J Am Med Assoc. 1941;116:36–8.

35. Paul O. Background of the prevention of cardiovascular disease. Circulation. 1989;79:1361–7.

36. Amanna IJ, Slifka MK. Wanted dead or alive: new viral vaccines. Antiviral Res. 2009;84:119–30.

37. Chobanian A. Personal communication to the author. 8 Mar 2013.

38. Wesselhoeft C. Weighted retractors for tracheotomy. J Am Med Assoc. 1933;101:365–6.

39. Wesselhoeft C. Hydraulic lift for patients with partial leg paralysis. J Am Med Assoc. 1948;136:56.

40. In Memoriam. Conrad Wesselhoeft. 1962. Unpublished document, provided by courtesy of Caroline Williams.

41. Letter from Conrad Wesselhoeft to his sister. July 12, 1940. By permission of Caroline Williams.

42. Wesselhoeft C. Personal communication to the author. 31 Mar 2013.

43. Kraft M. The Doctors Wesselhoeft. Boston University Medicine: celebrating the sesquicentennial. Boston University School of Medicine. 1998;6:13.

44. Robins N. Copeland's cure: homeopathy and the war between conventional and alternative medicine. New York: Knopf; 2005. p. 162.

45. Boyd LJ. New York Medical College, Flower and Fifth Avenue Hospitals. NY State Med J. 1957;57:575–9.

46. Yasgur J. Personal communication to author. 26 Apr 2012.

47. Manning S. Personal communication to the author. 7 Nov 2012.

48. McKeown LA. Eighty years later, a yearbook and a lost pin reveal an alum to his surviving family. Chironian – New York Medical College. 2008;Spring/Summer:22.

49. Boyd LJ. A study of the simile in medicine. Philadelphia: Boericke & Tafel; 1936.

50. Boyd LJ. Koetschau's scientific basis of homeopathy; simplified version. J Am Inst Homeopath. 1930;23:1156–62.

51. Boyd LJ. Some factors responsible for recent progress in homeopathy. J Am Inst Homeopath. 1931;24:1219–37.

52. Boyd LJ. Study of action of chelidonium. Bull New York Med College, Flower and Fifth Avenue Hospitals. 1939;2:149–61

53. Boyd LJ. Cocculus indicus: a review of the verification of its symptomatology. J Am Inst Homeopath. 1923;15:891–6.

54. Boyd LJ. Remarks upon the medical treatment of cirrhosis of the liver. J Am Inst Homeopath. 1923;15:814–20.

55. Boyd LJ. Heloderma: notes upon its effects and the explanation of the action of some of the snake venoms. J Am Inst Homeopath. 1922;14:803–10.

56. Boyd LJ. Remarks upon *Latrodectus mactans* and its use. J Am Inst Homeopath. 1922;15:406–9.

57. Obituary. Linn J. Boyd. The New York Times. 1981 Oct 6.

58. "Human Guinea Pigs" for Experiments: Studies to Eat Poison Pellets in the Interest of Science. The Milwaukee Sentinel. 1935 Nov 24; 20.

59. Spider not so deadly: a step further. The Literary Digest. 1935;June 22:19.

60. The Widow Again. The Spartanburg Herald. 1935 July 6:4.

61. Séror R. 2001. Latrodectus mactans [Internet]. Excerpted from Anshutz EP. New, old and forgotten remedies. 1900. [Cited 2012 Jul 14]. Available from: www.homeoint.org/seror/patho1900/latrodectus.htm.

62. Leeser O. Actions and medicinal uses of snake venoms. Br Homoeopathic J. 1958;74:153–71.

63. Hering C. Wirkungen des Schlangengiftes, zum aertzlichen Gebrauche zusammengestellt. Allentown. 1837. German.

64. Boyd LJ. A note on ancistrodon and lachesis. J Am Inst Homeopath. 1935;1:437–44.

65. Boyd LJ, Brody JG, Anchel D. Experimental treatment of cardiac arrhythmias. Proc Soc Exp Biol Med. 1929;26:570–2.

66. Medical Students Begin Poison Diet. New York Times. 1925 Jan 19. p. 10.

67. Swiderski R. Poison eaters: snakes, opium. Arsenic, and the lethal show. Boca Raton: Universal Publishers; 2010. p. 249–53.

68. Poisons fed to 72 in medical tests. New York Times. 1935 Jan 4. p. 25.

69. Pal SK, Gomes A, Dasgupta SC, Gomes A. Snake venom as therapeutic agents: from toxin to drug development. Indian J Exp Biol. 2002;40:1353–8.

70. Nash EB. Leaders in homeopathic therapeutics. Philadelphia: Boericke and Tafel; 1913. p. 111.

71. Peck SM, Rosenthal N, Erf LA. The value of the prognostic venom in thrombocytopenic purpura. J Am Med Assoc. 1936;106:1783–91.

72. Boyd LJ. A study of four thousand cases of aneurysm of the thoracic aorta. Am J Med Sci. 1924;168:654–7.

73. Gelvin EP, Kenigsberg S, Boyd LJ. Results of addition of liothyronine to a weight-reducing regimen. J Am Med Assoc. 1959;170:87–92.

74. Boyd LJ, Cammer L, Mulinos MG, Huppert VF, Hammer H. Meprobamate addiction. J Am Med Assoc. 1958;168:1839–43.

75. Howe HS, Boyd LJ, Cattell M, Goodfriend MJ, Greeley AV, Kolb LC, et al. Report on drug addiction. Bull New York Acad Med. 1955;31:592–607.

76. Epstein IG, Boyd LJ. The treatment of human pulmonary tuberculosis with cycloserine: progress report. Dis Chest. 1956;29:241–57.

77. Mersheimer WL, Glass GBJ, Speer FD, Winfield JM, Boyd LJ. Gastric mucin – a chemical and histologic study following bilateral vagectomy. Gastric resection and the combined procedure. Ann Surg. 1952;136:668–78.

78. Glass GBJ, Lillick LC, Boyd LJ, Gunnis C, Corti LG. Metabolic interrelations between gastric hematopoietic factor and vitamin B_{12}. Blood. 1954;9:1127–40.

79. Lange K, Boyd LJ. The use of fluorescein to determine the adequacy of the circulation. Med Clin North Am. 1942;26:934–52.

80. Greenglow [Internet]. TIME. 15 January 1942 [Cited 2012 Aug 10]. Available from: www.time.com/time/magazine/article/0,9171,795842,00.html.

81. Silverman D, Wagner FW. Prediction of leg viability and amputation level by fluorescein uptake. Prosthet Orthot Int. 1983;7:69–71.

82. Lange K, Boyd LJ, Loewe L. The functional pathology of frostbite and the prevention of gangrene in experimental animals and humans. Science. 1945;102:151–2.

83. Book reviews. Clinical electrocardiography, by David Scherf, M.D., F.A.C.P., and Linn J. Boyd, M.D., F.A.C.P. 3rd Edition. Heinemann. 1948. Postgrad Med J. 1948;24:612.

84. Boyd LJ, Huppert VF, Mulinos MG, Hammer H. Meprobamate in treatment of hypertension. Am J Cardiol. 1959;3:229–35.

85. Book review. The doctrine of the healing power of nature throughout the course of time, by Max Neuberger. J Nerv Ment Dis. 1934;80:374–5.

86. Duffy J. Otto E. Guttentag: an oral history (sound recording)/interviewed by John Duffy. 24 July 1968 [transcript] [Internet] [Cited 2012 Jul 5]. Available from: http://oculus.nlm.nih.gov.

87. James Stephenson: an oral history (sound recording)/interviewed by John Duffy and Martin Kaufman. 18 June 1968 [transcript] [Internet] [Cited 2012 Jul 5]. Available from: http://oculus.nlm.nih.gov/cgi/t/text/pageviewer-idx?c=oralhist;cc=oralhist;idno=2935125r;frm=frameset;view=image;seq=2;page=root;size=l.

88. McGavack TH. The homeopathic principle in therapeutics. Philadelphia: Boericke & Tafel; 1932.

89. Prodan L. Cadmium poisoning. J Ind Hygiene. 1932;14:132–5.

90. Opposes State and Socialized Medicine. Report of 93rd annual meeting, American Institute of Homeopathy, Boston. The Lewiston Daily Sun. 1937 Jun 18. p. 4.

91. McGavack TH, Hart CE. Kidney disturbances produced by heavy metal intoxications. J Am Inst Homeopath. 1938;XXXI:653–5.

92. McGavack TH. The thyroid. St. Louis: Mosby; 1951.

93. Book review. The thyroid. J Am Med Assoc. 1951;149:313.

94. Book review: The thyroid. Br J Surg. 1951;39:287.

95. Lorenze EJ. In Memoriam. Thomas Hodge McGavack, MD. April 7, 1898 – May 23, 1973. The Gerontologist. 1973;13:326.

96. McGavack TH. Remocreation – restoration of the chronically ill. J Am Geriatr Soc. 1965;13:967–72.

97. Record of the Hampden-Sydney Alumni Association [Internet]. Thomas H. McGavack 1917. A Remarkable Life [Cited 2012 Aug 17]. Available from: http://www26.us.archive.org/stream/recordofhampd-8012004hamp/recordofhampd8012004hamp_djvu.txt.

98. US vs. 60 28-capsule bottles, more or less, etc. [Internet] 211 F. Supp 207 (1962) United States District court D New Jersey September 27, 1962. [Cited 2012 Jul 28]. Available from: http://www.leagle.com/xmlResult.aspx?page=4&xmldoc=1962418211FSupp207_1384.xml&docbase=CSLWAR1-1950-1985&SizeDisp=7.

99. Griffith HR. The field of homeopathic remedies in scientific medicine. J Am Inst Homeopath. 1930;23:762–5.

Oncology

12

Oscar Auerbach

The discovery of a causative link between cigarette smoking and lung cancer is one of the twentieth-century medicine's greatest triumphs. It was a tale that took over 20 years to unfold, beginning with epidemiological studies in Germany, the United States, and Great Britain in the 1930s, 1940s, and 1950s. Richard Doll and Tony Bradford Hill are perhaps the best known of these early investigators [1, 2]. Despite their persuasive epidemiological findings, there was resistance from the tobacco industry and others, who argued that epidemiological associations failed to show any causative explanation. Data concerning possible mechanisms were based on animal studies, which were considered to be of limited relevance. Even Doll and Bradford at first thought the rise in lung cancer rates could be explained by air pollution.

The next stage in demonstrating a connection between tobacco and lung cancer began with Oscar Auerbach (1905–1997), a pathologist whose work is regarded as a major milestone in investigative pathology, ranked alongside the discoveries of smallpox vaccination and prevention of hospital sepsis [3] (Fig. 12.1). Auerbach neither completed high school nor undergraduate school, but was accepted into New York Homeopathic Medical College on the strength of passing its entrance exams. He qualified in 1929 and went to work at Halloran Hospital and Sea View, a tuberculosis hospital on Staten Island. He subsequently accepted a position in the Veterans Administration, where he conducted seminal work on lung cancer. For 12 years, Auerbach held a faculty position in the department of pathology at NYMC, and then in his later years at the New Jersey Medical School. His teaching left an impression on at least one student, Arthur Topilow, who recalled that in 1964 at NYMC, Auerbach asked all the assembled students to refrain from smoking in his class, whereupon several walked out of the room. In the words of Topilow, who forever gave up smoking after the lecture, they "missed a ground-breaking presentation" [4].

Auerbach was known as a tireless researcher who adhered to impeccable standards. He was extraordinarily productive:

while most of his colleagues examined 200 slides a day, Auerbach examined 2,000 [5]. Auerbach published two articles in the *New England Journal of Medicine*, which appeared in 1957 and 1961. The first report showed that among 117 deceased veterans, there was an increased degree of tissue change in proportion to the extent of smoking, as obtained from the medical history [6]. Auerbach's study was the first to examine this relationship directly by tissue histology and to relate it to patterns of smoking. In a second report [7], he extended his earlier findings in a larger sample and answered

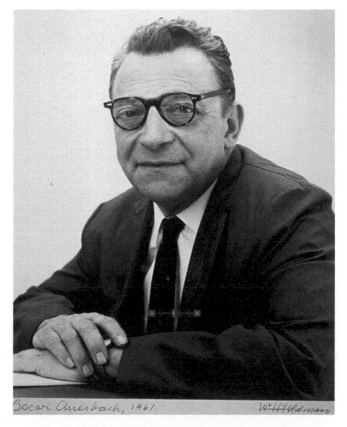

Fig. 12.1 Oscar Auerbach. Pathologist known for demonstrating a clear link between smoking and lung cancer (Image in the public domain, by courtesy of National Library of Medicine)

J. Davidson, *A Century of Homeopaths*,
DOI 10.1007/978-1-4939-0527-0_12, © Springer Science+Business Media New York 2014

an important methodological criticism of his previous report that concerned possible misclassification of the abnormal tissue findings. In this second paper, Auerbach concluded that "the histological evidence from this study greatly strengthens the already overwhelming body of epidemiological evidence that cigarette smoking is a major factor in the causation of bronchogenic carcinoma." An accompanying editorial in the journal seemed to agree with their conclusions [8]. In each study, Auerbach obtained over 200 samples from each subject, to represent the entire tracheobronchial tree – a monumental accomplishment. All of his ratings were conducted without knowledge of any other details about the patient, which had been coded separately.

In demonstrating a clear association between cellular change in the lungs and extent of smoking, Auerbach moved the debate about cancer and smoking beyond population statistics into the realm of tissue pathology, directly examined.

The impact of Auerbach's work cannot be overestimated. Lynch notes the "tremendous public health impact" of his studies, which were given prominence in the 1964 surgeon-general's report on tobacco that did so much to shape tobacco regulations on labeling and advertising.

Charles Cameron

Charles S. Cameron (1908–1998) was a 1935 Hahnemann graduate who later became an expert in the diagnosis and treatment of cancer (Fig. 12.2). He subsequently became dean of Hahnemann, where he shepherded a troubled institution away from its homeopathic past towards a future highly ranked allopathic medical school. Cameron was the first Hahnemann graduate to complete an internship at the prestigious Philadelphia General Hospital, where he developed an interest in cancer [9]. This led him to a Rockefeller Fellowship at Sloan-Kettering from 1938 to 1942 and then four war years in the Navy. From there, Cameron was appointed medical and scientific director and vice-president of the American Cancer Society (ACS). In addition, he served on the National Cancer Institute Study Section, and later as a member of the AMA National Board of Medical Examiners. Cameron authored a best-selling book *The Truth About Cancer*. He was a champion of public education about the disease, the need for early detection and treatment, and a strong advocate of the Pap smear before it was accepted as a standard screening test for cervical cancer. Another of Cameron's legacies was the journal *CA – A Cancer Journal for Clinicians* – which he founded in 1950 and which is still going strong 62 years later. As Cameron wrote in the first issue, the journal was designed to "condense authentic information about diagnosis, treatment, control, and research" for

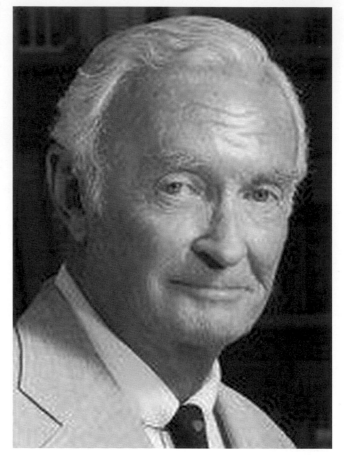

Fig. 12.2 Charles Cameron. Dean of Hahnemann Medical College and pioneer in cancer medicine (By permission, *CA: Cancer Journal for Clinicians*)

busy clinicians [10]. *CA* is the now most widely circulated oncology journal in the world, with a circulation of approximately 84,000. *CA* reaches a wide and diverse group of professionals and continues to fulfill Cameron's original vision of presenting information to these professionals about cancer prevention, early detection, treatment, palliation, advocacy issues, and quality-of-life topics. For his work with the ACS and for his book, Cameron has been acknowledged as a father of the national campaign against cancer (Fig. 12.3).

In 1956, Cameron was recruited back to Hahnemann as Dean of the College and later as president and chairman of the board of trustees. Notwithstanding the ups, downs, and conflicts that are an inevitable part of institutional change, under Cameron's leadership, the Hahnemann ship stabilized and prospered on its voyage to respectability as an orthodox medical school. As one who was trained in, and familiar with, homeopathy, Cameron wrote some perceptive accounts of the specialty and of its founder, Samuel Hahnemann (see Chap. 2) [11–13].

AMERICAN CANCER SOCIETY, INC.
47 Beaver Street
New York 4, New York

Statement of Dr. Charles S. Cameron
Medical and Scientific Director

The report of Doctors Hammond and Horn, and the exhibit summarizing their report are the first published data based on the large-scale survey of smoking practice among some 187,000 healthy men. The first of its kind ever attempted, it is being carried out with the assistance of 22,000 volunteers in 394 counties scattered throughout the United States, and is now in the 29th month. The correlation of the smoking practices of these many thousands of subjects - recorded while they were alive and in good health - with the causes of their deaths as they occur has provided important information in advance of the time schedule originally estimated. Furthermore, it is information so clearly valid - beyond any question of statistical error - that it appeared to warrant publication at this time. While the observed correlation between heavy cigarette smoking and the likelihood of death from cancer of the lung and from cardiovascular disease was perhaps not astonishing, the degree of that relationship was. In addition, deaths from forms of cancer other than the lung appear to be associated with heavy cigarette smoking, thus opening up new considerations of the mode of action of the carcinogen, if any, contained in tobacco smoke.

Personally I am not convinced that the Hammond-Horn theory of cause and effect relationship between heavy cigarette smoking and increased susceptibility to death from cancer in general is as yet entirely proved. One cannot at this time exclude the possibility that heavy cigarette smoking and the tendency to cancer are both expressions of a more fundamental cause of a constitutional or hormonal nature.

Whatever interpretation is put on the evidence brought forth by this study, the data themselves and the methodology employed to get them are sound. The results appear to be of first importance in consideration of the changing death rates of the past 25 years. If further validated, they point the way to the means of still further lengthening man's life-span.

June 17, 1954

Fig. 12.3 Letter from Charles Cameron to the American Cancer Society, June 17, 1954, regarding the association between tobacco smoking and lung cancer (Image by permission John W. Hill Papers, Wisconsin Historical Society Archives)

Howard W. Nowell

Homeopathy basked in warm sunshine in 1913, when the national press gave extensive coverage to research from the Evans Memorial Institute purporting to have identified a cause of cancer. The chief investigator of this study was Howard Wilbert Nowell (1872–1940), a 1911 graduate of Boston University who was appointed to the faculty as instructor of pathology (Fig. 12.4). He gained quick promotion and was granted extensive research support at Evans. Nowell surrounded himself with experienced collaborators, including Allen Rowe, J Emmons Briggs, and William H. Watters, as well as receiving administrative support from Drs. Sutherland, Richardson, and Mann, all of BUSM; he was also granted the services of two research assistants.

Nowell conducted extensive experiments on rabbits, into which he injected material from human carcinoma. The rabbits in turn developed tumors microscopically and macroscopically similar in character to the human tumor. He then injected into healthy rabbits serum obtained from those with tumors and found that antibodies were produced in the former group. In a third step, Nowell then injected into healthy rabbits a mixture of the tumor-inducing substance and antitumor antibodies. This last set of experiments demonstrated that tumors did not develop and led Nowell to consider the possibility that serum containing these antibodies would either prevent the development of human cancer or treat it when established. The results of Nowell's research, which had taken 3 years, were first presented at the 73rd Annual Meeting of the Massachusetts Homeopathic Society in April 8, 1913, and were extensively covered in the *New York Times* of April 20 that year [14]. Nowell wasted no time in testing his serum in humans with cancer, having administered it within a few weeks to 50 patients, many of whom noted a rapid reduction in pain such that they could lower the dose of their opiate analgesics [15]. In a third article about Nowell within a 2-month period, the newspaper quoted Nowell as saying "This work has progressed further than we had any idea it would go. In experimental work time has to elapse, and usually a long time, before definite results can be ascertained." The article reported that Nowell's experiments have been so successful that the Evans administration increased his laboratory space and personnel [16]. The senior administrators at Boston University Medical School hailed Nowell's work as groundbreaking.

What then became of Nowell and his work is unclear. His animal studies led to the logical next step of administering his "cancer antiserum" to patients with the disease, and Nowell commenced a highly ambitious 600-patient program, the ultimate outcome of which was negative [17]. Nowell seems to have left Evans rather sooner than might have been expected given the spectacular promise of his initial work. By 1915, he had relinquished his faculty appointment in pathology and in 1917 was elected a fellow of the American

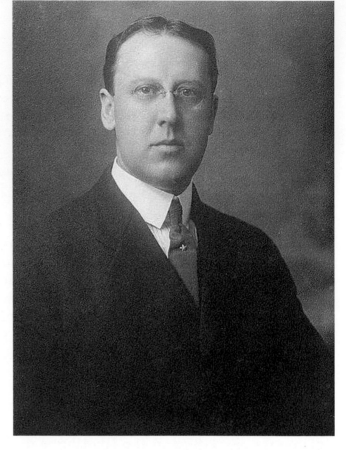

Fig. 12.4 Howard W. Nowell. Pathologist at Evans Institute who thought he had found a cause for cancer (Image in the public domain)

Public Health Association, somewhat of a change in direction for such a promising pathologist. His name appeared again in the American Public Health Association Yearbook of 1930–1931.

There are, however, some useful lessons to be learned from Nowell's work. (1) Firstly, Nowell and his associates were appropriately restrained about their findings; amidst all the excitement and intense press coverage, they took pains to explain that results of the initial animal studies should not be construed as providing a cure for cancer. (2) Secondly, in selecting patients for this new treatment, Nowell's team required either that the accepted treatment (i.e., surgery) must have been first tried or that patients were considered too high of a surgical risk and thus have few options left. In other words, they wisely adhered to the principle of balancing risk and potential benefit, by not exposing patients to a new treatment with all its possible side effects and unknown efficacy, unless they have received customary treatment or were unsuitable for it. (3) Nowell established an oversight board to guide the study and to select subjects, whose diagnosis of cancer had to be confirmed by the five-physician oversight panel. These moves were farsighted for the time and accord with the requirements of today's clinical trials.

Ita Wegman

Ita Wegman (1876–1943) was born into a Dutch colonial family in Karawang, Java, which was then part of the Dutch East Indies, where she resided until 1900 (Fig. 12.5). Wegman returned to Europe to study physical education and methods of massage based on Swedish massage. A biographical summary [18] of Wegman's life reveals that between 1906 and 1911 she studied medicine at the University of Zurich, and thereafter practiced gynecology. Wegman was profoundly influenced by the ideas of Rudolf Steiner, who became her mentor, friend, and, ultimately, her patient in his terminal illness. Early in Wegman's medical career, Steiner suggested that mistletoe (or *Viscum album* L, to give its botanical name) might be a useful treatment for cancer, and together they worked on its preparation as a medicinal agent. Between 1917 and 1920, Wegman used mistletoe in her Zurich practice. By 1922, commercial formulations of the drug were being made by the pharmaceutical company Weleda AG (under the name of "Iscador"™), and other companies have since followed suit. In 1921, Wegman set up a clinic near Basel, which still thrives today. Her initial work in cancer has stimulated further activity, much of which is carried out at the Lukas Clinic, a second AM center, established in 1963 in Arlesheim.

The research on mistletoe in cancer has been extensive, and while debate still continues about the extent of its therapeutic effect, there is good evidence that it has antitumor and anti-metastatic properties in animal experiments [19]. What is not in doubt, however, is the fact that mistletoe is now widely used in Central Europe. In 2007, for example, mistletoe products accounted for 23 % of all chemotherapy agents sold in Germany [20]. An extensive body of information on mistletoe is available at the National Cancer Institute website [21] and elsewhere [22].

Wegman was not a homeopath in the strict sense of the word, but is known for her collaboration with Steiner in introducing anthroposophical medicine (AM) as a new system [23]. AM incorporates homeopathy into its practice and more importantly perhaps has assimilated a basic principle underlying homeopathy, namely, that medicinal potency remains into highly diluted material [24, pp. 259–261]. The earliest research in AM, conducted by Kolisko in 1922, sought "to examine the behavio[u]r of matter on the way to and beyond the boundary of its ponderable existence" [24, p. 526]. AM and homeopathy can rightfully be seen as medical cousins.

Mistletoe is available in different strengths, including a homeopathic preparation of 30X, although for the most part, it is used at conventional doses, with initial doses being on the low side and then increased up to a point of side effects [25].

Wegman's other activities included the development of rhythmical massage, curative education for the disabled, and

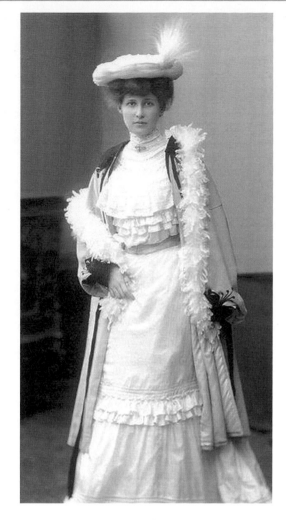

Fig. 12.5 Ita Wegman. Founder of anthroposophical medicine and advocate of mistletoe for cancer (Image in the public domain)

the AM movement in general. She was a cofounder of Weleda pharmaceuticals, which has grown into a global organization over the past 90 years. The worldwide Camphill School movement was begun by her pupil, Karl Konig. Wegman established a number of AM clinics in Europe, the best known being the clinic in Arlesheim, Switzerland, which is now named after her.

Edward Cronin Lowe

In 1933, the pathologist Edward Cronin Lowe (1880–1958) reported the development of a test to diagnose cancer. This publication appeared in the *British Medical Journal* and quickly generated correspondence and an attempt at replication by another group. Unfortunately this second study failed to support any value to the Cronin Lowe test, which eventually was abandoned. Lowe is better known for his work in influenza, as described in Chap. 13.

References

1. Doll R, Hill AB. Smoking and carcinoma of the lung. BMJ. 1950;221(ii):739–48.
2. Doll R, Hill AB. A study of aetiology of carcinoma of the lung. BMJ. 1952;225(ii):1271–86.
3. Lynch RG. Cigarette smoking and lung cancer. Milestones in Investigative Pathology. 2009;9–10. Originally published in American Society of Investigative Pathology Bulletin. 2003;6(2).
4. Arthur Topilow. When will people heed the Surgeon General's warning? [Internet]. HemOnc Today. 25 Mar 2009 [Cited 2012 Oct 21]. Available from: http://www.healio.com/hematology-oncology/news/print/hematology-oncology/%7B5c5d48bd-2372-4082-a357-c6a512aae210%7D/when-will-people-heed-the-surgeon-generals-warning.
5. Burkhart F. Oscar Auerbach, 92, Dies; Linked Smoking to Cancer. The New York Times. 1997 Jan 16.
6. Auerbach O, Gere JB, Forman JB, Petrick TG, Smolin HJ, Muehsam GE, et al. Changes in the bronchial epithelium in relation to smoking and cancer of the lung. N Engl J Med. 1957;256:98–104.
7. Auerbach O, Stout AP, Hammond EC, Garfinkel L. Changes in bronchial epithelium in relation to cigarette smoking and in relation to lung cancer. N Engl J Med. 1961;265:253–67.
8. Editorial. The great debate continues. New Engl J Med. 1961;265:294.
9. Rogers N. An alternative path: the making and remaking of Hahnemann Medical College and Hospital of Philadelphia. New Brunswick: Rutgers University Press; 1998. p. 179.
10. Holleb AI. A tribute to Charles S. Cameron, MD, CA's founding father [Internet]. CA Cancer J Clin. 1999;49:32 [Cited 2012 Oct 10]. Available from: http://onlinelibrary.wiley.com/doi/10.3322/canjclin.49.1.32/pdf.
11. Cameron CS. Homeopathy in retrospect. Trans Stud Coll Physicians Phila. 1959;27:28–33.
12. Cameron CS. Hahnemann: a second century look. Phila Med. 1957;53:83–7.
13. Cameron CS. Hahnemann and rush: a re-evaluation. Hahnemann Alumni News. Spring 1969. p. 16–21.
14. Thorne VB. Cause of cancer found at last by Boston Scientist. The New York Times. 1913 Apr 20.
15. Anonymous. Cancer alleviated by Nowell Serum. The New York Times. 1913 May 11.
16. Anonymous. Extends cancer study. The New York Times. 1913 June 16.
17. Nowell PG. What causes lymphocytic tumors? Cancer Invest. 1990;8:49–57.
18. Ita Wegman Biography. Anthroposophical Society of New Zealand. 2007 [Cited 2013 Mar 6]. Available from: http://www.anthroposophy.org.nz.
19. Kienle GS. The story behind mistletoe: a European remedy from anthroposophical medicine. Alt Ther. 1999;5:34–6.
20. Hamre HJ, Kiene H, Kienle GS. Clinical research in anthroposophical medicine. Alt Ther. 2009;15:52–5.
21. Mistletoe Extracts (PDQ®). [Cited 2013 Mar 6]. National Cancer Institute. Available from: http://www.cancer.gov/cancertopics/pdq/cam/mistletoe/patient/page1.
22. Die Mistel: Scientific Information. [Cited 2013 Mar 6]. Available from: http://wissenschaft.mistel-therapie.de/index.php5?page=52&lang=1.
23. Steiner R, Wegman IM. Extending practical medicine: fundamental principles based on the science of the spirit. [First published 1925]. Bristol: Rudolf Steiner Press; 2000.
24. Lehrs E. Man or matter. London: Rudolf Steiner Press; 1958.
25. Hamre HJ. Personal communication. 4 Mar 2013.

This chapter describes homeopaths who have contributed to gymnastics (Lewis), massage (Taylor), chemistry (Remsen), pediatrics (Fischer), Native American Indian health (Eastman), and immunization (Cronin Lowe).

Gymnastics, Education, Temperance, and Social Reform

Diocletian Lewis

From the purist's perspective, it may be argued that Diocletian ("Dio") Lewis (1823–1886) was not a fully qualified homeopathic doctor, but for all practical purposes, he can be regarded as legitimate under the rather loose training standards of the time (Fig. 13.1). To call him "no doctor," as did Okrent, seems an injustice [1]. Lewis entered Harvard Medical School in 1843 but dropped out, probably for financial reasons [2, p. 36]. He later entered the Cleveland Homeopathic Hospital College and was awarded an honorary MD degree. For some years, he practiced homeopathy and founded the lay journal *The Homeopathist*. By 1852, Lewis gave up full-time medical practice in order to pursue other health initiatives and social causes, some of which still reflect his influence. It is claimed that his wife's illness was a determining factor in Lewis' change of course: he was persuaded that she could regain her health by taking up a course of exercise [3]. Okrent likened Lewis to a "harvesting machine of causes and campaigns" [1], of which can be counted education, temperance, healthy eating, and gymnastics.

Lewis was a man of imposing presence brought to life by the following vivid descriptions: "Here is an original character. Nobody will ever mistake Dr. Dio Lewis for Dr. somebody else. His large, rotund body and well-formed head make him at once a striking and conspicuous figure. He stands nearly six feet high and weighs over two hundred pounds…. His nature is peculiarly sympathetic…. He is overflowing with good feeling, affection, charity, aspiration

and adoration…. He is, in brief, a live, original, energetic, enthusiastic, sympathetic, emotional gentleman. He is emphatically Dr. Dio Lewis." He was a compelling and confident orator. In speech, Lewis "stated his thought briefly, illustrated it with a spirited and pointed anecdote … or personal sketch, and stopped" [2, pp. 337–339, 372].

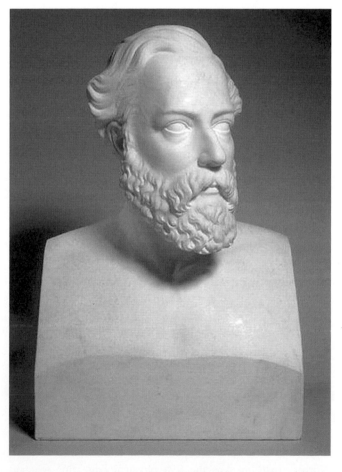

Fig. 13.1 Bust of Dio Lewis, 1868. By Edmonia Lewis, first African-American sculptor to gain national recognition (*Source*: Walters Art Museum, Baltimore. Image in the public domain)

J. Davidson, *A Century of Homeopaths*,
DOI 10.1007/978-1-4939-0527-0_13, © Springer Science+Business Media New York 2014

It is for his original work in physical culture, education, and temperance crusading that Lewis is best known. While in medical practice, Lewis originated a system of gymnastics that did not require the use of apparatus and which he taught to student teachers in gymnastics class. Lewis predicted that the Americans' increasingly sedentary lives would result in loss of physical fitness, and as a result, he set about promoting a user-friendly regime of exercise and gymnastics, which did not require expensive or unwieldy equipment [4]. His program used light, portable aids such as dumbbells, rings, and the beanbag: to Lewis goes credit for inventing the latter [1]. This work then took a backseat as Lewis immersed himself in the nascent temperance movement: in 1853, he gave his first public talk about temperance on *The Influence of Christian Women in the Cause of Temperance*. In the years that followed, the temperance movement gathered steam and, partly as a result of Lewis' efforts throughout the country, had driven more than 250 liquor businesses out of town within the first 3 months due to demonstrations. Of course, many saloons reopened once the protests stopped, but at least these efforts drew attention and garnered support for the temperance cause.

All the while, Lewis remained committed to improving physical fitness, and he therefore limited temperance work to Sundays, freeing up the week for other activities. In 1858, on a visit to Dixon, IL, he lamented not going the extra step in his temperance campaign, because "I was burdened with what I felt to be my life-work, that of urging upon the people their right to a 'sound mind in a sound body,' and the introduction of a new system of physical training into the schools of the country, and I therefore gave only Sundays to the temperance work" [2, pp. 66–67]. However, perhaps his greatest achievement on behalf of temperance occurred in 1874, when he founded the Women's Christian Temperance Union (WCTU), the outcome of a characteristically inspirational speech given in 1873 at Hillsboro, Ohio [5]. The WCTU continues in existence today, representing the basic principles on which it was founded and embracing over time other causes such as illegal drug use, gambling, pornography, and tobacco control. Information about the WCTU can be found at the organization's website [6].

Lewis advanced the cause of physical fitness education when he founded the Boston Normal Institute for Physical Education in 1861. The charismatic Lewis was able to recruit the president of Harvard, Cornelius Felton, to serve as president of the institute. Directors included John Andrew, the governor of Massachusetts, and Walter Channing, professor of hygiene at Harvard. None of these men would be remotely expected to sanction homeopathy, and Lewis was shrewd enough to keep his homeopathic sympathies to himself. The Normal Institute was the first physical education teacher-training school in the United States, and it gave rise to the nationwide spread of an educational system. Three years later, Lewis founded a girls' school in Lexington, Massachusetts, where he implemented his education philosophy, promoting informal relations between pupil and teacher and banning corporal punishment; one of its teachers was the well-known pioneer in women's education, Catherine Beecher. The school burned down in 1867 and was not rebuilt. Among the school's alumnae were Louisa Alcott and Una Hawthorne, daughter of Nathaniel Hawthorne. Those who attended the school attested to its rejuvenating effect as in the case of Lillie Chase Wyman, who said: "I attended his school worn out in body and mind and a mere bundle of damaged nerves, but gained there courage and strength to take up the battle anew" [3]. Several graduates went on to direct similar programs at Vassar, Smith, and Mount Holyoke colleges.

Even prior to opening of the Normal Institute, Lewis had widely promoted his system in books and pamphlets; he was a prolific writer – one book, *The New Gymnastics for Men, Women and Children*, went through 25 editions (Figs 13.2 and 13.3). In 1860, Lewis received a major boost when the leading educational authority of the time, the American Institute of Instruction (AII), endorsed his program [7]. At its annual meeting that year, a discussion of the following question was on the agenda: "Is it expedient to make calisthenics and gymnastics a part of school training?" Straightaway, Lewis took the institute's committee to see a demonstration of his methods and quickly persuaded them of its merits. On short order, the AII unanimously passed a resolution to introduce Lewis' gymnastic system into all schools. The program has been described in further detail by Welch, who credits Lewis as the first in this respect. He included in the teacher-training curriculum courses on anatomy, physiology, hygiene, gymnastics, and Swedish massage. The scientific content of Lewis' course provided a sound basis for the new field of study, and it "reveals a prototype upon which contemporary pedagogy is founded" [7, p. 31]. Although the institute had a short life, it graduated between 250 and 421 women [8], whose influence was profound. One well-known pupil, Adele Parot, was solely responsible for introducing Lewis' gymnastics into the California school system [9, 10].

The influential abolitionist, writer, and supporter of homeopathy, Thomas Wentworth Higginson acclaimed Lewis' ideas and called for their wider dissemination to colleges and seminaries [11]. Welch sees Lewis as the standard-bearer of physical education for women: "When American society embraced few career opportunities for women, Dio Lewis wrote and spoke of their abilities to succeed as teachers of gymnastics. His standards … led the way nearly a century and a half ago" [7, p. 34]. Blocker (2000) noted that, in style, Lewis was an individualist who rejected collective or organizational solutions to social problems. As a result, by the time of his death in 1886, his "voice no longer commanded assent," even though the causes he championed largely proved suc-

Fig. 13.2 Title page, The New Gymnastics by Dio Lewis (Image in the public domain)

THE

NEW GYMNASTICS

FOR

MEN, WOMEN, AND CHILDREN.

WITH A

TRANSLATION OF PROF. KLOSS'S DUMB-BELL INSTRUCTOR
AND PROF. SCHREBER'S PANGYMNASTIKON.

BY DIO LEWIS, M. D.,
PROPRIETOR OF THE ESSEX STREET GYMNASIUM, BOSTON.

WITH THREE HUNDRED ILLUSTRATIONS.

"By no other way can men approach nearer to the gods, than by conferring health on men." — CICERO.

TO

THE GIRLS AND BOYS

OF AMERICA,

WHOSE PHYSICAL WELFARE HAS BEEN THE STUDY OF HIS LIFE,

THE AUTHOR

MOST AFFECTIONATELY DEDICATES

This Work.

Fig. 13.3 Dedication page, The New Gymnastics (Image in the public domain)

cessful. Nevertheless, as is clear from this review, his influence has been enduring, for example, with respect to the WCTU and the educational approach to physical fitness in the nation's schools. Despite this long-lasting influence, Lewis has been practically forgotten, but in his day he was celebrated, fêted with testimonial dinners, and was the subject of an honorific novel written by Moses Coit Tyler called *The Brawnville Papers*. Lewis' concern with the perils of an increasingly sedentary society remains as relevant today as ever, and the alarm has again been sounded that its menace needs to be addressed: the solutions are simple [12].

Swedish Massage

Matthias Roth, George Taylor, and Charles Taylor

Swedish massage includes the application of kneading, stroking, stretching, and pressure. It was developed by the Swedish fencing instructor Per Ling (1776–1839), who combined established techniques with newly designed exercises. It is said that Ling, who was not a doctor, at first intended the exercises to remedy his stiff elbow and later for application in other diseases [13]. Ling had studied anatomy and physiology and based his massage on sound medical principles. Because he never qualified as a doctor and presented his ideas in somewhat mystical language, he was ignored by the medical profession for about 20 years. Ling was nonetheless awarded a license to practice, opened an academy in Stockholm, and successfully promulgated his methods via international lecture tours and training seminars. Ling's system became quite popular in Europe, being helped along in this process by translation of his works into English. Ling's influence is also evident in the work of Ita Wegman, who developed a modified form of rhythmical massage, partly based on Ling's methods (see Chap. 12).

As far as Britain and the United States are concerned, three physicians are of particular importance in spreading the gospel of Swedish massage: Mathias Roth and George Herbert Taylor, who were homeopaths, and George Taylor's younger brother, Charles Fayette Taylor, a non-homeopath.

Matthias Roth (1818–1891) was of Hungarian origin and settled in London, where he practiced orthopedics and homeopathy. As with Lewis in America, Roth championed the cause of physical education in British schools, claiming that without attention to physical education in the school system, the nation's health would surely deteriorate. Roth saw the benefits that came from Ling's massage and he translated one of Ling's essays into English, as well as writing his own book, *The Prevention and Cure of Many Chronic Diseases by Movements*. He became an activist for better physical health by lobbying the government, politicians, and army. He

attracted the attention of many, including the Taylor brothers, one of whom (Charles) came from the United States to train under Roth in London, while the other (George) travelled to Sweden to study at Ling's academy. Both returned to the United States, where they introduced Swedish massage in their practice and promoted its wider dissemination.

George Taylor (1821–1896) came from Williston, Vermont. As a youth, he was plagued by mysterious illnesses that were unsuccessfully treated. Taylor was self-taught and himself became a teacher at age 18, later becoming the town's school superintendent. For a period of time, he practiced hydropathic medicine and then furthered his medical studies at the New York Medical College, graduating in 1852. He entered medical practice as an allopath, but some time later, his wife fell sick with tuberculosis and was cured homeopathically by Dr. Federal Vandenburgh in Connecticut. After this experience, George Taylor was converted to homeopathy [14]. In 1858, Taylor travelled to study Swedish massage at the Royal Gymnastic Central Institute in Stockholm under Lars Branting, who had succeeded as director after the death of Per Ling. In 1860, Taylor published a book entitled *Exposition of the Swedish Movement Cure* and, over the next 30 years, at least five other books. One of these, *Diseases of Women*, extolled the virtues of mechanotherapy, or massage, for gynecological disorders and was the first book written about massage for gynecological problems [15]. Taylor also gained a reputation as a specialist in pelvic and hernia surgery and designer of exercise and mechanical massage equipment. George Taylor's views on massage and practice in general were in line with the teachings of homeopathy. He saw movement therapy as "a means of enabling the natural tendencies of the system … to act more powerfully and effectually" [16]. Taylor subscribed to the belief that with better education, patients could take more responsibility for their health, daily function, and quality of life [17].

In terms of historical attribution, it is of some interest that an editorial written in the *Journal of the American Medical Association* reported favorably on the benefits of Ling's massage and structured gymnastics yet, hewing to the allopathic line, nowhere referred to George Taylor or Dio Lewis, who introduced their techniques many years previously. Instead, the article applauded two later non-homeopaths in Germany, dating from 1876 to 1886, as though they were the first to communicate on the subject [18].

Charles Taylor (1827–1899) studied medicine at the University of Vermont and graduated in 1856. He immediately travelled to London for an instruction in Swedish massage from Matthias Roth and then returned to set up practice in New York as an orthopedic surgeon; he was the first to introduce Swedish massage to the United States. Charles remained true to the allopathic school. Although there is one reference to his being converted to homeopathy, this seems chronologically impossible, since Taylor would have been only 6 years old at the time [17]. Taylor invented various orthotics, including the Taylor Brace for spinal tuberculosis. Both he and his brother published papers and books on a variety of topics.

The brothers worked together for a time, setting up the Improved Movement Institute, where they incorporated exercise, massage, and hydrotherapy, as well as "common sense" psychotherapy [19, pp. 84–87, 20]. They were well respected, particularly among eclectic medicine circles, and attracted the patronage of celebrities such as Theodore Roosevelt, his sister Anna, and Mark Twain's wife Olivia ("Livy") Clemens. Although both Taylors have a hand in bringing about Livy's recovery, for some reason, Mark Twain gave all the credit to George [19, p. 93]. Both Taylors occupy a secure place in the popularization of Swedish massage, which remains in use today and is often referred to as therapeutic massage.

Chemistry and Administration

Ira Remsen

Ira Remsen (1846–1927) was a pioneer in chemistry and the food industry (Fig. 13.4). He began his professional life as a medical student at the New York Homeopathic Medical College, from which he graduated in 1865. Because Remsen had not yet attained the minimum age required by NYHMC as a condition of graduation, he was at first awarded only an MD degree, with the diploma to be withheld until he reached the proper age. Therefore, his name did not appear in the roster of graduates for 1863–1864, but it did appear the following year, along with mention that he had completed a graduation thesis on changes in the urine. In the college's Seventh Annual Prospectus and announcement for 1866 and 1867, Ira Remsen is listed as an assistant chemist, that is, a junior faculty member, with responsibility for the chemistry course. In 1869, the college trustees published a report from the committee of nominations who appointed three new professors, one of whom was Ira Remsen, professor of chemistry. (Although the term "professor" was used, it is likely that the position was at a more junior level comparable to an assistant or associate professor in today's academic rankings.) The report was officially accepted and confirmed, and the three new faculty members were duly elected to their positions.

From the above, it would seem clear that Remsen was a product of the homeopathic system, yet biographical accounts rarely make mention of his training at NYHMC, eliding this detail in favor of his later training at the Columbia College of Physicians and Surgeons. Remsen's own attitude to his homeopathic background was mainly one of denial, or at least minimization. In this, he was far from being alone as

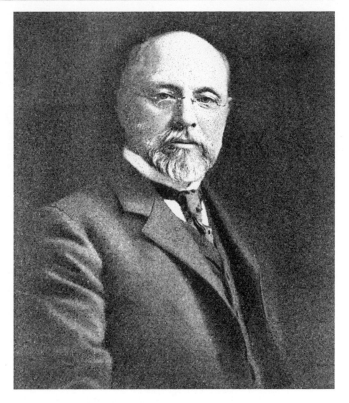

Fig. 13.4 Ira Remsen. Graduate of New York Homeopathic College and President of Johns Hopkins University (Image in the public domain. *Popular Science Monthly* 1901;(July):59)

many other onetime homeopaths renounced their medical heritage in order to gain wider acceptance. In Remsen's case, writing later, and with the benefit of half a century's reflection, he stated that while at the homeopathic college, he "became dissatisfied with the whole situation and decided to go over to the regular school" [21]. For a man of Remsen's ambition, this may not have been too surprising, given the shaky status of homeopathy. Moreover, there may have been family influences at work, since his entry into NYHMC was largely determined by Remsen's father and their family doctor, Dr. D.D. Smith, a homeopath and professor of chemistry at NYHMC. Smith was to be Remsen's preceptor, but from Remsen's account, he was not too happy with the arrangement. So as far as Remsen was concerned, in a letter written shortly before his death in 1926, he opined that "I do not know whether I am regarded as a graduate of the College or not but it is certain that I am not entitled to be so regarded." He claimed that the 1869 faculty appointment had been made while he was in Germany and that he never accepted it: "… I cannot in any sense be regarded as an early Professor of Chemistry there." Notwithstanding, in a 1916 issue of *The Chironian*, the student newspaper at NYHMC, under "Alumni Notes," the following announcement appeared: "Ira Remsen [1865 graduate], formerly Professor of Chemistry in the New York Homoeopathic Medical College in 1869, has recently resigned as president of Johns Hopkins University" [22]. Two different views prevailed. Even today, NYMC includes him in its list of distinguished alumni.

Considering late in life his connections to homeopathy, Remsen may have been colored by the exalted position which he reached in the world of regular medicine. He served as president of Johns Hopkins University which, under his leadership, set the standard for science-based and anti-sectarian medicine that swept across the United States. His vision of medical training as being heavily structured around laboratory research was a legacy of his time in Germany and fully in accord with his personal identification as a chemist rather than a clinician. With Johns Hopkins having been upheld in the Flexner Report as the model medical school, it is to be expected that Remsen would distance himself from any personal association with homeopathy. However, all was not ideal at Hopkins, and Sir William Osler, one of Johns Hopkins' most distinguished faculty, wrote a critical letter to Remsen on September 1, 1911, taking him to task both for Flexner's biased and incomplete presentation of their institution and more generally for the kind of medicine that Remsen stood for. It was Osler's fear that a medical school dominated by research and laboratory science would lead to the production of "clinical prigs, the boundary of whose horizon would be the laboratory, and whose only interest in human research" [23].

In 1884, Remsen was asked by the National Board of Health to investigate the best method of determining the character and amount of organic matter in the air, as well as researching the amount of "carbonic oxide" in furnace-heated rooms [24]. (As noted elsewhere, Tullio Verdi, another homeopath, served on this committee.)

Remsen achieved fame as the lead discoverer of saccharin in 1878, although he was excluded from the patent by his opportunistic Russian graduate student, Constantin Fahlberg, who presented himself as the sole discoverer. Remsen was displeased but did not challenge Fahlberg on the matter. In 1908, Remsen was appointed by President Theodore Roosevelt to chair a committee that addressed questions of food safety. This position was offered to Remsen in the wake of the 1906 Pure Food and Drug Act (PFDA), once it had become apparent that the latest scientific evidence should be considered in implementing the PFDA. Specifically, the pressing question at the time was whether sulfur dioxide and sodium benzoate were safe food preservatives. In 1909, the "Remsen Board" as it was known issued a report affirming the safety of these two preservatives, which set off a heated debate between those who supported the committee's ruling and those opposed to it, led by Harvey Wiley, chief chemist at the Department of Agriculture. Later, President Woodrow Wilson took a critical stance against the Remsen Board, largely for political reasons. Despite Wilson's opposition to benzoate, it has stood the test of time and remains in use today in some foods and drinks [25].

The board also ruled on the safety of saccharin after Harvey Wiley's Bureau of Chemistry had tried to impose a ban on the grounds that it was an adulterant. Wiley's challenge drew a testy reaction from Roosevelt, who enjoyed his daily saccharin [26].

Ira Remsen was appointed professor and chair of chemistry at Johns Hopkins in 1876 and later became president of the institution in 1901, a position he held until ill health forced his retirement in 1912. In 1879, he founded the *American Chemical Journal* and authored many papers and three textbooks, *Inorganic Chemistry*, *Organic Chemistry,* and *Theoretical Chemistry,* which remained standard for several years. He received numerous awards and honorary degrees from Europe and the United States, including the Priestley Medal, the American Chemical Society's highest award.

Pediatrics

Carl Fischer

Carl Fischer (1902–1989) graduated from Hahnemann in 1928 and went on to specialize in pediatrics, becoming departmental chairman and professor at his alma mater (Fig. 13.5). During 1961–1962, he served as president of the American Academy of Pediatrics. Fischer was the last of Hahnemann's "old guard" to retain departmental leadership, retiring in 1968. According to Barbara Williams [27], he was open-minded about homeopathy, telling her that "[at Hahnemann] we had the best of both worlds, could use whichever we needed, when we needed it."

Fischer's presidency of the academy took place in the wake of recommendations made by the reorganization committee in 1961. One outcome of this reorganization was the establishment of a committee on the infant and preschool child, which tackled the growing problem of child abuse, and resulted 5 years later in a report. Fischer issued a call to fellows of the academy to become involved in the ongoing legislation proposed by President John F. Kennedy, which addressed three issues concerning pediatrics: universal immunization, the creation of a separate child and developmental institute at the National Institutes of Health, and provision of improved services for those with mental retardation [28]. In the early 1960s, the academy, which had primarily been an organization of scholars, was threatened with a split among its members over the extent to which it should be involved in social and legislative aspects of pediatrics, a cause which was close to Carl Fischer's heart. The academy was able to avoid fragmentation and thereafter embraced social and legislative activities with more vigor, while still preserving its principal mission as a scientific and educational organization, rather than a guild or political body [29].

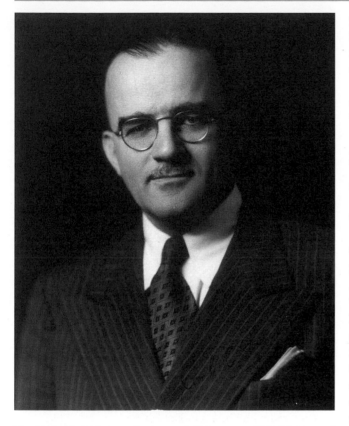

Fig. 13.5 Carl Fischer. Graduate of Hahnemann, Philadelphia, and president of American Academy of Pediatrics (Image courtesy of National Library of Medicine, in the public domain)

Shortly after the end of Fischer's term, a meeting took place between senior officials of the academy (including Fischer) and the secretary of the Department of Health, Education, and Welfare, the surgeon-general, and other government leaders. This meeting was important as it began a process of dialog between the academy and government, as well as heightening awareness within government of the academy's concerns.

Fischer authored a book on the physician's role in environmental pediatrics [30], in which he stressed that the physician had a broader responsibility than to the individual child's health, extending to the child as a member of the community and society. Chapters covered topics such as adoptions, accidents, adolescence, the handicapped, and school health. Fischer concluded with a call for the pediatrician to dedicate himself/herself to this newer concept of pediatrics. He had for some years been active in the local tri-county adoption program and the Pennsylvania State Governor's Committees on Children and Youth and on Handicapped Children. These experiences lead him to recognize that physicians too often steered clear of social and community aspects of pediatrics because they had not been adequately trained. To remedy this deficiency, he introduced a didactic course at Hahnemann and wrote the aforementioned book. Fischer continued to

publish in the homeopathic literature for many years, including papers on the thymus gland in infancy, a study of modern infant feeding trends, and the biochemistry of pediatric disorders [31–33].

Fischer was honored at Hahnemann in 1980 by its naming of the Carl C. Fischer, M.D. Neonatal Intensive Care Unit at the Hahnemann University Hospital.

The First Native American Indian in Modern Medicine

Charles Eastman

Charles Eastman (1858–1939) was a Native American Indian member of the Santee Sioux (Fig. 13.6). His birth name was Hadakh, which means "pitiful last," in recognition of the fact that Eastman's mother had died in giving birth. When, at a later date, Hadakh led his tribal lacrosse team to victory against another Indian tribe, his grandmother changed his name to Ohiyesa, or "the winner." At the urging of his father, Ohiyesa adopted the name by which he is widely known: Charles Eastman. Eastman aspired to great things and entered Dartmouth University, graduating in 1887. His undergraduate years were filled with athletic and academic success, and the university has perpetuated his name in the Chavez-Eastman-Marshall Dissertation Fellowship, awarded annually to promising students from underrepresented minority groups who have ambitions to pursue an academic life at Dartmouth. From there, he went on to medical school at BUSM, becoming in 1890 the first Native American Indian to obtain a regular medical degree. At BUSM, he distinguished himself and was selected by his classmates to present the graduation address, for which he chose the topic *The Comparative History of the Art of Healing*.

In October 1890, he took up medical duties on the Pine Ridge reservation in South Dakota. One of his first actions was to tighten up the clinic's practices by putting an end to the reckless way in which medicines have been dispensed and to conduct thorough physical examinations. He gained the respect of tribal healers, even though the form of medicine he practiced was not based on Indian tradition [34]. There is no evidence one way or the other as to whether he prescribed homeopathic remedies. At Pine Ridge, Eastman dispensed cod liver oil and alcohol mixtures and the salves, ointments, and cough syrups that the Indians favored. He also abolished the custom in which previous doctors have given medicine through a small portal in the wall without even seeing the patient, who had usually self-diagnosed their problem. Eastman insisted on an examination first. At Pine Ridge, Eastman instituted a number of important public health measures, including the removal of decaying animal carcasses from the streets, quarantining Indians when they

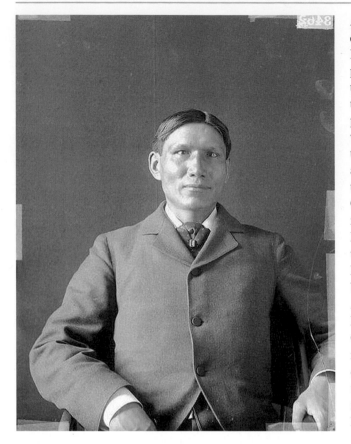

Fig. 13.6 Charles Eastman, first Native American to graduate from a US medical school (Image from Smithsonian Institute, in the public domain)

returned from tours to Europe, and improving living conditions in the overcrowded Indian school dormitories [35].

Eastman and his fiancée, Elaine Goodale, were present at the Wounded Knee Massacre, which took place December 28, 1890. Three hundred Indians were killed in a matter of minutes, as well as a number of US Seventh Cavalry troops. Eastman rode out to the snow-covered battlefield to recover the bodies and transported survivors to his hospital, where he treated Indians and cavalry alike. He also solicited food and clothing from Boston.

Eastman grew increasingly disenchanted with government corruption, found himself in conflict with authorities, and in 1891 left the Bureau of Indian Affairs. With his wife, Elaine, they moved to St. Paul to set up private practice. Business was slow, but while there, he became involved in the YMCA, organizing regional chapters for Indian youth. This was the start of a life of public service and lobbying that required extensive travelling and public speaking. Around 1910, Eastman played a leading part in formation of the Boy Scouts of America.

In 1897, Eastman began to lobby for Indian rights in Washington, DC. He spent years attempting to settle claims and treaty payments that have been promised to the Sioux.

Although these initial efforts bore little success, they did earn for Eastman a reputation as one of the most influential Indians in the white world. He later returned to medical practice in the Indian Service and embarked on a productive writing career about his life, Indian health, and education. In this, he was greatly encouraged by his wife, who played a seminal role – indeed, she contributed much of the writing herself. In 1903, President Roosevelt assigned him to help Sioux members regain or retain their allotted lands, and under President Coolidge, he was a US Indian inspector. Coolidge invited Eastman to serve on the Committee of One Hundred, a reform panel created to recommend on matters of health, civil rights, justice, and schools for Indians. The deliberations of this committee gave rise to the Meriam Report, which in turn was an anchor of Franklin Roosevelt's New Deal for the Indian. Among the honors bestowed on Eastman were invitations to represent the American Indian at the First World Races Congress in England in 1911 and again to speak in England at Oxford, Cambridge, and other universities in 1927. In 1933, he received the medal of the Indian Council Fire for the most distinguished achievement by an American Indian. Towards the end of his life, Eastman retired to the Canadian wilderness and once again took up the practice of medicine when he wintered with his son in Detroit.

Eastman has been misunderstood by some who have tended to view him pejoratively as an "apple," that is, red on the outside and white on the inside, and thus traitorous to the Indian cause, but this is far from the case. He was fully dedicated to rights and justice for his people, but could only do so much against a government that at best was ambivalent towards the American Indian. Milroy commented that Eastman had "the courage to accept new challenges and the determination to advance to successive heights of achievement" [36]. In similar vein, Graves wrote that "Dr, Charles Eastman … worked first to improve himself, something he did not least during his years at the Boston University School of Medicine, then to improve the condition of his people…. Though accomplishing less than he hoped, through a lifetime of disappointments Charles Eastman persisted in faith and works. One feels he represents a kind of success not measured by the common gauges" [37].

Pathology

Edward Cronin Lowe

Edward Cronin Lowe (1880–1958) was born in New Zealand and trained in London at Guy's Hospital, receiving his MD degree in 1905. He subsequently obtained homeopathic training and became a member of the British

Homoeopathic Society, taking up appointments as consultant pathologist at the Liverpool Homeopathic Hospital and the Southport Infirmary. Rather unusually, Lowe was able to blend homeopathic and allopathic identities together. For example, he sponsored the homeopathic Anglo-French homeopathic war hospital at Neuilly-sur-Seine in World War I and was later chair of the Southport division of the British Medical Association and its representative at two national meetings.

During World War I, he served as a captain in the New Zealand Expeditionary Force and was recognized with the award on an MBE (Member of the British Empire) medal for his work in reducing the toll of influenza. Lowe and his colleague John Eyre conducted an immunization program for New Zealand servicemen, by means of a compounded mixed catarrhal vaccine (MCV) which contained seven bacteria responsible for respiratory infections and reported their work in two Lancet publications. Their 1918 publication represented the first long-term observations of the effects of MCV in military personnel and demonstrated a much lower incidence of influenza in those who received inoculation [38]. A second article in 1919 presented a follow-up of the cohort through the ensuing influenza epidemic later that year: the results again showed lower morbidity and mortality in those who had been inoculated [39].

For many years, Lowe was known in British medicine as an authority on vaccines and published repeatedly in leading journals such as the *British Medical* and *British Dental Journals*. His work in cancer detection was less successful as he attempted to refine a diagnostic test which was in use. Lowe was known for pioneering contributions to blood transfusions. Although one source credits him with "inventing the concept of the blood bank" [40], this is not corroborated in any of the main historical accounts of the bank. Nevertheless, in an obituary, the *British Medical Journal* does credit Lowe in the following way: "In the early days of blood transfusion Dr. Cronin Lowe was the first man in the district to type donors and recipients and carry out transfusions in suitable cases" [41]. The obituary was fulsome in its praise, describing Lowe's personality as "vivid and lovable" and noting that Lowe was "an indefatigable research worker, always feeling for a deeper and wider understanding of disease and not afraid of being unorthodox." It observed that Lowe's MBE (Member of the British Empire) award was given for achievements in the 1918 influenza epidemic, and that his work on pathogen selection for vaccine preparation and creation of oral vaccines was well known. The obituary concluded that Lowe was deeply religious and actively involved in foreign missions: a significant reminder of family tradition, for Lowe's grandfather, *Edward Cronin* (1801–1882), a homeopath and medical missionary, was one of four founders of the Plymouth Brethren religious movement.

References

1. Okrent D. Last call: the rise and fall of prohibition. New York: Scribners; 2010. p. 13.
2. Eastman MF. The Biography of Dio Lewis, A.M., M.D. [Internet]. New York: Fowler & Wells Co; 1891 [Cited 2012 Mar 13]. Available from: http://books.google.com/books?id=J67qXsLvJOQC&pg=PA 1&img=1&zoom=3&hl=en&sig=ACfU3U1NfzNLTok0T81GB 5VD_lVzey0mkg&ci=512%2C19%2C439%2C724&edge=0
3. Fletcher DM. The pioneer of genteel gymnastics for ladies [Internet]. Sports Illustrated. 8 Mar 1965 [Cited 2012 Aug 23]. Available from: http://sportsillustrated.cnn.com/vault/article/magazine/MAG1076988/2/index.htm.
4. Blocker JS. "Lewis, Diocletian." [Internet]. American National Biography Online. Feb 2000 [Cited 2012 Mar 13]. Available from: http://www.anb.org/articles/15/15/-00410.html.
5. Vest EB. When Dio Lewis came to Dixon. J Illinois State Historical Society (1908–1984). 1947;40:298–312.
6. Women's Christian Temperance Union: welcome to the WCTU [Internet]. 20 Oct 2011 [Cited 2012 Mar 13]. Available from: http://www.wctu.org/.
7. Welch P. Dio Lewis' Normal Institute for Physical Education. J Phys Educ Dance. 1994;65:29–31.
8. Leonard FE. The 'new gymnastics' of Dio Lewis (1860–1868). Am Phys Educ Rev. 1906;11:87–90.
9. Barney RK. A historical reinterpretation of the forces underlying the first state legislation for physical education in the public schools of the U.S. Res Q. 1973;44:357–9.
10. Barney RK. Adele Parot: Beacon of the Dioclesian Lewis School of Gymnastic Expression in the American West. Can J Hist Sport. 1974;5(2):63–75.
11. Higginson TW. Gymnastics. The Atlantic Monthly. 1861;March:300. Cited in Welch, 1994.
12. Levine J. Move a little: lose a lot. New York: Three Rivers Press; 2009.
13. Swedish massage [Internet]. Fine Balance Bodyworks 2008 [Cited 2012 Mar 13]. Available from: http://www.finebalancebodyworks.com/swedish.html.
14. Young S. The Taylor surname and homeopathy [Internet]. 2008 [Cited 2012 Mar 13]. Available from: http://sueyounghistories.com/archives/2008/10/08/mathias-roth-1818-1891/.
15. Rutkow IM. The history of surgery in the United States 1775–1900, vol. 1. San Francisco: Norman Publishing; 1988. p. 301.
16. Taylor GH. Exposition of the Swedish Movement Cure. New York: S.R. Wells and Company; 1876. p. 29.
17. Haller Jr JS. The history of American Homeopathy: the academic years, 1820–1935. New York: Pharmaceutical Products Press: The Haworth Press; 2005. p. 48.
18. Editorial. Massage and methodical exercise. J Am Med Assoc. 1887;IX:529–31.
19. Skandera-Trombley LE. Mark Twain in the company of women. Philadelphia: University of Pennsylvania Press; 1994.
20. Slater L. The Taylor brothers bring massage to the USA [Internet]. 3 Apr 2011 [Cited 2012 Mar 14]. Available from: http://www.articlesbase.com/alternative-medicine-articles/the-taylor-brothers-bring-massage-to-the-usa-4529119.html.
21. Wershub LP. One hundred years of medical progress: a history of the New York Medical College, Flower and Fifth Avenue Hospitals. Springfield: Charles C. Thomas Publisher; 1967. p. 57.
22. Alumni notes. The Chironian. 1916;32:205.
23. Men and Books. Sir William Osler on full-time clinical teaching in medical schools. Can Med Assoc J. 1962;87:762–5.
24. Anonymous. Annual Report of the National Board of Health for the Year 1884. Washington: Government Printing Office; 1885. p. 13–4.
25. Jones R. Food safety and JHU's Second President. [Internet]. E-Libris. Sheridan Libraries of Johns Hopkins University. 18 Jun

2011 [Cited 2012 Jul 1]. Available from: http://elibris.jhu.edu/2011/01/18/food-safety-and-jhus-second-president/.

26. Merrill RA, Francer JK. Organizing federal food safety regulation. Seton Hall Law Rev. 2011;31:61–113.

27. Barbara Williams. Personal communication to author. 14 Sept 2011.

28. Fischer CC. President's message: President John F. Kennedy's health message to the congress. Pediatrics. 1962;30:157–8.

29. Hughes JG. American Academy of Pediatrics: the first fifty years. Evanston: American Academy of Pediatrics; 1980.

30. Fischer CC. Role of the physician in environmental pediatrics. New York: Landsberger Medical Books; 1960.

31. Raue CS, Fischer CC. The thymus gland in infancy. J Am Inst Homeopath. 1931;24:541–2.

32. Fischer CC. A study of the modern trend in infant feeding. J Am Inst Homeopath. 1931;24:1056–9.

33. Fischer CC. The bio-chemistry of disorders of children. J Am Inst Homeopath. 1936;29:76–8.

34. Eshman R. Stranger in the land. Dartmouth Alumni Magazine. 1981;Jan-Feb:20–3.

35. Steele VW. Charles Alexander Eastman, M, D. (Ohiyesa): a Sioux physician between two worlds. J West. 2007;46:40–9.

36. Milroy TW. A physician by the name of Ohiyesa. Minn Med. 1971;5:569–72.

37. Graves J. Ohiyesa. Bostonia. 1993;Spring:50–4.

38. Eyre JWH, Lowe CE. Prophylactic vaccinations against catarrhal affections of the respiratory tract. Lancet. 1918;2:484–7.

39. Eyre JWH, Lowe EC. Report upon the autumn influenza epidemic (1918) as it affected the N.Z.E.F. in the United Kingdom. Lancet. 1919;2:553–60.

40. Foreman L. Richard Arnell Obituary. [Internet]. The Independent. [Cited 2013 Apr 18]. Available from: http://www.independent.co.uk.

41. Obituary. E, Cronin Lowe, MBE, MB, BS. Br Med J. 1958;1:1126–7.

Royal Copeland observed that a healthy society depends on the good health of its leaders. One might take Copeland's quip further and stress that public health measures and legislation on the part of these leaders can promote health and well-being of the entire population.

Three homeopaths have provided medical care to US presidents, one of whom, Susan Edson, has been described in the section on women in homeopathy (Chap. 3). The others were Charles Sawyer and Joel Boone. Willis Danforth treated Mary Todd Lincoln following her husband's death. Sir John Weir set an unparalleled record of personal care to seven European monarchs. Royal Copeland, Jacob Gallinger, and Dickson Mabon have left their mark as elected politicians, and their accomplishments will be outlined.

that coordinated under one structure in the different federal hospital systems: Army, Navy, Public Health Service, Interior Department, Veterans' Bureau, Office of Indian Affairs, and St. Elizabeth's Hospital. The board was to function in an advisory capacity to the president, and its tasks included the initiation of studies to analyze and review activities and programs operated by these agencies, to determine need for existing or additional facilities and their locations, and to prevent unnecessary duplication of services. Interestingly, 5 of 16 persons at the initial planning meeting

Charles E. Sawyer

President Warren Harding is regarded by historians as one of the worst American presidents, mainly because of the extensive corruption and cronyism that characterized his administration. One of the beneficiaries of this cronyism was Dr. Charles Sawyer (1860–1924), homeopathic physician to the First Lady, Mrs. Florence Harding (Fig. 14.1). Sawyer had for many years been her personal doctor, and a strong bond was created between them. When Harding was elected president, his wife insisted on appointing Dr. Sawyer as the White House physician. Harding needed no convincing because his parents had been homeopathic practitioners, but to secure the appointment, incentives were offered, as it would require Sawyer to relinquish a lucrative practice in Marion, Ohio. These incentives came in the form of military appointment as Brigadier-General in the Army Medical Corps Reserve and as chairman of the soon-to-be-created Federal Hospitalization Board. Of the former, the diminutive Sawyer cut a comic figure riding the large cavalry horse that accompanied the position, and he has been called "the suddenest Brigadier-General in US History" [1]. Of the latter, the Federal Board was to become an influential body

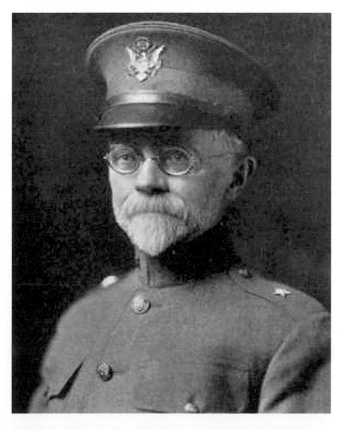

Fig. 14.1 Charles Sawyer. Presidential physician to Warren Harding (Image courtesy of Sylvain Cazalet, Homeopathe International, Montpellier, France)

J. Davidson, *A Century of Homeopaths*,
DOI 10.1007/978-1-4939-0527-0_14, © Springer Science+Business Media New York 2014

were homeopaths, as was one of the three members of the executive planning committee formed to implement the board [2].

Sawyer had built a reputation as a medical entrepreneur and respected homeopath. He originally qualified as a doctor in 1881 at the Cleveland Homeopathic Medical College and set up practice in Ohio. He became chairman of the American Homeopathic Surgical and Gynecological Association and president of the American Institute of Homeopathy. His diminutive 5 ft, 100 lb frame belied a man of ambition and entrepreneurial talent, which came to fruition in 1895 when he established the Sawyer Sanitarium for nervous dysfunctions in Marion. This facility grew into a substantial enterprise on 100 acres of land and became so well known that a special railroad spur was constructed to bring patients from all over the United States directly to the hospital. By 1900, Sawyer was prospering and his practice was organized with a capital stock of $450,000. With his psychiatrist son, Carl, the two men ran the sanitarium until Charles' death in 1924, and his son kept it going into the 1950s.

Sawyer came to the Hardings' attention in 1897 when he rescued the future president's mother, Mrs. Phoebe Harding, from a tricky professional situation. In her homeopathic practice, Mrs. Harding lost one of her patients allegedly because of malpractice. Dr. Sawyer was called to consult on the case, which he judged to have been managed appropriately, thus preserving Mrs. Harding's professional reputation. Thereafter, the Hardings and Sawyers became personal friends, and Dr. Sawyer was engaged as Mrs. Florence Harding's doctor. Florence Harding had chronic kidney disease resulting in a nephrectomy in 1905, and she became very dependent on Dr. Sawyer, convinced that only he could keep her alive. It was in the context of this background that Charles Sawyer found his way into the White House, and he was not shy to capitalize on such good fortune. (Later, when Sawyer was the official White House doctor, he stood fast against the opinions of two specialists who have been called in when Florence Harding was seriously ill. The specialists recommended removal of her one remaining kidney, which Sawyer stubbornly opposed, a judgment which turned out to be correct as Mrs. Harding recovered from her illness.)

Sawyer's record as chief coordinator of the Federal Board of Hospitalization was not particularly distinguished, but neither was it marred by incompetence nor scandal, in itself a stellar achievement given what we know about other Harding cronies. At its inception, the board was responsible for programs affecting 99 hospitals that provided 28,412 beds. In his 1922 report to the director of the US Budget Bureau, Sawyer referred to the painstaking work that went into setting up the program, and he mentioned that a major conference of government hospital commanders had produced "unanimity of purpose which has been of incomparable value to the operation of hospitals under Government control" [3]. The board also developed a standardized building plan for government hospitals and recommended the creation of postgraduate schools at St. Elizabeth's and other government hospitals.

A much more serious problem arose, one which demanded action by Sawyer. Director of the Veterans Bureau, Colonel Charles Forbes, was rumored to be embezzling millions of dollars, diverting hospital supplies intended for VA hospitals and receiving kickbacks from contractors, making land deals and denying huge numbers of disability claims from World War I veterans [4, pp. 554–557]. Sawyer investigated further and found there to be truth in these rumors. Unable to keep silent, he passed on his findings to Harding, who ordered Forbes to stop selling hospital equipment. This he refused to do, so Harding demanded Forbes' resignation. Forbes escaped to Europe for a time but returned to the United States, where he ultimately stood trial, was found guilty of defrauding the US government, and sent to jail [4, p. 629].

While the board fulfilled its charge during Sawyer's tenure, he was caught up in a public feud with Forbes, which antagonized the American Legion, who considered Forbes to be their advocate and saw Sawyer as obstructive of veterans' welfare, particularly those with "shell shock." However, Sawyer proved to be right in his handling of Forbes' indiscretions, and the removal of Forbes was obviously necessary to advance the welfare of veterans and the board's function. It was perhaps a good thing that Sawyer was a "thorn in the flesh" of the VA Bureau director [5].

Although Sawyer's term as chairman of Federal Board of Hospitalization lasted only a short time, over the course of its life, the board was considered to have "successfully accomplished the coordination of the peacetime responsibilities of the Federal Government" [6], and he played an important role in shepherding the board's transition from idea to reality. Sawyer was succeeded by the capable General Frank Hines, who accomplished much as leader of the board. After Harding's death, Sawyer's health declined, but he remained for a while as physician to President Coolidge, before resigning in June 1924. He then returned to Marion, where he lived for another few months, before dying in September 1924, shortly before his patient Florence Harding died.

Joel Boone

Joel Boone (1889–1974) came from a Quaker background, lost his mother to cervical cancer when he was 11, and was raised by his father and stepmother (Fig. 14.2). His childhood was one of hard labor and long days, as he was required to assist in running the family hay and grain business. His father was a heavy drinker and circumstances were not particularly happy. Fortunately for Boone, he was being sent to an excellent boarding school, which prepared him for entry

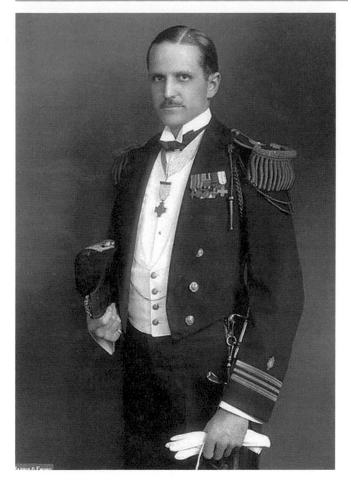

Fig. 14.2 Joel Boone. Physician to four presidents; director of the Veterans Administration (By courtesy National Library of Medicine. Image in the public domain)

into medical school. He was influenced in this decision by his uncle, Dr. George Boone, a homeopathic family doctor in rural Pennsylvania, who permitted young Joel to accompany him on his rounds.

Boone was accepted into Hahnemann Medical College in Philadelphia and graduated in 1913, going on to complete a 1-year internship there. He remained proud of his homeopathic training throughout his life and referred to it as an enhanced form of medical training that provided additional therapeutic options to doctors [7]. In 1914, Boone enlisted in the US Navy and began a career that brought great distinction, studded with bravery in war. Initially, Lieutenant Boone was assigned to Haiti as part of a Marine peace mission. Upon the outbreak of war, Boone was made assistant regimental surgeon to the Sixth Marine Regiment in France, a new experience for a homeopathic doctor, as homeopaths have previously been excluded from military medical practice. In 1918, President Woodrow Wilson awarded Boone the Congressional Medal of Honor for bravery in aiding wounded marines under enemy fire in the open field – something of a

rarity for a naval officer serving in the World War I trenches. In 1920, Franklin Roosevelt, as Secretary of the Navy, pinned on Boone the second of Boone's two *Croix de Guerres*. In 1931, French Marshal Pétain sent Boone a *Légion d'honneur* medal for bravery in France, although official acceptance of this medal had to await congressional approval, which was finally granted during the Eisenhower years. Boone was "reputed to have won more decorations, while serving with the Marines, than any other medical officer" [8].

In 1920, Joel Boone and his wife Helen received an invitation to the White House, where Mrs. Florence Harding, the president's wife, offered them tea. At the time, Boone had no idea why they had been invited, thinking perhaps it had to do either with his wartime distinctions or because of his friendship with the head of the Navy's Medical Corps. As it turned out, President Warren Harding had asked his wife to research Boone as a potential physician to *Mayflower*, the presidential yacht [9, p. 32]. This appointment required the incumbent to provide medical care to the ship's crew and to the president and First Lady when they were on board. Mrs. Harding, whose medical problems were documented previously, took a liking to Boone and would periodically request his presence at the White House for consultations. This eventually led to Boone's formal appointment as Assistant White House Physician [10].

Much has been said and disputed about the circumstances of President Harding's death while on a campaign trip in San Francisco. His senior doctor, Charles Sawyer, claimed it was due to food poisoning, a view not shared by any of the other doctors in his team. Dr. Boone had conducted a physical examination a few days before Harding died and found evidence of ventricular hypertrophy, or enlargement of the heart, which would point to heart failure as a likely diagnosis. Because Boone was the junior member of the medical team, he did not press his disagreements too strongly, although he did share with Sawyer what he found [9, p. 62]. However, Boone was determined not to remain a passive onlooker, so he separately appealed to Secretary of Commerce Herbert Hoover to request the consultation from Dr. Ray Wilbur, president of Stanford University, and another eminent local cardiologist, when Harding arrived in San Francisco. This was all to no avail as Harding died shortly afterwards, and without a postmortem, the exact facts of his case will never be known.

Although Boone and Sawyer were both homeopaths, little love was lost between them due largely to Sawyer's resentment of Boone's presence in the White House. Sawyer tried to insist that Boone should never treat the president without his knowledge, although Boone's response was typically to let Sawyer know that he viewed Harding as his commander-in-chief and thus gave higher priority to Harding's requests than to those of Sawyer. When Coolidge assumed the presidency, Boone was chagrined to learn that another physician,

James Coupal, was appointed as senior physician, with Boone continuing on as assistant. It did not help that Boone considered Coupal to be of inferior ability. This team of physicians provided care to the Coolidge family throughout the president's terms in office, and they dealt with the tragic death of the Coolidges' 16-year-old son. Drs. Boone and Coupal had to treat a chronic and incapacitating depression on the part of the president. Although the doctors did recognize Coolidge's changed behavior and hypochondriacal ways, they seemed unable to penetrate this illness, which ultimately caused Coolidge to stand down from office after his first full term. It is not known what treatments they recommended, but according to Ullman, when Coupal and Boone recommended different therapies, Coolidge favored Boone, saying that he knew best. Ullman went on to provide evidence that Boone used homeopathy in his practice, even though official reports were silent on the matter [11].

Following the Coolidge administration, Boone continued to serve the next president, Herbert Hoover, as principal medical officer. One of his chief accomplishments was to motivate Hoover to take up regular exercise with a medicine ball, so that he lost weight and became fitter. When Franklin Roosevelt was elected president in 1933, Boone was not retained, even though they had enjoyed cordial relations going back to the time of his *Croix de Guerre* award. After a few weeks as caretaker physician in the Roosevelt White House, Boone left service as presidential physician, having been intimately involved in delivering healthcare to three presidents over an 11-year period.

Boone's legacy as White House physician has been recognized by one of his successors, Dr. Connie Mariano, doctor to President Clinton. Mariano acknowledged that Boone (and Hoover) were first to obtain official recognition of the position and title of Physician to the White House through congressional legislation (Public Law 89–71 Congress (S. 2515)), which by statute established the office. This physician not only was responsible for care of the first family but also became director of the White House Medical Unit, an organization that has now grown far beyond anything Boone might have envisioned. Boone also was first to secure adequate office space in the White House to discharge the duties of presidential doctor. To Boone goes the credit for bringing an appropriate level of stature to the position of presidential doctor.

Important as his accomplishments were in respect to presidential care, Boone distinguished himself on a broader stage. Following his departure from the Roosevelt White House, Boone returned to regular naval duties. During the 1930s, he spent most of the time on the Pacific coast, responsible for medical aspects of amphibious landings [9, p. 157]. As World War II was drawing to a close and before the Japanese surrender, Boone was the first to land in the Tokyo Bay area to rescue allied prisoners, and he represented the Navy Medical Corps on the deck of the USS *Missouri* at the signing of the Japanese surrender [9, p. 165].

After World War II, new opportunities beckoned for Rear-Admiral Joel Boone. In 1946, President Truman authorized his secretary of the interior to take over the bituminous coal industry after a series of damaging strikes. Boone was to serve as medical adviser to the Federal Coal Mines Administration and direct a medical survey of the coal industry, focusing on hospital and community facilities and housing in the nation's coal mining regions. Having grown up in the anthracite mining area of Pennsylvania, and being somewhat familiar with the mining culture, Boone was a suitable choice for this role. The health and welfare of the country's coal miners had become a matter of considerable controversy and many mines had been taken over from private ownership by the government after crippling industrial action had threatened to affect the country's coal supply. Fourteen percent of mines in government custody were sampled, employing over 70,000 miners. The report received good marks for being impartial yet not holding back its punches and has been hailed by many as furthering miners' health. It found important deficiencies in about 75 % of hospitals and noted many homes to be substandard. The Boone Report was critical of the contract system in use for healthcare delivery, which was regarded as deplorable and prone to abuse. Initially, the report was suppressed until the United Mine Workers forced its release [12]. Arising from the committee's recommendations was the creation of 10 new hospitals and recruitment incentives for doctors to work in mining communities. Also created were a group practice structure, a new emphasis on rehabilitation medicine, a coordinating role of the physician as overseer of all aspects of medical care and introduction of the idea of "fee for time" rather than "fee for service." The report provided a road map for the newly created United Mine Workers' Association Fund to reform its healthcare program [13].

Not long after the completion of his report, Boone was again called upon by the federal government, this time to serve as executive secretary to a committee on Medical and Hospital Services of the Armed Forces. He was also under consideration for the post of surgeon-general, although this went to a younger candidate, but Boone had the backing of three four-star generals. He did not regret the outcome since it enabled him to accept the position of medical director of the Veterans Administration after he retired from the Navy in 1950. He served in this position for 4 years until ill health forced him to finally retire from all government service, at the rank of vice-admiral in 1955. For the remaining years of his long life, he wrote his memoirs. Six years after his death, the Navy honored Rear-Admiral Boone by naming a guided missile frigate after him, the *USS Boone*, a ship that was in active service between 1980 and 2010 (Fig. 14.3). His name is also perpetuated at the Admiral Joel T. Boone Branch Health Clinic at Joint Expeditionary Base in Virginia Beach, VA.

Fig. 14.3 USS Boone. Exercise "Trial Spartan Hammer 2006." NATO archive (Image by permission of NATO)

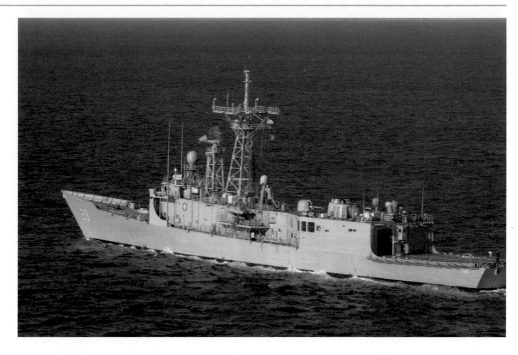

Willis Danforth

Willis Danforth (1826–1891) received his training from Rock Island Medical College, graduating in 1850. Ten years later, after having been successfully treated with homeopathy for resistant sciatica, he converted to homeopathy. His practice encompassed surgery, at which he was described as "safe and careful, though bold and fearless when there is occasion for the exhibition of such qualities" [14]. Danforth served as a cavalry captain, surgeon, and then medical director of the state of Kentucky during the Civil War. He later became professor of surgery at Hahnemann Medical College in Chicago. His claim to fame rests on the fact that for a period of time he was the personal physician to Mary Todd Lincoln during her time in Chicago. He played a critical role in the legal determination of Mrs. Lincoln's insanity. At her commitment hearing in 1875, Danforth gave testimony to her insanity, backing up this opinion with findings that Mrs. Lincoln was "possessed with the idea that some one was working on her head, taking wires out of her eyes … at times taking bones out of her cheeks and face, and detaching steel springs from her jaw bones … at other times she imagines that her scalp was being lifted by the same invisible power and placed back again." As the only one of several testifying experts who had actually examined Mrs. Lincoln, his words carried weight and helped jurors decide that she was incompetent to handle her financial affairs. It is also of interest that after the trial Danforth conveyed privately to a juror his belief that Mrs. Lincoln was not suffering from a primary psychological disorder but a disease of the brain, such as syphilis [15]. Whether or not Danforth was right, there is no question that unimaginable grief was a major factor behind the former First Lady's mental afflictions at this time, for by then she had lost three young sons to diphtheria, typhus, and tuberculosis and a husband to an assassin's bullet.

Six revealing letters to Danforth from Mrs. Lincoln and one from her son, Robert, came to light after a period of 117 years. In one letter, Mrs. Lincoln wrote that her problem was caused by addiction to chloral hydrate. In another, she begged Danforth to prescribe more powders for her constant nocturnal wakefulness. In a particularly poignant letter, written just before her first insanity hearing, she wrote to Danforth detailing her funeral instructions. Mrs. Lincoln was committed to a psychiatric facility in Chicago for a period of 3 months. At a second hearing in 1876, she was judged to have recovered and accordingly released from hospital [16].

In 1879, Danforth and his family abruptly left Chicago for Milwaukee, where he subsequently gained local prominence and was elected president of the Wisconsin Homeopathic Society. He died from complications of a fall in 1891 and was described in his obituary as "an ardent champion of homeopathy, capable surgeon, [an] opponent of bacteriology and relentless foe of quackery" [17].

John Weir: The Monarch's Doctor

John Weir (1879–1971) was a dominant figure in British homeopathy throughout the twentieth century. While he cannot be regarded as having contributed greatly to medicine (with one notable exception described later), his political skill and personal qualities led to an unmatched degree of royal patronage. He held appointments as Physician Royal to Edward VII, George V, Edward VIII, George VI, Gustav V (of Sweden), and Haakon VII (of Norway). In addition, Weir was physician to Queen Elizabeth II and her royal household, as well as to Queen Maud of Norway. Weir received multiple decorations and, in 1932, a knighthood. In 1949 he was awarded the Royal Victorian Chain from King George VI for "long and distinguished personal services" [18] and became only the twelfth living holder of this rarely bestowed decoration, whose other holders included the Archbishop of Canterbury, the king and queen, Queen Mary, and the Duke of Windsor. For service to the Norwegian King, in 1939 Weir was awarded the country's top honor, Knight Grand Cross of the Royal Order of St. Olav [19].

According to Julian Winston, Weir prescribed *ignatia* to five kings and three queens who were all attending the funeral of King George VI in 1952 [20]. Ignatia is often given as a remedy to cope with grief, and we can only suppose that Weir considered the level of grief in these eight sovereigns to be sufficiently painful to justify its use.

Weir and the cause of homeopathy were held in high approval by his royal patients. King George VI, for example, named one of his racehorses after the homeopathic remedy, *Hypericum*, and Queen Elizabeth II, when visiting the homeopathic hospital in London, looked directly at the portrait of Weir and declared that "he did a lot of good for my father" [21].

Through his connections and influence, Weir is largely responsible for parliamentary legislation which, in 1950, created the Faculty of Homeopathy Act, establishing homeopathy as a separately licensed medical specialty in the British National Health Service. By this act, the British consumer is assured of the option to obtain alternative (homeopathic) treatment.

As a homeopath, Weir evoked mixed reactions. He was variously seen as a kindly father figure and as a tiresome autocrat, determined to have his own way. Much of the polarization came about because of Weir's identification with the high-potency, single-remedy teachings of the American homeopath James Tyler Kent, which were anathema to many in the British homeopathic community. Perhaps the last word on Weir can be given to Kaplan [22], who opined: "In short, Weir may have achieved more as a homeopathic politician than as a lecturer or writer … To be described as 'able to talk to people in high places' is not to be taken lightly…. I believe we owe a great deal to people like Sir John Weir for finding the right political moves, making friends with the decision makers and generally speaking about homeopathy with exactly the right tone."

Homeopaths in Elected Office

Three homeopaths are conspicuous for their activities in national politics: senators Jacob Gallinger and Royal Copeland in the United States and the Rt. Hon. Jesse Dickson Mabon in the United Kingdom.

Jacob H. Gallinger

Jacob Gallinger (1837–1918) has the distinction of being the longest-serving physician in the US Senate and, along with Senator Bill Frist in the 1990s, the only physician to lead his party in the Senate [23, p. 114] (Fig. 14.4). Frist has described Gallinger's significant political accomplishments as reflective of what can be achieved when medical knowledge is applied to public health policy. Gallinger was known for inexhaustible energy and, for many years, the ability to combine clinical practice with a legislative career.

Gallinger was among the first to champion the protection of vulnerable human subjects (and animals) in medical research. He drew up some proposed rules for the field, although their political impact at the time was limited. He brought to congress' attention the fact that human vivisection was being carried out and that it was important to introduce greater regulation over animal and human experimentation. In 1900 and in 1902, Gallinger introduced Senate Bill 3424 to congress, which regulated human experimentation in the District of Columbia. This bill was designed to protect the

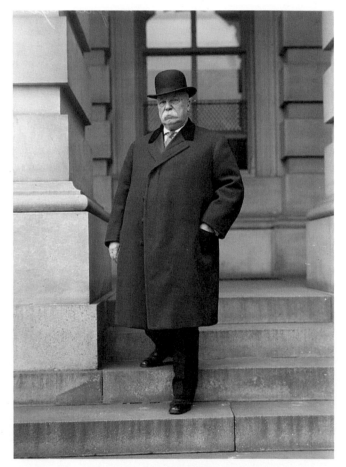

Fig. 14.4 Jacob Gallinger. US senator for New Hampshire, 1891–1918 and president pro tempore US Senate 1912–1913 (Image in the public domain, at www.senate.gov)

most vulnerable from exploitation, namely, infants, children, pregnant women, mentally ill, and charity patients. Investigators were to disclose the purpose of any nontherapeutic experiment on human subjects, to obtain written informed consent, and to furnish a post-study report no more than 6 months after completion of the project. Research on those incapable of giving consent was forbidden. Although the bill passed through committee, it was not enacted into law. It may now be seen as far ahead of their time, since many of its proposed measures have become standard practice [24]. With his commitment to protecting human subjects, one could make a case that, like Otto Guttentag, Gallinger was a homeopath who addressed bioethics long before others adopted the cause.

While Gallinger's efforts did not achieve all that he would have wished, his campaign was by no means unsuccessful: its proponents realized the chance of legislative success was slender, but they affirmed that education of the public about the ethics of experimentation and need for greater regulation were in themselves worthwhile goals [25]. As noted below with Guttentag, progress in the field of medical research ethics has been slow and suffered several setbacks during the twentieth century. The medical profession has responded very sluggishly to ethical issues. Even as late as the 1960s, the rights of human subjects were overlooked and abuses took place in many countries, including the United States. Illustrative of the Gallinger campaign's effect on public opinion was the unusual decision taken by Walter Reed in 1900 to obtain written consent for his yellow fever experiments being conducted in Havana. In this way, Reed no doubt was protecting himself from public criticism. As obvious as the need for these measures appears today, in the early decades of the twentieth century, the American Medical Association fought against their introduction and in 1916 rejected a proposal that investigators require written consent for human experimentation. It was not until 1946 that the AMA finally adopted such requirements [26]. Indeed, when passage of Senate Bill 3424 seemed possible, William Keen, president of the AMA, met privately with Gallinger to register his outrage and predicted that the medical profession would not take kindly to governmental restraint of their clinical and research freedom [27]. The bill had one main aim: to protect those who could not protect themselves. Yet, as uncontroversial as this principle appeared to be, the medical establishment was unready to accept it. It is clear that the AMA thought poorly of Gallinger, for in a 1914 commentary in *JAMA*, not only was his medical training belittled, but it was stated that he was not even taken seriously as a politician. This disparaging assessment reflected the commentator's view that Gallinger "opposes anything endorsed by the American Medical Association" [28].

Despite being known as a political conservative, Gallinger threw his support behind many liberal causes, of which anti-vivisection and patient rights have already been described. Other causes included temperance, women's suffrage, and Irish independence. In relation to the 18th (prohibition) and 19th (women's vote) amendments, Gallinger played an important part in the passage of legislation [29].

A brief review of Gallinger's life reveals that he was born in Canada and came to the United States at the age of 16 to work as a printer. Two years later, he entered the Eclectic Medical College in Cincinnati, qualifying in 1859. He later enrolled in the New York Homeopathic Medical College and obtained a homeopathic degree in 1869. He also studied abroad for 2 years and then settled in New Hampshire, where he prospered in general practice. Gallinger published in homeopathic journals and became surgeon-general of the state in 1879. He served in the New Hampshire House of Representatives between 1872 and 1873 and in the Senate between 1878 and 1880. He gave up medical practice in 1885 upon election to the House of Representatives in DC and later served in the US Senate between 1895 and 1918. He chaired a number of senate committees and was elected as president pro tempore during the 62nd Congress. As far as homeopathic activities were concerned, Gallinger was associate editor of the *New England Medical Gazette*, member of the American Institute of Homeopathy, and secretary of the New Hampshire Homeopathic Medical Society [30, 31].

Frist praised Gallinger's "profound impact on improving the practice of medicine in the federal district" and paid tribute to his efforts in tightening up regulation on medical practice and standardizing medical qualifications. His expertise "inspired the confidence of his colleagues and enabled him to mold broad consensus for his legislation." Frist characterized Gallinger as "an impressive model for future physician-legislators" and noted that "his ability to synthesize his medical training with public leadership demonstrates the unique contributions that physicians can make in the policy arena, by improving individual, communal, and national healthcare" [23, p. 114].

Royal S. Copeland

For many years, drug laws in the United States afforded the public little protection against the toxic effects of drugs or against false labeling. The 1906 Pure Food and Drugs Act banned interstate commerce of adulterated or misbranded drugs and required that dangerous ingredients be mentioned on the label, but did little more than that. Manufacturers, for example, were not required to disclose ingredients and directions for use or to warn against potential hazards. Apart from one minor modification to the act in 1918 and an unsuccessful attempt by Senator Rexford Tugwell in 1933, no further progress had taken place since 1906. It is of interest to note that Tugwell was thwarted by industry lobbying and finally

Fig. 14.5 Royal Copeland with Amelia Earhart at Senate hearings on aviation safety 1936. Copeland served as public health commissioner for New York City, dean of the New York Homeopathic Medical College, and US senator for New York (1923–1938). He was responsible for successful drug safety legislation in 1938 (Image in the public domain, accessed at Library of Congress)

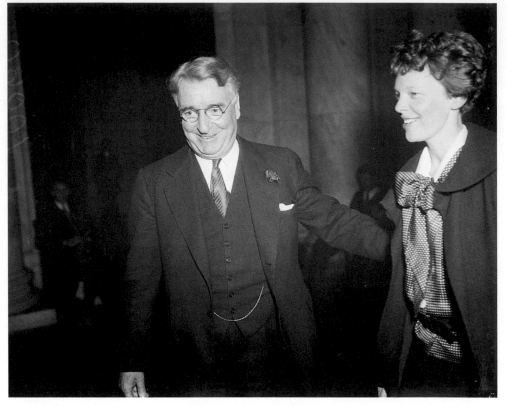

abandoned the cause [32]. This and other obstacles were to await anyone else who had the stomach for championing further revision of the 1906 Act.

Royal Copeland (1868–1938) has left an enduring mark on US health and drug safety legislation (Fig. 14.5). His major achievement in the eyes of many is the 1938 Food, Drug, and Cosmetic Act, which, as a democratic senator, he had taken over from Senator Tugwell and tirelessly crafted for 5 years until bringing it into law on June 2, 1938. Among other things, it protected the homeopathic pharmaceutical industry by including the Homeopathic Pharmacopeia of the United States (HPUS) as one of the legally recognized drug standards. But this was a minor aspect of legislation that became the centerpiece of drug regulation policy for over 50 years and did much to enhance the safety of drugs, foods, and cosmetics. As Frist says, passage of the bill "is a tremendous example of the enduring policy that can result from physician involvement in national politics" [23, p. 115]. Passage of the bill was anything but easy and, like its predecessors, was obstructed by industry opposition, professional resistance, and congressional stalling. It took an episode of mass poisoning to galvanize the community into demanding results when, in 1937, over 100 people died after taking a liquid form of sulfanilamide, an anti-infective drug. A follow-up investigation showed the presence of diethylene glycol in the medicine, which had been introduced to enhance dissolution of the active drug. At the time there was no requirement for the manufacturer to test for

safety, so this critical step never took place. Tragic as the incident was, its propitious timing hastened passage of the bill [33].

Copeland spent 15 years in the US Senate, chairing a number of committees and establishing a federally funded program to control sexually transmitted disease. Prior to senatorial service, Copeland was commissioner for Public Health in the city of New York between 1918 and 1923. In this role, he took action to contain the 1918 influenza epidemic, kept the schools open for purposes of morale, but came in for criticism owing to the death of 20,000 New Yorkers. Whether this was due to Copeland's response is debatable. He succeeded in doubling the per capita milk consumption, which led to a reduced infant mortality rate. Drug addiction became increasingly problematic in New York after World War I, and to deal with this, Copeland instituted a treatment center at Riverside Hospital in 1919 where war veterans could obtain free narcotics in order to bring them into treatment. This unprecedented experiment was too radical for the time and the practice was discontinued in 1920.

Copeland was a skillful communicator who wrote books for the public, including *Overweight? Guard Your Health: A Commonsense Book for Practical Persons, Healthbook* and *Dr. Copeland's Home Medical Book*. He hosted a radio show and from 1920 up to his last days, wrote a syndicated newspaper column on health, which reached over 11,000,000 readers and generated over 10,000 letters a week to his office. Arising out of this volume of mail was his *Healthbook*.

Frist notes Copeland to have been a natural leader, and from early in his life, Copeland knew that his calling was to be a physician who could use his training to bring about social change. To further this goal, he entered politics as a young man, serving as mayor of Ann Arbor between 1900 and 1903. He then campaigned (unsuccessfully) for a seat in congress and, later, became a parks commissioner in Ann Arbor and trustee of the board of education. Medically, he had qualified in homeopathy at the University of Michigan and then underwent specialty training in ophthalmology, spending some time in Europe. He became a well-respected surgeon, writing a textbook on refraction for medical students and, as already noted, earning fame as being the first to perform human-to-human corneal transplant surgery in the United States [34]. In 1913, he was elected fellow of the American College of Surgeons. Between 1908 and 1918, Copeland was dean of the New York Homeopathic and Flower Hospital Medical College, successfully steering the institution through the perilous waters of the Flexner Report, which came down harshly on homeopathic medical schools and resulted in the closure of most. Another feat worthy of mention was Copeland's leadership in establishing the first wartime army base homeopathic medical unit during World War I, United States General Hospital Number 5. This was no small achievement since (as noted) homeopathy had been excluded from military medical care during the Civil and Spanish-American Wars. Copeland overcame significant government opposition before finally triumphing. Despite admonishing his colleagues in the Senate against working themselves too hard, he failed to follow this advice himself and died, perhaps in part from overwork, shortly after passage of the Copeland Bill. A polite obituary appeared in the *JAMA* [35], making virtually no mention of his impact and ignoring his legislative record. In reality, over the years the AMA had found Copeland to be a tiresome maverick, but recognized his power and therefore trod carefully. However, when it came to Copeland's bill, the association fought it at every stage along the way.

J. Dickson Mabon

Jesse Dickson ("Dick") Mabon (1925–2008) was born in Glasgow, the son of a butcher. He grew up in that city and remained committed throughout his life to the interests of the Glasgow community and to those of Scotland in general. During World War II, he was assigned to work in the coal mines while the regular miners were performing military duty. Thereafter, he enrolled in medical school at Glasgow University, graduating with an MB, ChB degree. He practiced medicine on and off for much of his life, initially in Scotland and later in London, where he specialized in homeopathy. Mabon was board certified from the Faculty of Homeopathy and served as its president in 1995 and 1996.

Mabon's political career began early, with an unsuccessful run for election to parliament in 1951. When he was elected to parliament in 1957 at the age of 32, he was Labor's youngest MP. His 28-year career as a Labor party member of parliament included service in the cabinets of prime ministers Harold Wilson and James Callaghan, for whom he was minister of state for energy. In this post, he was responsible for the development of North Sea oil. He also advocated the use of nuclear energy and played a significant part in the successful 1975 referendum for the United Kingdom to remain in the European community. Although a medical doctor, he was not brought into healthcare to any great extent by his party. However, in the early 1960s, he was part of the Labor party opposition health policy commission and, in 1962, joined the front bench health team. He criticized the Tory party's record on hospital building. He also provided informal medical care to some of his parliamentary colleagues, including on one occasion Sir Winston Churchill [36, 37]. He voted against a bill for compulsory vaccination of children, perhaps illustrative of his belief in freedom of (parental) choice on matters of healthcare. In terms of medicine and social welfare, Mabon was proudest of his record in making available subsidized housing while minister for Scotland between 1967 and 1970. He later became chairman of UK section of SOS Villages, an international charity organization that enhances the lives of orphans. Unfortunately, his personal efforts to build two SOS homes in the Glasgow area were blocked by local opposition that refused to grant planning permission. Mabon was appointed to the Privy Council, a select group who advises the monarch, an honor reserved for distinguished politicians, judges, or senior church officials.

Other contributions to health affairs included vice-presidency of the Medical Practitioners' Union in 1964 and presidency of the faculty of the History of Medicine in 1990. His most substantial legacy, however, could be considered that of having twice helped rescue the Royal London Homeopathic Hospital (RLHH) (now known as the Royal London Hospital for Integrated Medicine (RLHIM)), which in the mid-1970s and again in 1991 was threatened with closure.

The first time Mabon intervened on behalf of the hospital was between 1974 and 1976, when moves were afoot to close the hospital. The then Minister of Health, David Owen, was influenced by a strong letter written by Mabon that proved to be a factor behind Owen's decision against closure. As Owen puts it, he believed that dissenting views should be tolerated and that an option that "focused on small quantities and natural products would be a worthwhile counter [to the pharmaceutical industry]" [38].

Nearly 20 years later, the hospital was once again threatened when, at a time of cost-cutting, the local health authority saw the RLHH as too small to be viable and set a date for closure in April 1992. As Fisher wrote, "… it really looked like the end of the road" [39]. For the homeopathic community, the loss of its flagship hospital would have been incalculable, given the critical role it had played for 150 years in providing care and as a center of research, education, and training. Indeed, given the international reach of the RLHH, which draws trainees and researchers from all over the world, the repercussions would have been far-reaching.

The Royal London Homeopathic Hospital

During the Margaret Thatcher administration, British politics saw the emergence of National Health Trusts, which empowered certain hospitals to negotiate with the primary care sector for funds to provide secondary (specialist) care. Under Mabon's leadership, the RLHH successfully applied for status as an NHS Trust, and Mabon became its first chairman in 1993, holding this position until 1997. Fisher pays tribute to Dickson's "shrewd reading of the situation, his political skill and connections and, above all, his robust optimism." Beyond rescuing the RLHH, Mabon's involvement with British homeopathy included modernizing the faculty of homeopathy and serving as vice-president and trustee of the Blackie Foundation Trust, an organization that promotes research into, and teaching of, homeopathy. As far as the RLHH/RLHIM is concerned, the English health system should count itself fortunate to offer this valuable option in the country's healthcare – many other countries, including the United States, are sorely lacking such facilities. Not only has the RLHH provided high-quality homeopathic care and training by experienced physicians with advanced medical qualifications, but it has notched up a number of "firsts" in British healthcare, including the first NHS complementary cancer treatment program (1960s), first acupuncture (1977), first complementary and alternative allergy and environmental medicine clinics (1977), and first manual therapy, autogenic training, and integrated antenatal care programs [40]. Its Missionary School of Medicine (MSM) also deserves mention. Founded at the RLHH in 1903, it continues today under another guise as the Medical Service Ministry (also abbreviated as MSM). The MSM provided education for missionaries working in countries that were then under British rule and provided courses in homeopathy, first aid, tropical medicine, and outpatient clinic teaching. Today, the MSM survives on a small scale as a limited grant-making body that enables indigenous providers and other candidates to train in child health, community healthcare, disaster relief, midwifery, palliative care, and tropical medicine. The history and scope of the MSM has been well summarized by Davies [41] and illustrates how valuable a resource the RLHH has been. Quite evidently, the hospital has gone beyond the confines of homeopathy to offer a more comprehensive program of CAM and to serve as role model in this respect. When seen in this context, Mabon's rescue efforts may be considered important.

References

1. Trani EP, Wilson D. The Presidency of Warren G. Harding. Lawrence: University of Kansas Press; 1977. p. 45.
2. Editorial. The proposed reorganization of federal health activities. Science. 1923;57:168–9.
3. Sawyer CE. Annual Report Federal Board of Hospitalization. In: Report to the President of the United States by the Director of the Bureau of the Budget. July 1, 1922. Washington: Government Printing Office; 1922.
4. Russell F, Warren G. Harding in his times. New York: McGraw-Hill Book Company; 1968.
5. Stevens R. Can the government govern? Lessons from the formation of the Veterans Administration. J Health Polit Policy Law. 1991;16:281–305.
6. Hines FT. Federal Board of Hospitalization. United States Government Manual, 1st ed [Internet]. Division of Public enquiries. Office of War Information. 1945 [Cited 2012 May 21]. Available from: www.ibiblio.org/hyperwar/ATO/USGM/FBH.html.
7. Boone JT. Centennial commencement address of the Hahnemann Medical College of Philadelphia. Hahnemann Hospital Tidings. 1948;LIII;89–132.
8. Rogers N. An alternative path. The making and remaking of Hahnemann Medical College and Hospital of Philadelphia. New Brunswick: Rutgers University Press; 1998. p. 294.
9. Heller Jr FM. The Presidents' doctor. New York: Vantage Press; 2000.
10. Deppisch LM. The White House physician: a history from Washington to George W. Bush. Jefferson: McFarland and Company, Inc. Publishers; 2007. p. 79.
11. Ullman D. The homeopathic revolution. Berkeley: North Atlantic Books; 2007. p. 196–8.
12. Forrestal F. Widows' walk rooted in decades of struggle by coal miners [Internet]. The Militant. 2002;66:14 [Cited 2012 Jun 20]. Available from: www.themilitant.org.
13. A brief history of UMWA health and retirement funds [Internet]. Triangle: United Mine Workers of America; 2008 [Cited 2012 Jun 17]. Available from: www.umwa.org.
14. Cleave E. Cleave's biographical cyclopaedia of homeopathic physicians and surgeons. Philadelphia: Galaxy Publishing Company; 1873. p. 245–6. [Internet]. Presented by Sylvain Cazalet [Cited 2012 December 26]. Available from: www.homeoint.org/history/cleavee/d/danforthw.htm.
15. Hirschhorn N, Feldman RG. Mary Lincoln's final illness: a medical and historical appraisal. J Hist Med. 1999;54:511–42.
16. Mitgang H. Sealed with sorrow: Mary Lincoln in letters. The New York Times. 1999 Sept 9.
17. Matile R. Dr. Danforth: the most famous local doctor you never heard of [Internet]. The Oswego Ledger-Sentinel [Cited 2012 December 27]. Available from: www.ledgersentinel.com/article.asp?a=8387.
18. The King Decorates Sir John Weir. The Glasgow Herald. Friday, June 19, 1949, p. 6, column 3.
19. Sir John Weir, G.C.V.O., M.B., Ch. B. Obituary. BMJ. 1971; 1:282–3.
20. Winston J. The faces of homoeopathy. Tawa: Great Auk Publishing; 1999. p. 206–7.
21. Lipman F. The King's homeopath? [Internet] [Cited 2013 Apr 27]. Available from: www.homeopathynearyou.co.uk/upload/The%20King's%20homeopath.doc.
22. Kaplan B. Homeopath to Kings and Queens – John Weir [Internet]. [Cited 2013 Apr 27]. Available from: http://www.drkaplan.co.uk/drk/spec_fea/weir.htm
23. Frist WH. Physician leadership in the United States senate: lessons from the past, a vision for the future. In: McKenna MK, Pugno PA, Frist WH, editors. Physicians as leaders: who, how and why now? Seattle: Radcliffe Publishing; 2006.

24. Lederer SE. Children as guinea pigs: historical perspectives. Account Res. 2003;10:1–16.

25. Lederer SE. Hideyo Noguchi's lutein experiment and the antivivisectionists. ISIS. 1985;76:31–48.

26. Lederer SE. Advisory Committee on Human Radiation Experiments [Internet]. Public Meeting, 18 May 1994 [Cited 2012 Jul 20] [Cited 2007 Jul 7]. Available from: http://www.gwu.edu/~nsarchiv/radiation/dir/mstreet/commeet/meet2/trnsca02.txt.

27. Vogel E. Perspectives on the experimentation of Udo J. Wile: insights into the past and considerations for today [Internet] [Cited 2012 Jun 18]. Available from: http://www.umich.edu/~historyj/pages_folder/articles/F06_MedicalExperimentation.pdf.

28. Old Doc Gallinger. J Am Med Assoc. 1914;62:1354–5.

29. Jacob Harold Gallinger Memorial Addresses. Washington: Prepared Under the Direction of the Joint Committee on Printing; 1919. p. 10.

30. Gallinger, Jacob Harold, (1837–1918) [Internet] [Cited 2007 Aug 15]. Available from: http://bioguide.congress.gov/scripts/biodisplay.pl?index=G000023.

31. Cazalet S. History of homoeopathy biographies [Internet] Source: Cleave's Biographical Cyclopædia of Homœopathic Physicians and Surgeons By Egbert Cleave [Cited 2007 Aug 17] Available from: http://homeoint.org/history/bio/g/gallingerjh.htm.

32. Davidson JRT, Dantas F. Senator Royal Copeland: the medical and political career of a homeopathic physician. Pharos Alpha Omega Alpha Honor Med Soc. 2008;71:5–10.

33. Ballentine C. Taste of raspberries, taste of death. The 1937 elixir sulfanilamide incident [Internet] [Cited 2008 Mar 8]. Available from: http://www.fda.gov/oc/history/elixir.html

34. Robins N. Copeland's cure. Homeopathy and the war between conventional and alternative medicine. New York: Knopf; 2005. p. 116.

35. Deaths. Royal Samuel Copeland. J Am Med Assoc. 1938;110:2169.

36. Obituary. J Dickson Mabon [Internet]. The Daily Telegraph. 14 April 2008 [Cited 2012 Jun 22]. Available from: http://www.telegraph.co.uk/news/obituaries/1585087/J-Dickson-Mabon.html.

37. Obituary. Dr Jesse Dickson Mabon. The Scotsman. 14 April 2008 [Cited 2012 Jun 22]. Available from: http://www.scotsman.com/news/obituaries/dr-jesse-dickson-mabon-1-1163880.

38. Lord David Owen. Personal communication. Email to the author. 11 Nov 2012.

39. Obituary. J Dickson Mabon. Homeopathy. 2008;97:163–4.

40. Anonymous. History of the Royal London Hospital for Integrated Medicine [Cited 2012 Nov 25]. Available at: www.uchl.org/OURSERVICES/OURHOSPITALS/RLHIM/Pages/historyofrlhim.aspx.

41. Davies AE. The history of MSM – homeopathy and natural medicines. Homeopathy. 2007;96:52–9.

After World War II, clinical research became an increasingly important in medicine. Randomized placebo-controlled, double-blind, clinical trials made their appearance, and the medical researcher became a more common breed. Many doctors saw themselves as researchers rather than healers as they moved into positions supported by readily available government and industry grants. A development of a more sinister kind took place during the 1940s and came to light in the aftermath of the World War II as shocking details of the brutal Nazi experiments were revealed. Both of these developments – the general growth of medical research and its appalling abuse – raised urgent ethical questions, to which the medical community awakened all too slowly. Jonsen wrote that in the 1940s and 1950s, "… many researchers had little interest in the ethics of research," and that there were "few medical men who spoke out publicly" [1, p. 140]. Worse still, and incomprehensibly, many German physicians were unconcerned about the horrifying Nazi medical experiments and even sought to justify them in some cases [1, p. 138].

One of the few physicians to squarely address these ethical concerns and place them in the forefront of debate was Otto Guttentag, a homeopathically trained doctor who devoted many decades of a long and productive life to this topic (Fig. 15.1). Guttentag has been described as "an often underappreciated figure in the development of medical ethics" [2], and his story is well worth telling since he has had a far-reaching influence.

Personal Background and Training

Otto Ernest Guttentag (1900–1992) was born in Germany to a family with three generations of physicians to its name. Otto followed in the family tradition and became a fourth-generation doctor when he qualified at Hallé in 1924. After further training there with his mentor, the distinguished nephrologist Franz Volhard, he moved to Frankfurt where he remained until 1933, when the Nazis came to power. Along

the way, he also studied biochemistry and pharmacology to better equip himself for a clinical research career. In Frankfurt, he directed a 50-bed homeopathic research ward, where he oversaw double-blind trials. Because of political events, in 1933 he left Germany for California to take up a research position with the Homeopathic Foundation of California, where he conducted more clinical research, publishing some of his results. In 1936, the Homeopathic Medical College of the Pacific merged with the University of California San Francisco (UCSF) Medical School, which offered Guttentag an endowed chair of homeopathy in the Department of Medicine. (This endowment still exists at

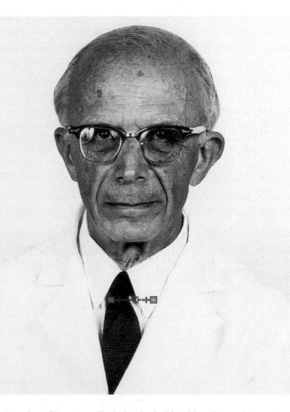

Fig. 15.1 Otto Guttentag. Early leader in bioethics (Image by courtesy of National Library of Medicine)

J. Davidson, *A Century of Homeopaths*,
DOI 10.1007/978-1-4939-0527-0_15, © Springer Science+Business Media New York 2014

UCSF, as the Samuel Hahnemann Professor of Medicine and Medical Philosophy, but today is completely divorced from homeopathy.) Guttentag continued to take an interest in subsequent homeopathic developments and published further articles on the topic, although his main interests were directed towards nephrology, the study of obesity, and the development of medical ethics. He remained active on the UCSF faculty until the end of his life, with two interruptions during World War II, when he served in the US army, participating in the D-Day landings, and shortly after the war when on an extended assignment in Germany. This second tour of duty took place in 1947, when he was granted leave of absence from his university to consult for the US military government in reforming and rehabilitating German medical education. Among the results of this effort was the formation of a medical education council (*Ausschluss für die Ausbildung und Fortbildung von Aertzen*) [3].

Academic Career

Although Guttentag is best known for his work in medical ethics, other details about his medical career will also be described. A homeopathic background did not prevent Guttentag from rapidly assimilating into the general UCSF academic community, where he became a much loved faculty member. He was frequently sought after as a mentor and course teacher on topics of homeopathy, the "medical attitude," and the role of the attending physician, which he continued to teach until the final months of his life. Guttentag established the first renal and obesity clinics at UCSF and cultivated an interest in physical anthropology and somatotypes.

Guttentag acquired national fame as an obesity expert and was consulted by the pharmaceutical industry as it developed new drugs for this particular problem. In 1957, the director of clinical investigation at Abbott Laboratories, Dr. George Berryman, approached Guttentag with a request that he evaluate the company's new formulation of methamphetamine hydrochloride (Desoxyn). Abbott was planning to obtain FDA approval for this once-daily formulation, which they hoped would be superior to their already-approved three times a day product. Guttentag reported to Abbott that he gave the drug to five patients, of whom two preferred the old drug, two had no preference, and one preferred the new drug. Guttentag had been advised by Dr. Berryman that the company was looking for a positive testimonial and this was not what Abbott had wanted to hear, yet Guttentag's disappointing evaluation did not stop the FDA from approving the product by the end of 1957. Of note, Guttentag told Abbott that these kinds of testimonial reports were not reliable and that larger trials with adequate statistics were called for [4]. This experience caused Guttentag to write a paper on the use of statistics in clinical medicine.

Guttentag received awards from UCSF, including its highest tribute, the UCSF Medal, and the Gold-Headed Cane Society membership, an honor bestowed for significant contributions to teaching and medical practice. He also received the annual award of the Society for Health and Human Values in 1978 [5].

Guttentag as Homeopath

Guttentag's first introduction to homeopathy occurred in Frankfurt, Germany, when he observed a patient with hyperthyroidism who had not responded to conventional treatment but in whom homeopathy produced recovery. Impressed by this therapeutic triumph, Guttentag resolved to train in homeopathy and moved to Stuttgart, where a homeopathic hospital had been established. For some years, Guttentag held a fellowship initially in Stuttgart and later in Frankfurt under the supervision of Dr. Josef Schier. He became familiar with the teachings of homeopathy and participated in research projects, although he did not conduct significant clinical practice beyond his research [6]. At the Stuttgart center, he conducted double-blind-controlled trials – at that time something of a rarity in medicine. Guttentag's interest in homeopathy was initially driven by its idiographic orientation, but he was far more skeptical about the much-vaunted benefits of high-dose dilutions. In other words, he subscribed to the *similia* principle as the core tenet of homeopathy, but not to belief in the potency of highest dilutions [5, 7]. In Germany, he became acquainted with other prominent homeopaths, including Karl Koetschau (see below), and in 1927 began studies to evaluate homeopathy in collaboration with Dr. J. Schier, which were interrupted but then resumed in 1930.

In 1933, Guttentag accepted an invitation from the Californian Homeopathic Foundation to conduct homeopathic research. After the merger between Hahnemann Medical College and the University of California, the nature of his work changed somewhat, although he never abandoned his commitment to homeopathy. According to his son, Christoph Guttentag, this commitment arose in part from the gratitude he felt towards homeopaths for bringing him to the United States when conditions became perilous in his home country [8].

Among his homeopathic achievements, Guttentag helped to "rescue" the 6th edition original of Hahnemann's *Organon* which, as the result of Hahnemann's family, had been languishing in obscurity under lock and key for decades. In cooperation with the manuscript's custodian, Guttentag arranged for its transfer to the UCSF Library in 1972. At a homeopathic society meeting later that year, Guttentag displayed this manuscript. The UCSF Library continues every year to receive many pilgrims wishing to study this almost-sacred manuscript, which contains numerous revisions in the hand of the author, for example, on high potencies and post-natal treatment [9].

Guttentag taught homeopathy to UCSF medical students for many years, attended meetings of the local homeopathic society, and wrote occasional publications. His 1940 paper offers a good review of the homeopathic renaissance that occurred in Germany during the 1920s and 1930s, following August Bier's call for reappraisal. Guttentag summarized the highlights of the revival and its appearance on the stage of German academia, noting that it arose from the concerted effort by a number of important figures, of whom Bier was the most prominent. Chairs of homeopathy were established in the universities of Berlin and Jena, and other programs started in Stuttgart, Frankfurt, and the Rudolf Virchow Hospital in Berlin.

In his review, Guttentag referred to the distinction between exploratory and explanatory approaches to medicine. The former is often known as "Hippocratic" or "empirical" medicine, representing medicine as an art and seeing the patient as an individual. The explanatory approach stresses medicine as a science with measurement as a key element: it has been called the "rational" approach. Alternative terms are, respectively, idiographic and nomothetic medicine. Guttentag places homeopathy in the idiographic camp and ranks Hahnemann with William Withering and Edward Jenner at a time in history around 1800 when medicine was in one of its idiographic periods.

Contributions to Bioethics and Medical Humanities

During his postwar secondment, Guttentag was shocked at the indifference of German medical colleagues towards Nazi medical abuses, and there is little doubt that experiences from his visit propelled him into the world of medical ethics. Of Guttentag's early work in this field, a federal committee said the following: "… among US physicians, Dr. Guttentag was nearly unique … in raising such problems in print." Jonsen refers to him as among "the boldest of the concerned physicians" [1, pp. 137–138]. As a prominent member of the United Church of Christ, Guttentag was able to forge successful collaborations with theologians, pastors, and physicians as they all tackled the common cause of ethical practice and research in medicine. In 1959, Guttentag and his UCSF colleague, Paul Sanazaro, began informal meetings with students at UCSF to discuss human problems related to medicine. Out of these humble beginnings, similar programs in medical humanities spread to other US medical schools and culminated in 1969 with formation of the Society for Health and Human Values (SHHV), an organization for which Guttentag can take much credit. In 1998, the SHHV merged with the Society for Bioethics Consultation to form the

American Society for Bioethics and Humanities, an association that is still thriving. In a 1960 publication, Guttentag argued for the inclusion of ethics courses in medical schools [10].

As made clear in his obituary, Guttentag's stature and his writings on medical philosophy and ethics influenced the national debate, particularly in respect of biotechnology and its impact on patient welfare [5]. His reputation was further strengthened as the result of a conference on human experimentation that he co-chaired with his colleague, Michael Shimkin, a cancer researcher at UCSF. This conference was held in 1951 at UCSF and was followed in 1953 by publications in the journal *Science*. Guttentag's presentation introduced key concepts that influenced many medical scientists as they began to understand medical research [1, p. 138]. According to Lederer, "Although it may have been difficult for researchers to confront the differences between therapeutic and nontherapeutic studies on human subjects, Guttentag, a homeopath by training, directly explored the tensions in clinical investigation." Distinguishing the "physician-friend" from the "physician-experimenter," Guttentag worried that the experimenter would be unable to resist taking advantage of a patient's distress in the interests of advancing knowledge [11]. Guttentag proposed separating the functions of physician as healer/advocate and physician as researcher [12]. This paper has been described as "seminal … one of the first to address these issues in a scholarly manner and to make recommendations for dealing with this essential part of medicine" [5]. The distinction between the two types of doctoring, when put so clearly, proved a key guiding concept. While it may now seem a statement of the obvious, at the time Guttentag's view was novel, and there was something of the emperor's new clothes in his stark message, reflective of Guttentag's characteristic style. Guttentag believed that we stumble not because of failure to understand the complex, but because we fail to "stop and analyze the obvious and the simple… Guttentag forces us to attend to the rarely articulated but fundamental question, 'Who and what is medicine all about?'" [13] Cassell and Siegel thought so highly of Otto Guttentag that they held a conference in his honor at Cornell University Medical College in 1979 and published its proceedings in the above-referenced book [14].

Guttentag obtained funding from the National Institute of Health in 1963 to survey medical educators about the impact of medical science on medical morality and ethics. Guttentag was the principal investigator of this project, the results of which were duly published in a book by Earl Babbie [15].

From his time in Germany, Guttentag experienced first-hand how state policy can affect the disadvantaged by enforcing utopian programs to maintain a healthy "national body" as defined by the state. He became one of a few stalwarts who championed protection of the poor, the mentally ill, the mentally handicapped, and the chronically sick from the depredations of such policies [16]. The important concluding words of Guttentag's paper in *Science* are no less relevant today than when they were written 60 years ago: "It is not the conquest of nature but the re-evaluation of man that appears to be the basic problem of our times. It is the re-evaluation of man as – to express it in old yet valid terms – created in the image of God and tempted by the devil.… We must be alert with ourselves lest, in our zeal for truth, we create healthy bodies at the cost of morally dulled minds" [12].

References

1. Jonsen AR. The birth of bioethics. New York: Oxford University Press; 1998.
2. Fox RC, Swazey JW. Observing bioethics. New York: Oxford University Press; 2008. p. 34.
3. Guttentag OE. Further notes on medical education in Germany. J Am Med Assoc. 1948;138:380–1.
4. Carpenter DP. Reputation and power: organizational image and pharmaceutical regulation at the FDA. Princeton: Princeton University Press; 2010. p. 201–2.
5. Brown E, Petrakis NL, Crede RH. Otto Ernest Guttentag, Medicine: San Francisco [Internet]. 1992 [Cited 2012 Mar 31]. Available from:. http://texts.cdlib.org/view?docId=hb7c6007sj&doc.view=frames&chunk.id=div00022&toc.depth=1&toc.id=.
6. Nossaman N. Personal Interview with Otto Guttentag, Spring 1990. Transcript sent to the author, April 9, 2012.
7. Guttentag OE. Trends toward homeopathy, present and past. Bull Hist Med. 1940;8:1172–93.
8. Guttentag C, Ph.D. Conversation with the author. 2 Apr 2012.
9. Mix LA, Cameron K. From Hahnemann's hand to your computer screen: building a digital homeopathy collection. J Med Library Assoc. 2011;99:51–6.
10. Guttentag OE. A course entitled 'The Medical Attitude.' An orientation in the foundations of medical thought. J Medl Educ. 1960;35:903–7.
11. Lederer S. The cold war and beyond: covert and deceptive American Medical Experimentation. In: U.S. Office of the Surgeon General, Department of the Army. Textbook of military medicine. Military medical ethics, vol. 2. Washington: Office of the Surgeon General, Department of the Army, United States of America; 2003. p. 507–33.
12. Guttentag OE. The physician's point of view. Science. 1953;117:207–10.
13. Cassell EJ, Siegler M. Introduction: understanding the future of medicine. In: Eric J, Cassell EJ, Siegler M, editors. Changing values in medicine. Frederick: University Publications of America; 1985. p. 7–9.
14. Duncan AS. Book review: changing values in medicine. J Med Ethics. 1986;12:95–101.
15. Babbie E. Science and morality in medicine: a survey of medical educators. Berkeley/Los Angeles: University of California Press; 1970.
16. Pross C. The attitude of German émigré doctors towards medicine under National Socialism. Soc Hist Med. 2009;22:531–52.

Less Is More: Finding the Right Dose

It is not difficult to make microbes resistant to penicillin in the laboratory by exposing them to concentrations not sufficient to kill them, and the same thing has occasionally happened in the body.

Sir Alexander Fleming, Nobel Lecture,
December 11, 1945

It is commonly assumed that if a drug is not effective, then the dose should be increased. This view is often, but not always, correct – sometimes the dose may have been too high, in which case the proper course of action would be to lower it. The relationship between dose and response is complex, and various explanatory models have been applied, including threshold, linear, and nonlinear models.

1. According to the threshold model, which dominated pharmacology for many years, a dose produces no real effect until a threshold is passed, beyond which the effect increases as the dose increases.

2. In the linear model, a direct linear relationship exists whereby an effect starts at the lowest dose and continues to increase as the dose is raised. This model, when used in toxicology, assumes that a harmful substance can be toxic at any dose and has been adopted by regulatory agencies in determining the dangers of carcinogenic (cancer-inducing) substances in the environment. This "safety-first" thinking is concerned not to overlook the possibility of danger even at very low doses. More recently, however, toxicologists have acknowledged that nonlinear relationships (see next paragraph) "should not be dismissed" [1].

3. There are nonlinear biphasic models, sometimes termed the "U-shaped" or "inverted U-shaped" dose-response curve. Nonlinear effects have also been referred to as non-monotonic dose-response curves (NMDRC). The essential feature of these curves is that, as the dose increases, the effect of a substance can change direction, for example, from producing less to producing more of an effect or vice versa. The U-shaped curve describes the situation in which a drug produces more of an effect at the low dose, less of an effect in the midrange, and an increase at higher doses. If the U is inverted (upside down to look like an arch), then as the dose is increased from a low starting point, the response increases with the dose up to a point where it then begins to decrease as the dose rises even further. Such relationships are common in pharmacology, and, historically, they have been invoked by homeopaths as a biological explanation of small dose effects [2].

Homeopathy stresses the value of a low dose in stimulating the system, but in the eyes of many, this has been taken to an absurd degree when applied to enormous dilutions of medicine. The work of Rudolf Arndt and Hugo Schulz has been used by homeopaths to explain drug effects. Following a summary of their work, this chapter will then take this information as a point of departure to discuss other concepts of drug action, such as hormesis, sensitization, nanomedicine, and intermittent dosing. Additionally, the discussion will address the recent unexpected detection of source drug in extremely high dilutions and inconsistencies in the drug manufacturing process. Terminology will be explained where necessary. (Compared to other chapters, there is less of a focus on the biographies of homeopaths and more a presentation of concepts and description of research which is germane to the question of drug effect in homeopathy.)

While neither Arndt nor Schulz was a homeopath, they were receptive to what homeopathy had to offer, and Schulz experimented with substances at homeopathic dilutions. Wapler described the work of Arndt and Schulz as a "great deed because both workers cleared away a dogma which had ruled school medicine since Galen's time: that is the belief … a weak dose acts correspondingly weak and a larger one correspondingly stronger" [3]. Later input into the debate was provided by the homeopath Karl Koetschau, which is reviewed below. The work of these individuals will be set in a broader context and the concept of sensitization then introduced, with reference to much later research, which finds common ground with some of homeopathy's teachings, including (1) potency of the low dose, (2) drug effect on body reactivity, (3) possible enduring effects from acute dosing, (4) the benefit of intermittent ("pulse") dosing rather than long-term daily dosing, and, more broadly, (5) the ability of a drug to produce effects that are not fully explained pharmacologically but which takes into account host reactivity or "secondary processes." Lastly, this chapter will discuss inconsistencies in preparing homeopathic remedies, the unexpected persistence of trace drug amounts in dilutions that were presumed not to contain any original drug, and possible explanations for these findings.

Rudolf Arndt

Rudolf Arndt (1835–1900) was a well-known nineteenth-century German psychiatrist. Besides making his name in psychiatry, authoring papers, and writing two major textbooks, Arndt is known today for his observations on the relationship between dose and response, as embodied in the Arndt-Schultz law, a term that still appears in the literature.

Most of Arndt's career was spent at the University of Greifswald, where he was professor of psychiatry and director of the local state asylum. Among his teachers was Heinrich Damerow, an influential psychiatrist who had homeopathic sympathies. However, although Arndt has been referred to as a "homeopathic physician" [4], this is probably not an accurate characterization.

As a psychiatrist, Arndt was known for his writings on psychiatry and research into the normal and pathological anatomy and histology of the nervous system. Aubrey Lewis placed Arndt in the company of leading contemporaries like Kraepelin, Wernicke, and Krafft-Ebing as one of several German psychiatrists who made contributions to the conception of paranoia [5]. Shorter identifies Arndt as one who contributed to "major steps in the panic story." In 1872, at a congress presentation, and again in an 1874 publication, Arndt described panic attacks, which he called "melancholic" anxiety attacks, and suggested they were associated with disordered nerves of the heart. Although tradition accepted the existence of anxiety attacks, it is thought that Arndt was the first to present this formally in Germany [6].

In 1871, Arndt wrote a 130-page volume on the use of electricity to treat psychopathology [7]. This account was reviewed by Hammond, who considered it to be one of the more important scientific contributions on the topic. Arndt noted that electrotherapy worked best for depression with vegetative (i.e., physical) symptoms, which corresponds to current experience. However, the method of application would have borne no resemblance to electroconvulsive therapy as it is now applied in psychiatry. Arndt also found that electrical treatment made some psychotic patients worse [8].

Arndt's *Textbook of Psychiatry* was published in 1883 and reviewed favorably in the *American Journal of Insanity* [9]. The reviewer commented on Arndt's spirited, expressive style and his graphic clinical illustrations and expected that the book would be received in the United States as it was in Germany, "with applause and satisfaction." The book was comprehensive in its coverage and embraced, among other things, Arndt's progressive view that criminal behavior could be the result of psychological disorder and that "each criminal is a diseased human being and deserves our sympathy rather than contempt." An important thesis in his book was that all forms of insanity represented one underlying process, but with different phases being present, a position held by other German psychiatrists at the time. Arndt believed that morbid mental processes were subject to the same physiological laws that governed the activity of overexerted, fatigued, or dying nerves, as per the findings of physiologists such as Pflüger and Wundt. He therefore concluded that the different phases of psychotic illness were a reflection of these laws, with melancholia, mania, and stupor being reactions to weak, medium, and strong provocation of the system. With respect to Arndt's view of psychoses, described above, he realized that the full evolution through all phases did not always occur. Arndt's schema have not left any lasting effect on psychiatric thought, but his interest in the effects of stimulus strength as a determinant of response proved to be of importance both for Arndt and for others, in particular Hugo Schulz (see below).

Arndt was in the thick of lively debates about military psychiatry around the time of the Franco-Prussian War of 1870–1871, and he believed that war resulted in higher rates of mental illness, with a peculiar type of "military psychosis" or "war psychosis" often being seen. Arndt also authored a standard German book on neurasthenia, *Die Neurasthenie* [10], a condition closely associated with war neurosis and that literally means weak or tired nerves [11]. For present purposes, *Die Neurasthenie* is important as the text where Arndt first presented his theory about the inverse dose-response relationship, which he considered to be a basic law (*Grundgesetz*) of biology. Arndt outlined his basic law of biology in the following manner: any foreign substance, drug, or external stimulus could affect the system in two ways, a weak stimulus promoted cellular activity, often in ways which were beneficial, while a strong stimulus (e.g., high dose of a drug) was inhibitory or toxic to the organism. Four phases were defined where weak stimuli have a mildly excitatory effect on living processes, moderate ones promoted them further, strong stimuli inhibited, and very strong ones destroyed them – a variant of nonlinear or NMDRC patterns in current parlance.

Arndt's interest in the biphasic dose-response found a ready audience in Hugo Schulz, who was a medical doctor and pharmacologist at the University of Greifswald. The two men became friends and collaborators, and Schulz recalled a walk they took in 1885, during which Arndt outlined his ideas. For Schulz, this readily explained some anomalous findings from his own work on the effect of compounds upon yeast, as described below, and influenced the course of his subsequent career. According to Schulz, Arndt received little recognition for this part of his work and was marginalized on account of his association with homeopathy (as was Schulz): he thus gave credit to his psychiatrist colleague by posthumously adding his name to what has become known as the Arndt-Schulz law. Schulz encountered great difficulty in publishing his monograph on *Rudolf Arndt and the fundamental law of biology*, and as a result it appeared as a University of Greifswald publication following several journal rejections [12].

Arndt was not a homeopath, nor did he receive any training in that discipline: his major interest lay in the effects of electrical stimulation rather than the effects of drugs [13]. Yet he was not above trying to reconcile his findings with the beliefs of homeopathy. In 1889, for example, he wrote that his basic biological law could open the possibility of a *rapprochement* between the two schools of therapy [14], a statement that was to haunt him, since it led to scorn from his peers who were hostile to homeopathy. In defending his view, Arndt later wrote "*Difficile est, satiram non scribere!*" ("It is difficult not to write a satire"), in commenting on the depreciative attitude of his colleagues [15]. The psychiatrist Willy Hellpach described Arndt as "a strange psychiatrist" [16], referring to his open-minded attitude towards homeopathy; even Schulz described Arndt's personality as being "idiosyncratic" [12], and other historians and contemporaries view Arndt as a loner.

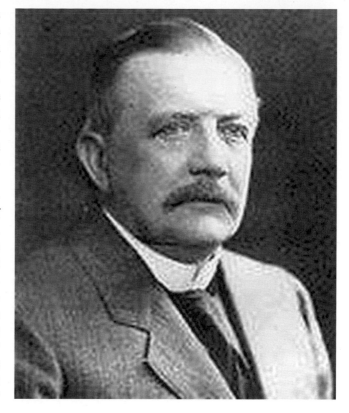

Fig. 16.1 Hugo Schulz. Pharmacologist who formulated the Arndt-Schulz law (Image by permission of Edward J. Calabrese, PhD. International Dose-response Society)

Hugo Schulz

The life of Hugo Schulz presents an illuminating example of how good scientific work can be held hostage to politics and belief. Schulz's findings were appropriated by the homeopathic community. They saw his (and Arndt's) theories as biological confirmation of Hahnemann's teachings about the power of small doses as well as the *similia* principle. By linkage with homeopathy, no matter how tenuous, Schulz became suspect to medical orthodoxy. Although he was neither a trained nor self-declared homeopath, he did experiment with homeopathic doses of substances and was open to what homeopathy had to say. Towards the end of his life, Schulz elaborated in greater detail about his proclivity towards homeopathy, as well as his reservations, in an apologia [17] where he stated that "I have succeeded in offering to the homeopathic school a scientifically founded basis in place of the necessity of being forced to work with more or less speculative material" [17, p. 14]. Of interest is that Schulz gives credit to Arndt for reviving the idea of taking into account the constitution when selecting the proper drug [17, p. 16]. As lead-in to an editorial in the *Journal of the American Institute of Homeopathy*, the journal editor Linn J. Boyd

commented on the profound influence of Schulz in homeopathic circles, noting that "His papers have been mentioned repeatedly in the columns of the JOURNAL and there is rarely any contribution to scientific homeopathy which does not quote the work of Schulz, particularly in reference to the Arndt-Schulz law" [17, p. 5, Editorial note by Linn J. Boyd].

Only of late has the story of Schulz and homeopathy been told in full [18].

The bare facts of his career reveal that Hugo Schulz (1853–1932) studied medicine initially at the University of Heidelberg and finally at Bonn, where he passed his qualifying examination around the year 1876 (Fig. 16.1). Schulz is almost exclusively known today as a pharmacologist, so it is perhaps surprising to note that as a junior doctor, he served as a house officer in the Hertz Mental Hospital, which he regarded a valuable experience, and that one of three teachers from whom he "gained the most" was a psychiatrist, Dr. Dittmar. Schulz's time in psychiatry was short-lived, but his friendship and contact with Rudolf Arndt were long-lasting and, as noted already, shaped his career profoundly.

Soon after completing medical training, Schulz embarked on his chosen path of pharmacology (the study of drug effects). He journeyed to Karlsruhe for 1 year to deepen his knowledge of chemistry and while there investigated the effects of arsenic and arsenic poisoning. In 1878, he returned to Bonn, now qualified to teach pharmacology at the Bonn Institute of Pharmacology. The thrust of his early work was (1) to demonstrate that living tissue converted arsenious acid into arsenic acid, (2) to study eucalyptus oil as an antiseptic, and (3) to evaluate whether carbon dioxide could break down alkaline chlorine compounds into free hydrochloric acid. While conducting these studies over a period of about 3 years, Schulz continued to work in clinical practice. In 1882, he accepted a professorial position in pharmacology at the University of Greifswald.

At first, it was quite a struggle, for Schulz was kept short of space by the university administration: indeed, as he put it, "it was not possible to bestow the respected title of Institute of Pharmacology on a single room on the Institute of Pathology, which had one window, two gas burners, but no water" [19], and there was not even a functioning weighing scale present. He elaborated that it was bad enough to drive him to despair but that "nothing sensible has ever come out of such a mental attitude" and that he "strived to do what could be done, since my pleas to the university curators at first remained totally unsuccessful." One might be tempted to see this as an example of the usual roadblocks met by incoming faculty, but Schulz persisted and after 25 years ultimately won his turf battle. More pertinent perhaps was his positive attitude, which would sustain him in dealing with the hostile attacks that yet awaited him.

Schulz' early pharmacological work at Greifswald took two directions. In the first instance, he studied processes of fermentation and decomposition. One substance that Schulz studied was formic acid, a compound known to inhibit the yeast-induced production of carbon dioxide (CO_2). To his surprise, he found that low doses provoked yeast fermentation, as shown by the increased production of CO_2. Schulz initially regarded his findings as anomalous and due to methodological error. But successive experiments repeatedly confirmed his original result, yet he remained unable to interpret the findings. As he put it, he "still did not realize that I had experimentally proved the first theorem of Arndt's fundamental law of biology" [19, p. 301]. So here was confirmation of the principle that low doses of inhibitory drugs can produce an opposite and stimulating effect – a so-called biphasic dose-response. A similar observation was later made by Sir Alexander Fleming in his pioneer work with penicillin, where low doses stimulated resistant strains while high doses killed the organisms.

A second thrust of Schulz' work was to study very dilute doses of veratrine, a drug derived from the white hellebore plant and which at the time was used to treat salmonellosis. Schulz tested low doses and found, as with formic acid, a paradoxical action whereby veratrine actually increased the colony count of salmonella bacteria. Other experiments involved the use of antiseptics in yeast cultures at low

dilutions of the order of 1:700,000 mercury bichloride and 1:600,000 potassium iodide, again showing the stimulating effects on fermentation at low doses [20, p. 458]. For his work with high dilutions, Schulz was derisively given the moniker *Greifswald homeopath*, a name that did not sit well with him since at that stage he had little desire to be seen as a follower of Samuel Hahnemann. However, he was becoming very interested in medical history and realized the importance of keeping an open mind towards iconoclasts like Hahnemann, whose views went against the grain of conventional medicine. In Schulz' opinion, to disdain such people could "signify a loss for drug therapy" [19, p. 303].

Four years after joining the Greifswald faculty, Schulz was given more space, which enabled him to broaden the scope of his experimental and theoretical work. With reference to the former, he undertook a series of homeopathic provings, in which he tested extremely low doses of sulfur, iron, quinine, and silicic acid on healthy volunteers. These studies were conducted single-blind (i.e., the participants did not know what they were taking) against an inert control, according to the best methods of the day. Results were mostly published as dissertations. With one substance, sulfur, Schulz was very cautious and waited 10 more years before he repeated (and replicated) his original results with the drug, only then announcing his results. Schulz was undeterred that his dalliance with homeopathic proving would be useful ammunition for colleagues who wished to discredit his work.

The second group of studies in 1908 was undertaken after Schulz had met Rudolf Arndt and was facilitated by the availability of further laboratory space, which finally permitted Schulz to build the kind of program he had envisioned from the beginning. His self-appointed task was to prove or disprove Arndt's basic biological law. To do so, he painstakingly undertook many experiments, using yeast fermentation as his model; all possible care was taken to reduce experimenter bias or equipment-related artifacts. He used a variety of drugs, including oleander, caffeine, and alcohol, and published the results of his studies in *Pflügers Archiv*, a leading journal of the time. Schulz remained a popular lecturer and drew students from many European countries. For some decades, the Arndt-Schulz principle was acknowledged by medical authorities, as illustrated in the textbook of therapeutics by Solis-Cohen and Githens [21], who referred to the biphasic action of castor oil, which had a primary laxative action followed by secondary constipation. The renowned Paul Ehrlich also referred to the "well-known biological principle … that substances which, in large quantities kill, bring about, in small doses, an increase of vital functions" [22]. Confirmation of the same principle was given by Fleming, who observed that bacteria that were killed by high doses of penicillin were "stimulated" into resistance when exposed to low doses [23].

Despite Schulz' popularity as a teacher and a degree of acceptance in medical circles, his long-term pursuit of Arndt's law was largely ignored by the scientific community, with the notable exception of August Bier. With a tinge of sadness perhaps, Schulz prophetically remarked "perhaps in the changes of time sooner or later an internist will take a closer interest in my work … regardless of whether it enjoyed the approval and understanding of renowned and unrenowned critics or not" [19, p. 316].

Calabrese has conducted a fascinating and meticulously researched piece of historical detective work regarding Schulz, how his findings were received and how his reputation suffered at the hands of professional rivals. The different kinds of dose-response curves have been alluded to above. Calabrese described the steps leading to the prevailing view of the dose-response, which is generally known as the threshold model and which has dominated pharmacology and toxicology for almost a century [18]. He indicates that this view, which has never been completely validated, originated as a reaction by medical orthodoxy to the "scooping" by homeopathy of Schulz' biphasic dose-response model (the Arndt-Schulz law). For a marginalized group like homeopathy to propose anything on the basis of science immediately called into question the integrity of the underlying scientific method – and that is exactly what happened. Firstly, Schulz was ostracized by many of his colleagues after his 1885 publication, which proposed that low doses of a drug promoted an adaptive (excitatory) effect. Indeed, for the remaining 50 years of his academic career, he remained an outsider, subject to constant criticism and prejudice. At his retirement, a colleague asked rhetorically what law he had broken to deserve such scientific boycott and character distortion [24]. As stated above, Schulz was not a card-carrying homeopath, but an open-minded seeker of the true facts as he saw them. As a result of such open-mindedness, he was willing to explore the relationships between his work and homeopathy. One matter about which Schulz was quite clear is that he did not believe in the ultramolecular, high dilution form of homeopathy, and to the extent that he connected his work to homeopathy, it was to the low potency dilutions that contained material substance. He agreed with Goethe's maxim *"Wo nichts ist, kann auch nichts warden."* ("Where there is nothing, nothing can be.") [25] But these fine distinctions were utterly overlooked by his allopathic opponents. As far as the high ultramolecular dilutions go, homeopathy may be unjustified in borrowing Schulz to affirm their validity. Although Schulz used extremely dilute doses of antiseptics in his yeast studies, these dilutions were in the range of 1:40,000 (arsenic) to 1:700,000 (mercuric chloride), which still contain molecules of the drug [20, p. 458].

As described by Calabrese, the response of orthodoxy was to advance an alternative proposal, stripped of any connection with homeopathy. The main champion was Arthur J. Clark, a prominent and well-respected British pharmacologist and author of an influential textbook in the 1930s. Clark promoted the threshold model and attempted to discredit Schulz through selective citation of his negative studies, while ignoring the positive ones. In Calabrese's opinion, Schulz' standing was damaged by this assault, as was the development of pharmacology, toxicology, environmental health, and risk assessment as a whole [18, p. 2661]. All would be forgiven if the threshold and linear models have convincingly proved themselves, but despite their merits, evidence has kept emerging to support the biphasic dose-response curve, and in head-to-head comparisons, it has gained the better over its rivals [18, p. 2668]. By 1940, Schulz had become a historical footnote, and his name was recognized by few, so when in 1943 a group of mycologists (i.e., scientists who study fungi) independently stumbled across a similar effect of red-cedar heartwood on wood-decaying fungi, they were unaware of the work by Arndt and Schulz and coined a new term, hormesis, to describe their observations. This word is derived from the Greek word *hormein*, which means "to set in motion" or to "excite" [26].

Hormesis

Subsequent work, most notably by Calabrese and his group, has provided considerable evidence to support hormesis [27, 28], and variants of this model are now widely used in the commercial development of new drugs by the pharmaceutical industry [29]. Different terminologies have been introduced to account for some subtle differences in the hermetic dose-response curve or to reflect different theoretical perspectives, such as parabolic, U-shaped, inverted U-shaped, J-shaped dose-response curves, and preconditioning, but the bottom line is that hormesis may be seen as a general (although not invariant) principle affecting cells, organs, and the individual as a whole, which takes account of drug action and the host's innate plasticity (i.e., powers of adaptation or resilience). It can be applied not only to the cure of disease but to the prevention, for example, exercise and caloric intake have been proposed as examples of hormetic effects [29, p. 610]. As Calabrese writes: "The dose-response explanatory principle of Schulz, so strongly rejected by the medical community nearly a century ago, underlies much of the success of the modern pharmaceutical industry in an ironic twist of scientific fate and promises to be even more significant in the future" [18, p. 2668]. Schulz was not alone in preaching the message. At the same time, the eminent bacteriologist, Ferdinand Hueppé (1852–1938) independently discovered a similar phenomenon and in his textbook, *Naturwissenschaftlichte Einführung in die Bakteriologie*, gave credit to Schulz as being first to report the biphasic effect. Hueppé was better known than Schulz, perhaps due to the fact that he studied with Robert Koch, who gave his blessing to Hueppé's work. His discovery became known as the Hueppé Rule and was taken more seriously. (Hueppé is also known to posterity as the first president of the German Football Association, an appointment created in 1900.) To all intents and purposes, the Hueppé Rule, the Arndt-Schulz law, and hormesis overlap. However, dose-response relationships are not set in stone as might be implied when the terms "law" and "rule" are used. There are too many exceptions for this to be the case, but there is no doubt that biphasic effects do often occur, that they have in the past been overlooked, and that they carry therapeutic implications. Low doses are believed to stimulate (or "excite") an adaptive, defensive, or reparative response within the host. In contrast, higher doses are more likely to attack the disease process directly (e.g., an antibiotic that kills the infectious organism).

Were Schulz and Arndt the first to discover hormesis? An awareness of the biphasic principle had been demonstrated centuries earlier by Hippocrates, Terence, and Paracelsus [30] and was known to William Shakespeare, as expressed in the following lines from Romeo and Juliet (Act 2, Scene 3):

> Within the infant rind of this small flower
> Poison hath residence and medicine power….
> ….Two such opposed kings encamp them still
> In man as well as herbs – grace and rude will

Hormetic effects were first demonstrated through a scientific experiment by Virchow in 1854, when he noticed that low doses of sodium hydroxide stimulated hair activity in the tracheal lining, whereas high doses were suppressive [31]. The effects of drugs on cellular function dominated medical research in the mid-nineteenth century, and Virchow's work may well have influenced Schulz, even though Virchow himself travelled no further down this road. However, homeopathy was known to Virchow, who paid tribute to Hahnemann as being the first to empirically test the effects of drugs on healthy people and for his concept of the minimum dose. He credited Hahnemann's theory of homeopathy as stimulating new investigations in chemistry and flirted closely with homeopathy in a paper on the relationship between cholera and arsenic poisoning [32].

Eduard Pflüger was a noted physiologist who played a seminal role in shaping Schulz' thinking. As a medical student, Schulz volunteered to be a subject in Pflüger's experiments and was well acquainted with the fact that Pflüger had shown that low and high amounts of electrical stimulation produced opposite effects on nerves. (Coincidentally, Pflüger had also been a major influence on Arndt as he formulated his own laws of biological activity.) So, while not being the first to detect the biphasic dose-response, Schulz was perhaps the earliest to make this a serious focus of study, and many of his contributions in this respect have withstood the test of time.

Limitations of the Arndt-Schulz Law

G.K. Chesterton once wrote that "Dogmas are not dark and mysterious. Rather a dogma is like a flash of lightning – an instantaneous lucidity that opens across a whole landscape." As a means of providing simplicity and certainty, there is always the temptation to accept dogma. However, such illumination can be false. Hormesis by no means provides a final or complete answer regarding drug effects. As medical students are taught, "there is no always and no never" in medicine. In keeping with this axiom, it is unwarranted to regard the Arndt-Schulz "law" or Hueppé "Rule" as dogma. Such a simplification would belie the more complex nature of drug activity and the behavior of the receptors on which drugs act. For example, while hormesis usually assumes that low doses stimulate and high doses suppress, the reverse pattern can be found, as in the case of inhibitory receptors in the body that are sometimes more sensitive to low doses of a drug, while excitatory receptors are activated at higher doses. Advocates of hormesis tend to view low-dose properties as beneficial and high-dose properties as harmful, but this is not always so – it is possible that adverse effects can occur at all points along the non-monotonic dose-response curve [33]. Clearly, the example of penicillin fits in here, where low doses can be potentially devastating, whereas high doses have a desirable effect.

Boyd has drawn attention to other shortcomings of the Arndt-Schulz law. He pointed out, for example, that the effect of a drug depended on the organ involved and that one drug could have opposite effects at the same dose according to other conditions, using as an example adrenaline, which could either constrict or dilate blood vessels according to the amount of calcium present [34]. Arndt and Schulz placed less emphasis on the impact of time as opposed to dose, but duration of treatment may also lead to switching of effect from one pole to the other. A good example in current drug therapy comes from the antidepressant drug fluoxetine (also known as Prozac™), which causes initial weight loss but eventually causes weight gain after longer-term treatment, even if the dose is unchanged. Such phenomena speak to the body's adaptive powers, which may be positive or negative, according to the nature of the response. Here, the work of Karl Koetschau comes into consideration.

Koetschau advanced the type-effect hypothesis, which posited that drug effects may alter over time, as in fact he demonstrated. Koetschau found that a small dose led to weak stimulation (which he referred to as Curve A), a moderate dose produced initial stimulation followed later by a reversible depression (Curve B), and a high dose led to brief intensive stimulation followed by irreversible depression (Curve C) [35]. In order to detect these patterns, it is necessary to follow drug response over time, otherwise false conclusions may be drawn. Koetschau's work excited the attention of contemporary pharmacologists, most notably Edouard Rentz from the University of Latvia, who found that low and high doses of cocaine had monotonic (linear) effects whereas intermediate doses had a biphasic, oscillatory effect. Such a complex dose-response pattern could not have been explained by the Arndt-Schulz law, and Rentz recognized Koetschau in saying "it is the great honor of Koetschau, through the hypothesis designated by him as the type-effect hypothesis, to have proposed correcting alterations in the Arndt-Schulz rule" [36, 37].

Besides needing to take into account time since initial dose, and/or effect of chronic drug administration, there is also a need to consider the baseline state of the organism. Thus, Wilder proposed what he called the law of initial value, which described the different effects of a drug according to the condition of the subject. Adrenaline was found to increase blood sugar in nondiabetics but does not demonstrate a "paradoxical" lowering in those with high glucose levels [38]. Another good example of the law of initial value occurs with chromium which, in diabetic subjects with high blood glucose, can improve the body's sensitivity to glucose, but will not do so in healthy nondiabetic individuals with normal glucose. Another recent example from large national cohorts totaling thousands of subjects showed that selenium supplementation might reduce mortality rates in those with selenium levels <122 µg/l, but could increase it in those with levels above this threshold. As Rayman put it, "the crucial factor that needs to be emphasized is the inextricable U-shaped link with selenium status: additional selenium intake … may well benefit people with low status. However, people of adequate or high status could be affected adversely.… This observation is a particular case of a general principle recognized by Paracelsus as long ago as 1567" [39].

Thus, while nonlinear relationships do exist between drug dose and response, the relationship is complex, being affected by a variety of factors besides dose, and cannot be reduced to simple rules or laws; the word "hypothesis" is more suitable perhaps, as it invites testing. But there are clearly some important implications to nonlinearity, which go beyond the scope of this book. To take an example of hormesis, substances that are carcinogens at higher doses could at low doses have the potential to lower risk of cancer (i.e., to have the opposite effect). At present, it is assumed that a carcinogenic substance is potentially toxic at all doses, with risk rising in linear manner as the dose increases; hormesis and NMDRCs make different predictions.

Another question that arises is how to identify the lowest dose of a drug compatible with therapeutic activity. It has been shown that ultralow dilutions can be associated with biphasic (opposite) effects even at such infinitesimal levels, such as for histamine when used to inhibit basophil activation (the basophil being a type of white blood cell). In this model, a histamine dilution of 10^{-16} served as the dividing point, with opposite effects on either side of this value. Similar results have been found for aspirin, which increases bleeding at conventional doses but which increases clotting at homeopathic dilutions [40]. The story of low-dose pharmacotherapy has not been fully told, and it arouses little interest on the part of drug developers because infrequent use of drugs at low dose offers little commercial benefit, as compared to longer courses of treatment at higher doses using patentable drugs. The minimum dose that produces healing effects (Curve A) and not the maximum tolerated dose (Curve C) should be the goal of drug treatment according to Koetschau, but this is rarely recommended in allopathic practice. Hormesis is not without its critics, who rightly point out the need for a uniform definition, more understanding of its generalizability, basis for mechanism, and shortage of rigorous studies [41].

Yet another difficulty comes about from oversimplification. Thus, it is possible for one drug to simultaneously have opposite effects in different parts of the brain. For example, the antidepressant drug tianeptine has one set of (NMDA-inhibitory) effects on stress response in a region of the brain known as the amygdala and an opposite (NMDA-enhancing) effect in an adjacent area referred to as the hippocampus, both of which play a role in stress responses [42]. Therefore, when pharmacologists talk about drugs stimulating at certain doses and inhibiting at other doses, these more nuanced effects should be considered – a drug can at once be inhibitory or stimulatory depending on which region is being referred to.

Drugs: To Be Given Every Day or Intermittently?

Frequency of drug administration needs to be taken into account: it is possible that equally good responses can occur in some disorders with infrequent use of low doses, compared to conventional daily doses at higher levels. For example, in treating depression, it is held that optimum results come from daily use at the maximum tolerated safe dose for some antidepressants. An alternative therapeutic approach of pulse loading and intermittent administration of a drug may be as effective. Pollack and colleagues conducted a study in which two single doses of the antidepressant clomipramine were given once a day to patients with major depression and followed for two weeks; response was substantial and continued to increase after the drug levels had become so low as to be unmeasurable [43]. In a second study, the same group repeated the design but for longer and against two double-blind control groups, finding the same results [44]. A study with electroconvulsive therapy (ECT) has demonstrated that a single treatment was as effective as six weekly treatments for depression, and similar results were obtained with respect to mental reaction time in a series of three studies of triazolam, a very short-acting hypnotic, when given once a week for 6 weeks. In these three trials, the drug-induced impairment of cognitive and psychomotor functions increased over 6 weeks even though there was no drug present during most of this period [45, 46]. Other reports indicate that a single dose of LSD can lower the rate of relapse for up to 12 months in alcohol and heroin use disorders [47]. Antelman ascribes such results to the phenomenon of time-dependent sensitization (TDS), wherein the effect of a drug (or any foreign substance) continues to grow with time from a single treatment. He further opines that traditional treatment regimens involving daily doses may not always be necessary, and he refers to the concept of sensitization, which can lead to enhanced response to stimuli of diminishing intensity. He draws an analogy between TDS and immunological memory, even though the immune system does not seem to mediate TDS. It is the "foreignness" of a drug that evokes a defensive reaction for which the organism prepares itself through a process of sensitization and not in a way that depends on the pharmacology of the stimulus. Such responses can be long-lasting, even from a single exposure, for example, acute severe sunburn in childhood can lead to malignant melanoma decades later [48], and the long-lasting effects of a single dose of LSD were noted above.

Time-Dependent Sensitization

As to TDS, Antelman et al. [49] state that "drugs may have been given the wrong way for centuries." Homeopaths would agree and perhaps can now find some scientific support for their longstanding beliefs about the power of low and infrequent dosing. The similarities between homeopathic prescribing and TDS are striking, and may be two faces of the same coin. Where they perhaps depart is over the matter of ultralow-dose effects, but even the TDS model assumes sensitivity to very low doses. Indeed, Antelman asserts that increased sensitization causes a smaller dose to evoke the same therapeutic response. As he and his colleagues point out, "TDS is a phenomenon in which less is better." Such could be the mantra of homeopathy. Apropos of the ability of very low or even ultramolecular doses to induce TDS, there has been at least one study by Bell showing that remedies diluted to 6, 12, and 30C most likely produce their effects by sensitization [50].

Antelman and Gershon [46] raise some unanswered questions about TDS that are similar to those raised by the work of Arndt, Schulz, and Koetschau, including the need to determine (1) the minimal dose of the therapeutic agent, (2) the optimal time interval between doses, and (3) when and whether to decrease or stop maintenance therapy. Advantages of prescribing according to the principle of TDS include

(1) less exposure to the side effects of a drug, (2) lower likelihood of tolerance (i.e., loss of effect) developing, (3) lower cost, and (4) greater adherence to medicine, in itself a major factor related to drug response. Strikingly, just as has occurred for homeopathy, the advocates of therapy based on principles of TDS acknowledge its heretical status. Not unlike the findings of Arndt and Schulz, TDS can result in a stimulating/excitatory effect when the dose is low and an inhibitory response when it is high.

The term TDS was coined by Antelman and Chiado in 1981 [51], but it has also been called pulsed therapy, a form of treatment used in homeopathy and advocated by Bier and Walbum, as well as by Hahnemann himself [52]. TDS represents an experimental rediscovery of one of Hahnemann's great insights. August Bier (quoted in Boyd) wrote of this question, "By reading Hahnemann's work one reads with astonishment that all these things were known to him as a general rule … to give similar remedies and not to give a second until the effect of the first had passed … Each actual progressive improvement in an acute or chronic case is a condition which, as long as it lasts, excludes any further application of the drug whatsoever. Each new administration of any drug would disturb the improvement" [53].

Whatever conclusions one may draw about TDS, the effects of drugs are sometimes based on more than simple pharmacology or direct pharmacological action (which Hahnemann termed "primary" effect). It may well be that TDS invokes an adaptive response by the organism to a threat or change in the environment and that the drug when given at low dose according to the *similia* principle activates the "secondary" process as it was called by Hahnemann.

Despite the complex relationships that exist between dose and response, and the multiple other factors that can influence drug effect, there still exists the notion that very small doses can be effective through activating the host's innate healing response, or, stated differently, by restoring to normal those processes that have become poorly regulated. Just how low this dose can be remains to be seen, but the most recent research supports the idea that extremely high dilutions of medicine are not inert. As Luc Montagnier has said, they are "not nothing," despite what Goethe and hundreds of others have claimed. The building blocks have been put into place over the past 150 years by individuals like Arndt, Schulz, Koetschau, and, more recently, Calabrese, Antelman, and Bell. Setting aside the vexed question of ultramolecular dilutions, the conclusion at this stage might be that there is scientific support for using low doses intermittently according to the *simile* principle. Many questions remain to be answered, only a few of which have been identified here. One important and, until recently, almost completely overlooked problem will be touched on – whether the claimed composition of the remedy matches up to information on the label.

Does the Label Tell the Truth? How Much Medicine Is Really There?

A reason for concern about labeling comes from at least three sources. Kerr and Saryan [54] set out to test the widely held belief that homeopathic drugs contained negligible amounts of their major ingredients. The investigators purchased six reputable over-the-counter commercial brands of *Arsenicum album*, at labeled doses of 3X, 6X, or 12X, which would be expected to contain measurable amounts of drug. Perhaps to the authors' surprise, in four cases the measured amount in their own laboratory differed significantly from what was on the labels, sometimes being more than double in quantity. In case one is tempted to think that the actual amounts were still too small to matter, the authors showed that if two of the six remedies were to be taken at the recommended daily doses for a long time, the amount of arsenic would be at levels associated with malignant tumors, hypertension, infant death, and neurological diseases. While this was a small study conducted many years ago, and it is possible that better quality control now holds true for homeopathic medicines, the report raises some disquieting questions about the actual dose vs. the labeled dose, as well as the assumed safety of homeopathic products. Further reason to consider whether remedy traces exist in high dilutions comes from Ives et al., who demonstrated measurable amounts of substance in 30C dilutions [55], finding that solutions prepared in glass retained the original substance to greater degree than solutions prepared in plastic containers.

A third study suggests that the question has not yet been laid to rest. Chikramane and colleagues [56] studied ultramolecular doses of six metal remedies: *Aurum metallicum, Cuprum metallicum, Stannum metallicum, Zincum metallicum, Argentum metallicum, and Platinum metallicum*, made by respected manufacturers. These remedies were given at dilutions between 30C and 200C, in other words at doses where no original substance was expected to remain. Surprisingly, the authors found that, in several of the remedies, there was measurable substance up to a level of 4 ng/ml, at which a pharmacological effect is possible. Again, as with the earlier study, there was a disturbing degree of variance, which was up to 40 % within one batch of the same brand and up to 1,550 % across brands. We clearly need to know a lot more about the measured doses in homeopathic products. How much medicine is really in the pill? Is one pill in a batch identical to another? More fundamentally, as far as the philosophy of homeopathy goes, the Chikramane study indicates that ultramolecular dilutions may contain quantities of drug that produce pharmacological effects and thereby explain how it is that such high dilutions can work. On the other hand, if the variability is so great, then one cannot depend reliably on these preparations to work consistently unless and until manufacturers can achieve better

standardization. Ives, Jonas, and Frye [57] have noted that dilutions that were made from the top layer, where nanocomplexes (see below) congregate, may yield different amounts than dilutions taken from the walls or bottom of the vial. So, after 200 years, the ability to produce homeopathic products in a consistent manner, and in a way that assures a known amount of substance, may still be in question. But what has been uncovered is the remarkable possibility that even the most infinitesimal dilution carries a pharmacological punch. How this can be is now the subject of inquiry by Iris Bell and others.

In brief, Bell has proposed that mechanical grinding or vigorous shaking (referred to by homeopaths as trituration and succession, respectively) generates sufficient disruptive force to create nanoparticles of specific remedy substance, which survive the process of multiple dilutions that has traditionally been thought to remove all traces of the remedy. Nanoparticles are between 1 and 100 nm in diameter, have a large surface area relative to their size, and differ chemically, thermally, and magnetically from bulk forms of the same material. Nanoparticles and homeopathic remedies are capable of inducing hormesis and altering epigenetic, genetic, metabolic, inflammatory, and stress-response activities [58]. These intriguing ideas, which are sure to be pursued further, open up the possibility of a new understanding about ultralow dose ("homeopathic") treatment and offer promise of a more constructive dialog between the different stakeholders in therapeutics.

References

1. Birnbaum LS. Environmental chemicals: evaluating low-dose effects. Env Health Perspect. 2012;120:143–4.
2. Helmstädter A. "Is there a tonic in the toxin?" The Arndt-Schulz law as an explanation for non-linear dose-response relationships [Internet]. Max-Planck-Institut für Helmstädter Wissenschaftsgeschichte. In: Balz V, von Schwerin A, Stoff H, Wahrig B, editors. Precarious matters. The history of dangerous and endangered substances in the 19th and 20th centuries. 2008. p. 29–37 [Cited 2012 Jul 10]. Available from: http://www.mpiwg-berlin.mpg.de/Preprints/P356.PDF.
3. Wapler H. The incorporation of homeopathy into united medicine. J Am Inst Homeopath. 1931;24:3–22.
4. Calabrese EJ, Baldwin LA. U-shaped dose-responses in biology, toxicology, and public health. Ann Rev Pub Health. 2001;22:15–33.
5. Lewis A. Paranoia and the paranoid. Psychol Med. 1970;1:2–12.
6. Shorter E. A historical dictionary of psychiatry. New York: Oxford University Press; 2005. p. 203.
7. Dukakis K, Tye L. Shock: the healing power of electroconvulsive therapy. New York: Penguin Group; 2007, Chapter 4.
8. Hammond WA. Review: electricity in psychiatry, by Rudolf Arndt. Arch für Psychiatrie. II Bd. U. 3. Heft, und Psychiatrisches Centralblatt. 1871. Journal of Psychological Medicine: A Quarterly Review of Diseases of the Nervous System, Medical Jurisprudence and Anthropology. 1871;5:590–91.
9. Anonymous. Lehrbuch der Psychiatrie. Am J Insanity. 1884;40:504–8.

10. Arndt R. Die Neurasthenie (Nervenschwaeche): ihre Wesen, ihre Bedeutung und Behandlung von anatomisch-physiologischen Standpunkte für Aertze und Studirende. Wien u.a; 1885.

11. Lengwiler M. Psychiatry beyond the asylum: the origins of German military psychiatry before World War I. Hist Psychiatry. 2003;14: 41–62.

12. Schulz H. Rudolf Arndt und das Biologische Grundgesetz. University of Greifswald. Greifswald. 1918. p. 6–7.

13. Eric J. Engstrom. Email communication to author. 30 Jan 2012.

14. Arndt R. Das Nervenerregungs-beziehentlich biologische Grundgesetz und die Therapie. Berl Klin Wochenschr. 1889;26: 949–53.

15. Tischner R. Geschichte der Homöopathie, vol. 4. Leipzig: Willmar Schwabe; 1939. p. 694–5.

16. Hellpach W. Grundlinien einer Psychologie der Hysterie. Leipzig: Verlag von Wilhelm Engelman; 1904. p. 61–2.

17. Schulz H. My attitude towards homeopathy. J Am Inst Homeopath. 1931;24:5–17.

18. Calabrese EJ. Toxicology rewrites its history and rethinks its future: giving equal focus to both harmful and beneficial effects. Environ Toxicol Chem. 2011;30:2658–73.

19. Hugo Schulz, translated by Ted Crump. NIH Library translation. NIH-98-134: Contemporary medicine as presented by its practitioners themselves, Leipzig, 1923: 217–250. Nonlinearity in Biology, Toxicology and Medicine. 2003;1:295–318.

20. Coulter HL. Divided legacy. Twentieth-century medicine: the bacteriological Era, vol. IV. Berkeley: North Atlantic Books; 1994.

21. Solis-Cohen S, Githens TS. Materia medica and drug action. New York: D. Appleton & Co.; 1928. p. 311.

22. Paul Ehrlich. The collected papers of Paul Ehrlich. Himmelweit F, editor. Three volumes. London: Pergamon Press; 1956–1960, p. 509.

23. Fleming A. Penicillin. Nobel Lecture. 1945, p. 92–3 [Cited 2013 Mar 10]. Available from: http://bbc.co.uk/news/health_21702647? print=true.

24. Martius-Rostock F. The Arndt-Schulz axiom. Munich Medical Weekly News. 1923;70:1–4.

25. Schulz H. Grenzen der Arzneiwirkung. Ärtzliche Rundsch. 1902;12:145–9.

26. Southam CM, Erhlich J. Effects of extracts of western-red cedar heartwood on certain wood-decaying fungi in culture. Phytopathology. 1943;33:517–24.

27. Calabrese EJ, Baldwin LA. Toxicology rethinks its central belief. Nature. 2003;421:691–2.

28. Kaiser J. Sipping from a poisoned chalice. Science. 2003;302: 376–80.

29. Calabrese EJ. Hormesis and medicine. Br J Clin Pharmacol. 2008;66:594–617.

30. Rozman KK, Doull J. Paracelsus, Haber and Arndt. Toxicology. 2001;160:191–6.

31. Virchow R. Uber die Erregbarkeit der Flimmerzellen. Virchows Arch. 1854;6:133–4.

32. Review. Virchow R. Resemblance to cholera in the symptoms of arsenic poisoning. Virchows Archiv. 1869;47:3–4. Br J Homoeopath. 1870;28:202–5.

33. Vandenburg LN, Colborn T, Hayes TB, Heindel JJ, Jacobs DR, Lee D-H, et al. Hormones and endocrine-disrupting chemicals: low-dose effects and nonmonotonic dose responses. Endocr Rev. 2012;33:378–455.

34. Boyd LJ. Kötschau's scientific basis of homeopathy. J Am Inst Homeopath. 1930;23:1156–62.

35. Koetschau K. The type-effect hypothesis as a scientific basis for the simile principle. J Am Inst Homeopath. 1930;23:207–295 and 971–1046.

36. Wapler H. The incorporation of homeopathy into united medicine. Citing Eduard Rentz, "On the phasic introductory and release actions of the cocaine group on vessel preparations in an attempt at a general evaluation of phasic events in general. Inaugural dissertation, University of Riga. J Am Inst Homeopath. 1931;24:3–22.

37. Rentz E. On phasic introductory and release effects of the cocaine group on vessel preparations and an attempt at a general appraisal of phasic effects. Ann Intern Med. 1931;5:811–2.

38. Wilder J. The law of initial value in neurology and psychiatry. J Nerv Ment Dis. 1957;125:73–86.

39. Rayman MP. Selenium and human health. Lancet. 2012. doi:10.1016/S0140-6736(11)61452-9.

40. Fisher P. Does homeopathy have anything to contribute to hormesis? Hum Exp Toxicol. 2010;29:555–60.

41. Mushak P. Hormesis and its place in nonmonotonic dose–response relationships: some scientific reality checks. Environ Health Perspect. 2007;115:500–6.

42. Pillai AG, Anilkumar S, Chattarji S. The same antidepressant elicits contrasting patterns of synaptic changes in the amygdale vs hippocampus. Neuropsychopharmacol. 2012. doi:10.1038/npp.2012.135.

43. Pollack BG, Perel JM, Shostak M, Antelman S, Brandom B, Kupfer DJ. Understanding the response lag to tricyclics. I. Application of pulse-loading regimens with intravenous clomipramine. Psychopharmacol Bull. 1986;22:214–9.

44. Dube S, Perel JM, Miewald J, Kupfer DJ. Antidepressant response to oral pulse loading with clomipramine. Biol Psychiatry. 1996;39:623.

45. Kroboth PD, McAuley JW, Derry CL. Time-dependent sensitization to triazolam? An observation in three studies. J Clin Psychopharmacol. 1995;15:192–6.

46. Antelman SM, Gershon S. Clinical application of time-dependent sensitization to antidepressant therapy. Prog Neuropsychopharmacol Biol Psychiatry. 1998;22:65–78.

47. Krebs T, Johansen P-B. Lysergic acid diethylamide (LSD) for alcoholism: meta-analysis of randomized controlled trials. J Psychopharmacol. 2012. doi:10.1177/0269881112439253.

48. Elwood JM, Jopson J. Melanoma and sun exposure: an overview of published studies. Int J Cancer. 1997;73:198–203.

49. Antelman SM, Levine J, Gershon S. Time-dependent sensitization: the odyssey of a scientific heresy from the laboratory to the door of the clinic. Mol Psychiatry. 2000;5:350–6.

50. Bell IR, Howerter A, Jackson N, Brooks AJ, Schwartz GE. Multiweek resting EEG cordance change patterns from repeated olfactory activation with two constitutionally salient homeopathic remedies in healthy young adults. J Altern Complement Med. 2012;18:445–53.

51. Antelman SM, Chiado LA. Repeated antidepressant treatments induce a long-lasting dopamine autoreceptor subsensitivity: is daily treatment necessary for clinical efficacy? Psychopharmacol Bull. 1981;17:92–4.

52. Boyd LJ. Some factors responsible for the recent progress in homeopathy. J Am Inst Homeopath. 1931;24:1219–37.

53. Boyd LJ. A study of the simile in medicine. Philadelphia: Boericke & Tafel; 1936. p. 364.

54. Kerr HD, Saryan LA. Arsenic content of homeopathic medicines. Clin Toxicol. 1986;24:451–9.

55. Ives JA, Moffett JR, Arun P, Lam D, Todorov TI, Brothers AB, et al. Enzyme stabilization by glass-derived silicates in glass-exposed aqueous solutions. Homeopathy. 2010;99:15–24.

56. Chikramane PS, Suresh AK, Bellare JR, Kane SG. Extreme homeopathic dilutions retain starting materials: a nanoparticulate perspective. Homeopathy. 2010;99:231–42.

57. Ives JA, Jonas WB, Frye JC. Do serial dilutions really dilute? Homeopathy. 2012;99:229–30.

58. Bell IR. Nanoparticles, adaptation and network medicine: an integrative theoretical framework for homeopathy [Internet]. HRI Research Article. 2012. 17:1–2 [Cited 2012 Oct 1]. Available from: www.homeoinst.org.

Three Charlatans

As with other branches of the healing arts, homeopathy has its share of ne'er-do-wells. Some of these figures (Pratt, Abrams, and Koch) achieved notoriety for flagrant profiteering from questionable treatments. Other homeopaths (Robert Reddick and his Maryland cronies; Gregory Miller in New York) violated professional ethics and exposed patients to risk by issuing medical licenses to unqualified people. One individual (George Simmons) began his professional life as a homeopath but renounced and then attacked it, while turning America's biggest medical association into a personal fiefdom: his professional life was surrounded by scandal and charges of unethical conduct. Lastly, there are the homeopaths who willfully applied their medical knowledge to take life (Hawley Crippen and Luc Jouret).

Edwin Hartley Pratt

The popular notion of "fatigue" in nineteenth-century medicine was used to explain a number of health problems; it gave rise, for example, to the fashionable disease of neurasthenia, a diagnosis that proved to be the bread and butter of many sanitaria that sprang up in America and Europe. One of the more unusual theories involving fatigue arose from homeopathic surgeon Edwin Pratt (1849–1930), who argued that good health depended on good blood circulation, which, he taught, was solely determined by vigorous sympathetic nerve function. Fatigue of the sympathetic nervous system caused stagnation of the blood, leading in turn to disease. Pratt further opined that muscles controlling the function of body orifices, such as the rectum and genitalia, were richly innervated by sympathetic nerves and that any dysfunction of these sensitive areas (such as hemorrhoids, tight foreskin, or redundant skin over the clitoris) caused muscle spasms that then exhausted sympathetic nerves and caused blood stagnation. For Pratt, the logical conclusion was that "weakness and power of the sympathetic nerve lies at the orifices of the body" [1] and that surgery could provide benefit by opening and smoothing these orifices. More bizarrely (to present-day thinking at least), Pratt held that orificial disorders such as cervical lacerations and rectal folds could account for more remote problems like epilepsy and asthma. The zeal with which Pratt promoted the orificial movement gave rise to many ramifications, including books, a journal, a society, annual meetings, stock purchase options, and so on (Figs. 17.1, 17.2, 17.3, and 17.4).

There appears to be nothing about orificial practice that derives from homeopathy, other than the fact that Pratt was a homeopath, and even the homeopathic establishment remained cool towards the practice. In reality, as explained by Gollaher [2], orificial surgery paralleled similar practices that had been introduced to regular medicine a decade earlier by Lewis Sayre and others. Sayre was a highly regarded orthopedic surgeon who, in 1870, was requested by J. Marion Sims (an equally prominent New York surgeon) to consult in the case of a young boy with muscle paralysis. Sayre believed that in this boy "excessive venery is a fruitful source of physical and nervous exhaustion, sometimes producing paralysis." He recommended and carried out circumcision, with outstanding results. Thereafter, he incorporated this procedure into his practice, advocating it enthusiastically for many conditions, including epilepsy, orthopedic problems, and insanity; he even operated on 67 institutionalized children at the Randall's Island Insane Asylum, although results were sadly disappointing. For his contributions to the field, Sayre was admiringly called "Columbus of the prepuce" by Peter Remondino, a prominent public health physician. By 1912, Frank Lydston, a high-profile member of the AMA, avowed that parents who failed to have their sons circumcised were guilty of negligence. For all that Sayre and Lydston promoted such ideas, they did match Pratt's excessive passion.

Pratt established the American Association of Orificial Surgeons, which drew into its ranks almost 300 members. By the early 1890s, they had collectively performed tens of thousands of operations, with Pratt himself taking credit for over 1,000 of them. The association held annual conferences

J. Davidson, *A Century of Homeopaths*,
DOI 10.1007/978-1-4939-0527-0_17, © Springer Science+Business Media New York 2014

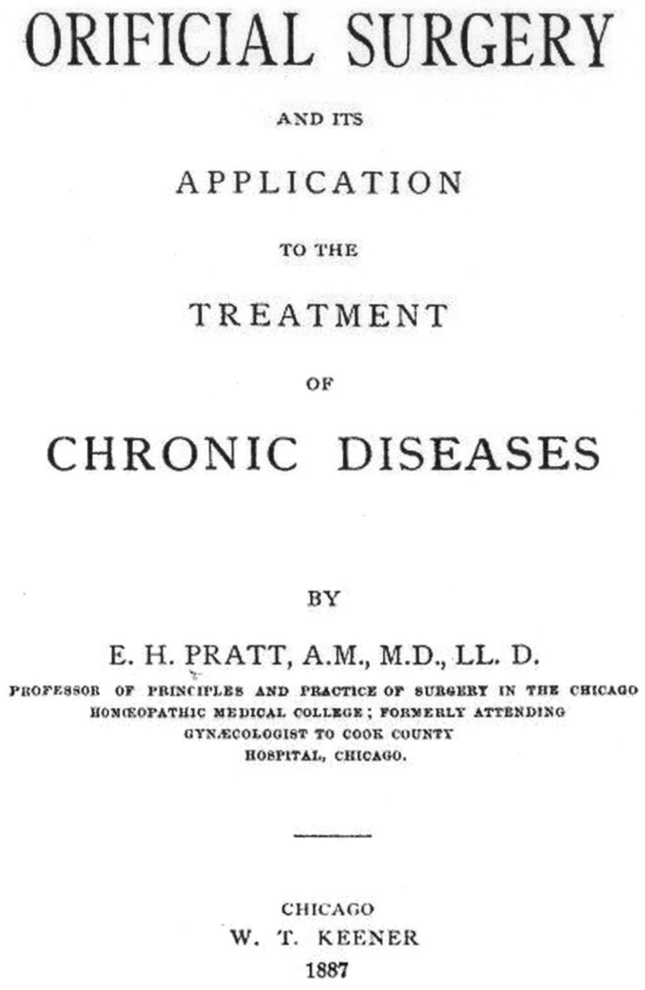

ORIFICIAL SURGERY

AND ITS

APPLICATION

TO THE

TREATMENT

OF

CHRONIC DISEASES

BY

E. H. PRATT, A.M., M.D., LL. D.

PROFESSOR OF PRINCIPLES AND PRACTICE OF SURGERY IN THE CHICAGO
HOMŒOPATHIC MEDICAL COLLEGE ; FORMERLY ATTENDING
GYNÆCOLOGIST TO COOK COUNTY
HOSPITAL, CHICAGO.

———

CHICAGO
W. T. KEENER
1887

Fig. 17.1 Book title: *Orificial Surgery and its Application to the Treatment of Chronic Diseases* by Edwin Pratt. 1887 (Image in the public domain)

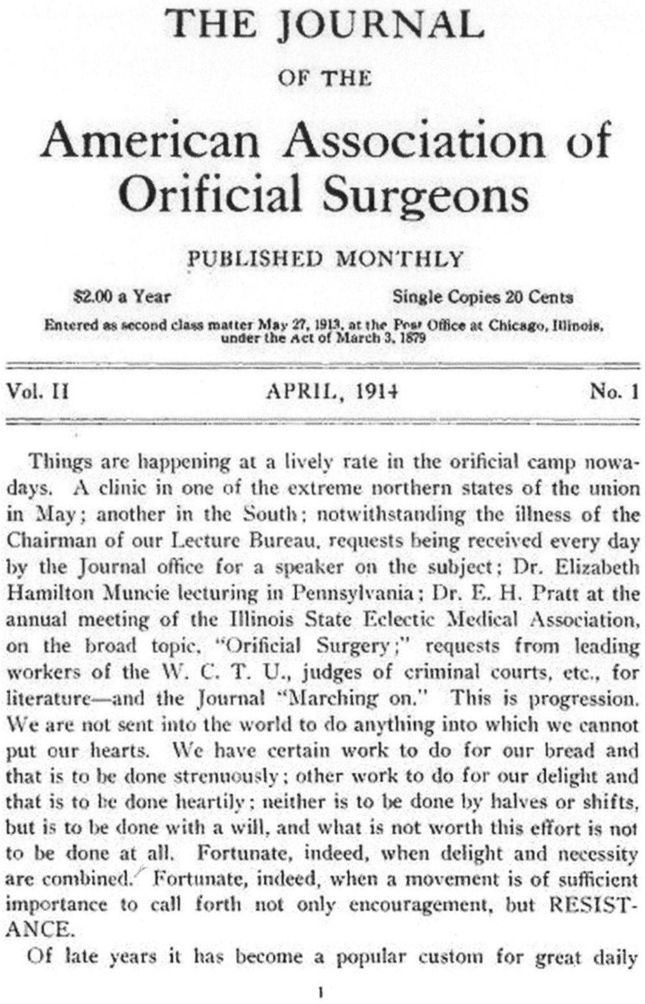

THE JOURNAL

OF THE

American Association of Orificial Surgeons

PUBLISHED MONTHLY

$2.00 a Year   Single Copies 20 Cents

Entered as second class matter May 27, 1913, at the Post Office at Chicago, Illinois,
under the Act of March 3, 1879

Vol. II   APRIL, 1914   No. 1

Things are happening at a lively rate in the orificial camp nowadays. A clinic in one of the extreme northern states of the union in May ; another in the South ; notwithstanding the illness of the Chairman of our Lecture Bureau, requests being received every day by the Journal office for a speaker on the subject ; Dr. Elizabeth Hamilton Muncie lecturing in Pennsylvania ; Dr. E. H. Pratt at the annual meeting of the Illinois State Eclectic Medical Association, on the broad topic, "Orificial Surgery ;" requests from leading workers of the W. C. T. U., judges of criminal courts, etc., for literature—and the Journal "Marching on." This is progression. We are not sent into the world to do anything into which we cannot put our hearts. We have certain work to do for our bread and that is to be done strenuously ; other work to do for our delight and that is to be done heartily ; neither is to be done by halves or shifts, but is to be done with a will, and what is not worth this effort is not to be done at all. Fortunate, indeed, when delight and necessity are combined. Fortunate, indeed, when a movement is of sufficient importance to call forth not only encouragement, but RESISTANCE.

Of late years it has become a popular custom for great daily

1

Fig. 17.2 *Journal of American Association of Orificial Surgeons,* April 1914 (Image in the public domain)

---

in Chicago between 1892 and 1901 and published the *Journal of Orificial Surgery*, of which Pratt was chief editor. Hemorrhoidectomy was performed for a wide range of conditions, including arthritis, tuberculosis, and psychosis. As Rutkow put it, "no mouth, penis, rectum or vagina was safe from a manipulation or scraping," and that Pratt was "the quintessential medical charlatan" [1, p. 98], who turned orificial surgery into one of America's more popular late-nineteenth-century medical specialties.

Pratt amassed fame and wealth and established his own hospital in Chicago, the Lincoln Park Sanitarium, which offered one of the region's earliest nurse training programs. He was appointed head orificial surgeon at the Cook County Hospital and belonged to Chicago's most prestigious clubs. The journal continued intermittent publication between 1892 and 1918 under different names, but by the mid-1920s, orificial surgery had become a footnote in history. Most of its surgeons were well qualified and transitioned comfortably to the practice of general surgery.

Although orificial surgery remained a homeopathic specialty, and drew few of its members from the allopathic profession [3], when seen in historical context, it may best be understood as an outgrowth of surgery that was practiced in the regular medical world through the influence of doctors like Lewis Sayre, but which was carried to greater extremes by Pratt.

Albert Abrams

According to a history of Stanford University School of Medicine [4], Albert Abrams (c.1863–1924) "was the most ingenious and notorious quack to be found in the practice of American medicine during the first quarter of the twentieth century" (Fig. 17.5). He has been called by Wilson the "cool prince of fakery." While he was neither trained in nor a fully committed practitioner of homeopathy, he did experiment with low doses of drugs and came to embrace a basic tenet

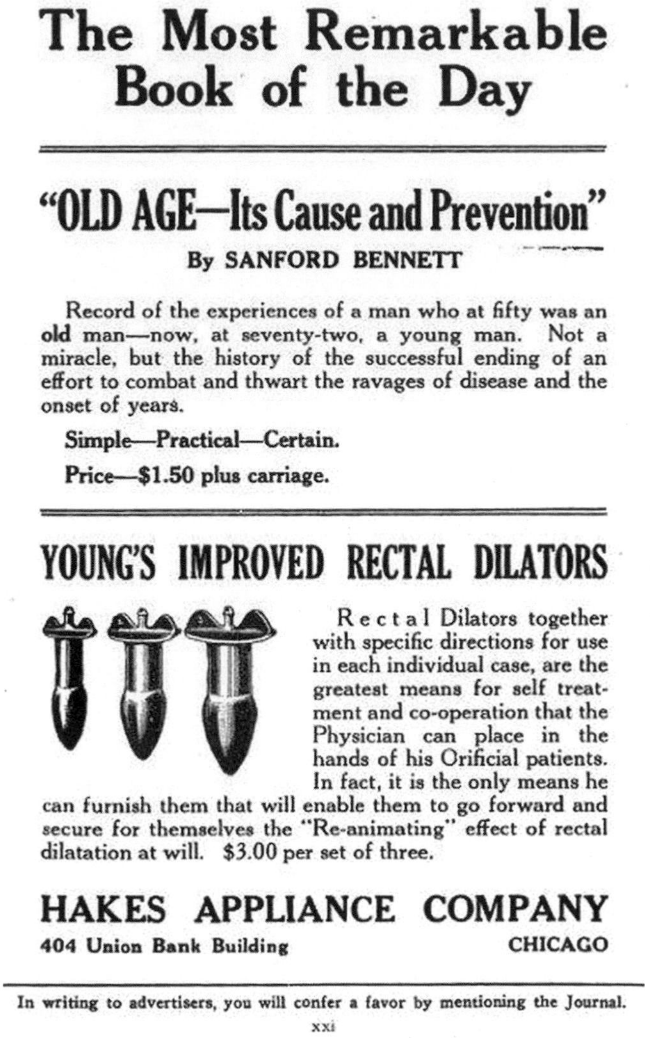

The Most Remarkable Book of the Day

"OLD AGE—Its Cause and Prevention"

By SANFORD BENNETT

Record of the experiences of a man who at fifty was an old man—now, at seventy-two, a young man. Not a miracle, but the history of the successful ending of an effort to combat and thwart the ravages of disease and the onset of years.

Simple—Practical—Certain.

Price—$1.50 plus carriage.

YOUNG'S IMPROVED RECTAL DILATORS

Rectal Dilators together with specific directions for use in each individual case, are the greatest means for self treatment and co-operation that the Physician can place in the hands of his Orificial patients. In fact, it is the only means he can furnish them that will enable them to go forward and secure for themselves the "Re-animating" effect of rectal dilatation at will. $3.00 per set of three.

HAKES APPLIANCE COMPANY

404 Union Bank Building CHICAGO

In writing to advertisers, you will confer a favor by mentioning the Journal.

xxi

Fig. 17.3 Advertisement claiming benefits of rectal dilators (Image in the public domain)

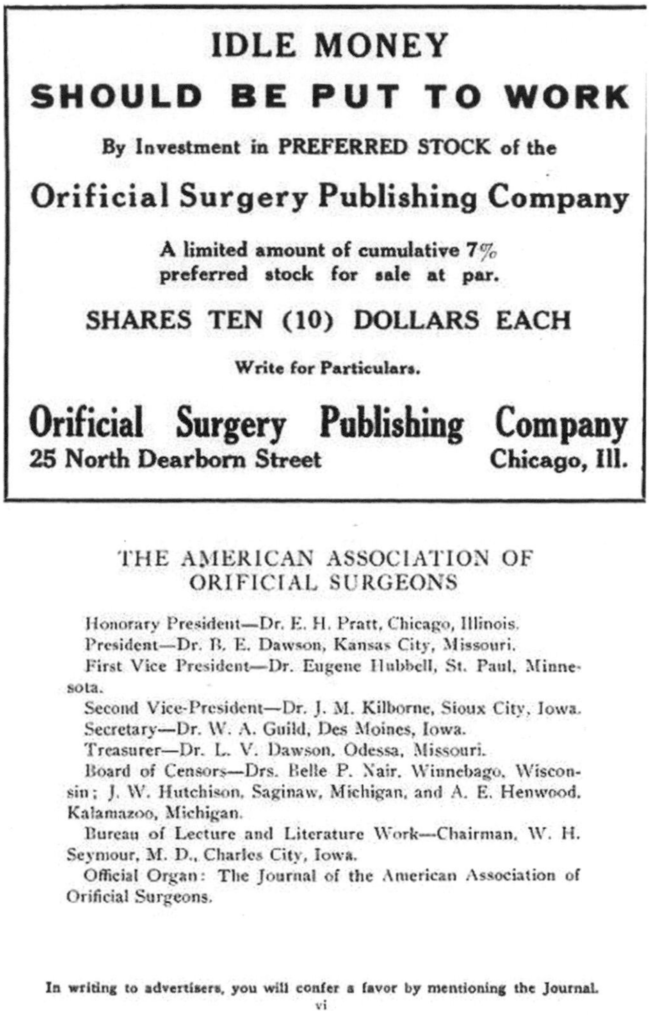

IDLE MONEY

SHOULD BE PUT TO WORK

By Investment in PREFERRED STOCK of the

Orificial Surgery Publishing Company

A limited amount of cumulative 7% preferred stock for sale at par.

SHARES TEN (10) DOLLARS EACH

Write for Particulars.

Orificial Surgery Publishing Company

25 North Dearborn Street Chicago, Ill.

THE AMERICAN ASSOCIATION OF ORIFICIAL SURGEONS

Honorary President—Dr. E. H. Pratt, Chicago, Illinois.

President—Dr. B. E. Dawson, Kansas City, Missouri.

First Vice President—Dr. Eugene Hubbell, St. Paul, Minnesota.

Second Vice-President—Dr. J. M. Kilborne, Sioux City, Iowa.

Secretary—Dr. W. A. Guild, Des Moines, Iowa.

Treasurer—Dr. L. V. Dawson, Odessa, Missouri.

Board of Censors—Drs. Belle P. Nair, Winnebago, Wisconsin; J. W. Hutchison, Saginaw, Michigan, and A. E. Henwood, Kalamazoo, Michigan.

Bureau of Lecture and Literature Work—Chairman, W. H. Seymour, M. D., Charles City, Iowa.

Official Organ: The Journal of the American Association of Orificial Surgeons.

In writing to advertisers, you will confer a favor by mentioning the Journal.

vi

Fig. 17.4 Solicitation for purchase of stock in Orificial Surgery Publishing Company (Image in the public domain)

of homeopathy, namely, the activity of extreme dilutions [5]. He contended that the vibratory rate of homeopathic drugs became increasingly apparent as their potency (or dilution) increased. Moreover, his work captured the attention of several homeopaths, a few of whom adopted his beliefs and even undertook further research along similar lines, such the emanometer research of the Scottish homeopath William Boyd.

Abrams improperly represented his professional credentials. He claimed a medical degree from Heidelberg University, another degree from the University of Portland, and a doctor of laws degree from an unspecified institution. He also claimed to have a degree from Cooper Medical College (which later merged with Stanford University). According to van Vleck [6], the facts appear to be that Abrams did receive an MD degree from Cooper in 1883, but the degree from Portland was fictitious since no such place ever existed, and the LL.D. degree was also imaginary. Regarding his Heidelberg claim, although the Stanford account says otherwise, the AMA did in fact vouch for this degree, which was given to Abrams when he was 20 years old [7]. Between 1885 and 1898, Abrams served on the Cooper College faculty as demonstrator and later professor of pathology. On May 16, 1898, Dr. Abrams submitted his resignation, which was accepted by the college's board of directors in November, but without any expression of appreciation for his services. The record is silent about the reasons for his resignation, but it is assumed to have been the result of his controversial practices. Despite severing his connection with Cooper, Abrams continued for years to capitalize on his prior relationship with the institution, even implying an affiliation with Stanford that had never occurred, since Abrams left Cooper before its merger with Stanford University. Abrams' claims evoked strong protest from the university's president, who wrote, "It seems to me bad enough for such a responsible institution as the Associated

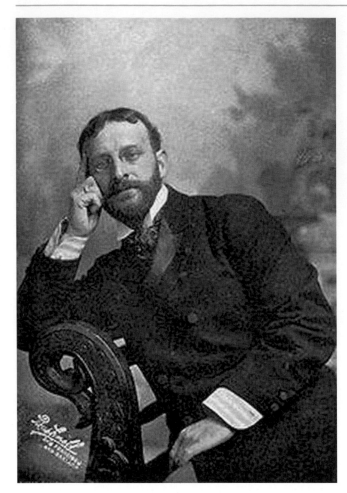

Fig. 17.5 Albert Abrams. Inventor of treatment known as Electronic Reactions of Abrams (ERA) (Image in the public domain)

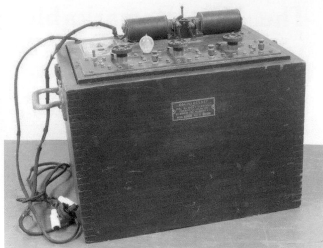

Fig. 17.6 The Oscilloclast, used for diagnosing and treating illness (Image in the public domain. Source: Library of Congress American Memory)

Press to herald far and wide the scientific rubbish of Dr. Abrams, and worse still to connect the name of the University in any way with such absurdities" [8].

Abrams was a prolific writer who enthusiastically advocated his brand of "electronic medicine." In 1904, he published *The Blues – Splanchnic Neurasthenia,* followed in 1909 by *Spinal Therapeutics*, and, in 1910, *Spondylotherapy*. In 1916, he published *New Concepts in Diagnosis and Treatment*, where he introduced the concept of electronic reactions and sound vibrations which, he asserted, could be used to diagnose disease and just about anything else, including sex and religious belief. An interesting illustration of Abrams' claims was given in the *Lancet* by Humphris [9], who diagrammed areas of dullness to abdominal percussion which, it was asserted, differentially characterized Catholics, Methodists, Seventh-Day Adventists, Theosophists, Protestants, and Jews. As described by Wilson, other outrageous claims included the use of Samuel Pepys' and Edgar Allen Poe's signatures to make a diagnosis of congenital syphilis.

Lacking the slightest touch of humility, Abrams referred to his new medicine as the "Electronic Reactions of Abrams"

or ERA. He followed up his book with a journal entitled *Physico-Chemical Medicine* and designed medical devices by which it was possible to make diagnoses. Initially he used the "Dynamiser" to identify vibrations by percussing the subject's abdomen to locate areas of dullness. More remotely (and more absurdly), Abrams claimed that diagnosis could be reached by abdominal percussion of an intermediary who represented the subject by holding something that belonged to that person, for example, a sample of blood, saliva, handwriting, etc. Later, Abrams devised another machine, which he called the Oscilloclast, a device set to the vibrations obtained from the Dynamiser and then applied by the Oscilloclast as a form of treatment over several sessions (Figs. 17.6 and 17.7). Both of these instruments were extremely simple, yet Abrams required users to sign an agreement that they would refrain from tampering with the box, make a down payment of $250 and then weekly payments of $5 for use of the box. ERA practitioners charged as much as $200 for "guaranteed cure" of syphilis, tuberculosis, cancer, and sarcoma. Large fortunes were made with ERA.

Abrams was a master of self-promotion. At the peak of ERA, thousands of doctors were using Abrams' devices, and ERA had grown into a cult in America and Britain. Not surprisingly, Abrams became the focus of scrutiny by medical and governmental establishments. He declined an offer by two respected San Francisco physicians to join them in testing his samples; he was investigated by several organizations, including the AMA, the British Air Ministry, the journal *Scientific American*, and even by homeopaths themselves, through the International Hahnemannian Association (IHA) under the leadership of Dr. Guy Stearns. IHA was unable to replicate any results and eventually distanced themselves from Abrams' claims: as of 1924, no homeo-pathic organization had endorsed Abrams' methods of diagnosis or treatment [10]. Stearns subsequently pursued this line of work further, but without the master's showmanship. In Britain, a committee under the chairmanship of Sir Thomas

Horder found neither scientific basis nor ethical justification for the use of electronics, yet some felt that the Horder report was "annoyingly non-committal" [11], as it left the door slightly open to the ERA community's claims by its receptive attitude to the potential of Boyd's emanometer studies (Figs. 17.8 and 17.9).

At the time of his death in 1924, Abrams was a wealthy man (although part of that came from a family inheritance). Even though no convincing evidence has yet surfaced to support Abrams' work, there are still some believers, such as those who practice radionics and dowsing. There are two sides to every story, and not surprisingly some homeopaths are aggrieved at the way Abrams was investigated, likening it to the Jacques Benveniste witch-hunt that occurred in France half a century later [5]. While perhaps there were some superficial similarities in the manner with which the two individuals were investigated, the analogy is a poor one, as significant differences existed between the two men and the way in which they conducted their work. There were too many misrepresentations on the part of Abrams, whose chief motive appears to have been making money. Moreover, there were cases of fakery and outlandish, unproven claims on the part of Abrams. His probity was (correctly) questioned as

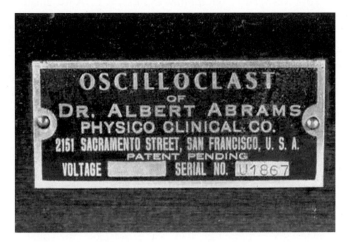

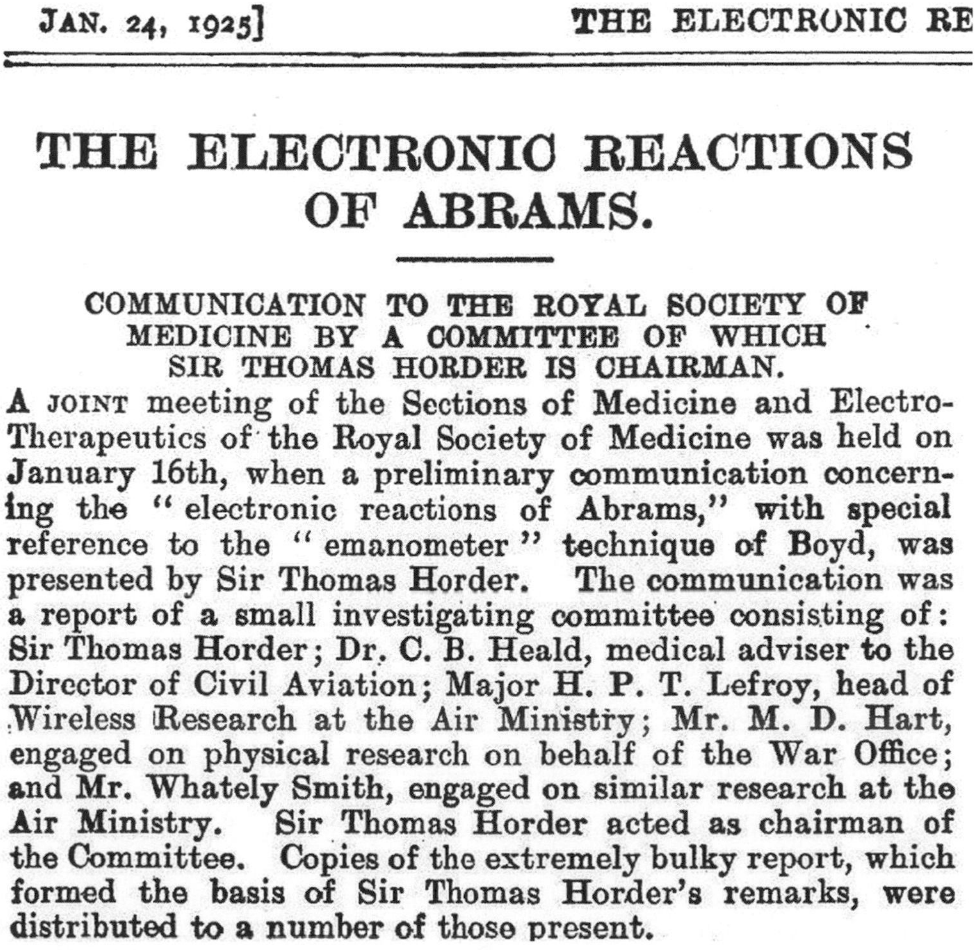

Fig. 17.7 Oscilloclast label (Image by permission of Nicholas Lindan, the Lindan Collection)

Fig. 17.8 Report of the Horder Committee which reviewed the Electronic Reactions of Abrams, *British Medical Journal*, 1925 (Image in the public domain)

JAN. 24, 1925]   THE ELECTRONIC RE

THE ELECTRONIC REACTIONS OF ABRAMS.

COMMUNICATION TO THE ROYAL SOCIETY OF MEDICINE BY A COMMITTEE OF WHICH SIR THOMAS HORDER IS CHAIRMAN.

A JOINT meeting of the Sections of Medicine and Electro-Therapeutics of the Royal Society of Medicine was held on January 16th, when a preliminary communication concerning the "electronic reactions of Abrams," with special reference to the "emanometer" technique of Boyd, was presented by Sir Thomas Horder. The communication was a report of a small investigating committee consisting of: Sir Thomas Horder; Dr. C. B. Heald, medical adviser to the Director of Civil Aviation; Major H. P. T. Lefroy, head of Wireless Research at the Air Ministry; Mr. M. D. Hart, engaged on physical research on behalf of the War Office; and Mr. Whately Smith, engaged on similar research at the Air Ministry. Sir Thomas Horder acted as chairman of the Committee. Copies of the extremely bulky report, which formed the basis of Sir Thomas Horder's remarks, were distributed to a number of those present.

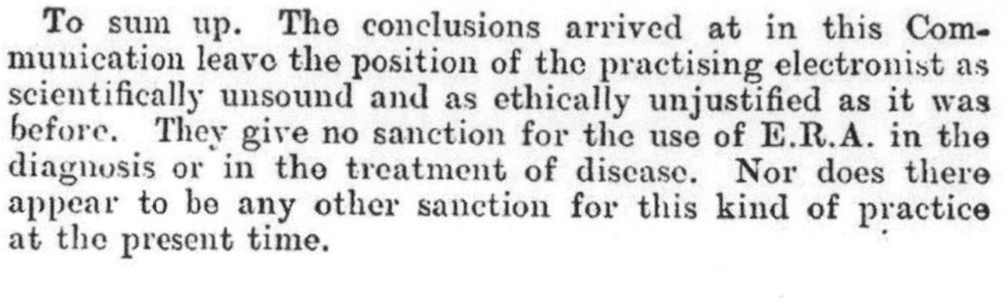

To sum up. The conclusions arrived at in this Communication leave the position of the practising electronist as scientifically unsound and as ethically unjustified as it was before. They give no sanction for the use of E.R.A. in the diagnosis or in the treatment of disease. Nor does there appear to be any other sanction for this kind of practice at the present time.

Fig. 17.9 Summary of the Horder Committee report, *British Medical Journal*, 1925 (Image in the public domain)

early as 1898 by a Cooper College medical student, Wilbur, who subsequently became president of Stanford University, and dishonesty seems to have dogged Abrams throughout his life. In the case of Jacques Benveniste, a principled scientist was hounded by an establishment driven by prejudice as much as by science.

William Koch

William Frederick Koch (1885–1967) studied at the University of Michigan, where he obtained a PhD in 1910. Following graduation, Koch took a faculty position as instructor in the departments of histology, embryology, and physiology. At one point, he attended classes in homeopathy, given by Professor W.A. Dewey at the University of Michigan Homeopathic College. He was subsequently appointed professor of physiology at Detroit Medical College, where he enrolled in medical school, graduating as MD in 1918 [12–14].

Owing to the loss of his father to cancer, Koch dedicated himself from the start to finding a cure for the disease. Within 1 year of opening practice, he claimed to have found a specific cure (or "antitoxin" as he called it) and spent the rest of his life promoting this remedy, which later came to be known as glyoxylide, along with two other kindred substances to be called malonide and benzoquinone. Koch believed that cancer cells could not survive in an oxygen-rich environment and claimed that his medicine cured cancer by producing such an environment. Merely treating cancer was insufficient for Koch who, encouraged by his successes, expanded his claims to be able to cure asthma, leprosy, syphilis, and tuberculosis with his proprietary remedies. Any form of experimentation to test his approach was scorned by Koch, who was unwilling to go further than publishing successful case reports, an approach that is very limited and generally confirms preexisting biases.

Word of Koch's clinic in Detroit spread and he received many referrals. Further, he established a group of at least 40 physicians who paid for the right to administer Koch's antitoxin – these physicians were required to charge patients $300 for the initial injection, an exorbitant sum at the time. Eventually, about 5,000 medical practitioners, many of whom were naturopaths or osteopaths, were using Koch's treatments. In 1926, Koch established the Koch Cancer Foundation, among whose patrons were disciples of Albert Abrams. After 1930, Koch turned his attention away from direct treatment of patients towards the general promotion of his approach to cancer. Like Abrams, Koch became the subject of investigation, but for many years, the FDA was unable to demonstrate any violation of law. By 1943, however, the agency was sure that Koch had fallen afoul of the 1938 Food, Drug, and Cosmetics Act (the Copeland Bill) by fraudulently misrepresenting the ingredients of his medicine, which had been found independently to contain nothing more than distilled water. Despite the government's best efforts, and at great cost to the taxpayer, two trials in 1943 and 1946 failed to find Koch guilty of any crime, although the Federal Trade Commission did succeed in restricting his ability to advertize. Koch moved to Brazil in 1950, where he continued to promote his cause; he even resumed medical practice and published another book, *The Survival Factor in Neoplastic and Viral Disease*s, in 1961. Through an osteopathic colleague, glyoxylide was also made available in Tijuana, Mexico. The Brazilian authorities finally caught up with Koch's practices and began efforts to shut down his clinic. His death in 1967 closed the chapter however, although the Koch family continues to protect his reputation [14].

Koch's connections to homeopathy were varied. As noted, he studied some homeopathy as a premedical student in Michigan. Early in his campaign against cancer, Koch put the dean of Michigan's homeopathic college on his payroll and consulted with him in preparing homeopathic antitoxin. Dilutions as high as 10^{-12} (one part in a trillion relative to the original tincture) were obtained. At his 1946 trial, Koch said that the greater the dilution, the "more serviceable" the medicines became. Not infrequently, sources have referred to glyoxylide as a homeopathic product, even if it has not been assimilated into homeopathy to any great extent.

License Fraud

In the mid-twentieth century, two homeopaths were associated with bogus license schemes, which enabled virtually anyone who paid the requisite fee to practice medicine, even though they were untrained and unqualified by any recognized medical school.

Robert Reddick

Improbable, ingenious, opportunistic, nefarious, fraudulent, and reprehensible – all of these words describe the scheme set up in the 1950s by Robert Reddick, a 1937 graduate of Hahnemann Medical College, who went on to specialize in psychiatry. He was employed for a time at the Gowanda Homeopathic State Psychiatric Hospital, then in 1951 became chief of service at the Eastern Shore State Hospital in Maryland. His clinical work was regarded as quite satisfactory and it was not on this account that he ran into serious trouble. Outside of his psychiatric activities, Reddick embarked on a quixotic adventure selling bogus medical licenses that enabled untrained holders to practice medicine in the State of Maryland and the 25 other states and territories of the United States that offered reciprocity.

To achieve his goals, Reddick seized control of the moribund Maryland State Homeopathic Medical Society, a once-lively organization that had dwindled away as its members died off. The society had historically been empowered to issue licenses, which entitled homeopathically qualified physicians to practice medicine in the state of Maryland, but over time it had ceased to be a meaningful organization and was largely forgotten. After its president, Dr. Evans, died in 1951, the society held no meetings until 1954, although there was an elected president, Dr. Julius Chepko, a Hahnemann graduate. In 1954, Dr. Reddick made a move to acquire influence in the society and succeeded in being legitimately elected as secretary and treasurer of the society as well as one of eight board members. Unbeknownst to any of the members, Reddick began holding "examinations" in 1955 that granted licenses to those who passed. At the first sitting in December 1955, there were 23 candidates, none of whom had received adequate training. Applicants paid $400–$500 to Reddick, ostensibly for the protection and maintenance of homeopathy, but Reddick retained full control of how this money was used. Dr. Chepko eventually became aware of what was happening and conveyed his alarm to the Maryland attorney-general, who advised Chepko to invalidate Reddick's actions. Meanwhile, Reddick attempted to overthrow Chepko and four other board members, whom he replaced with four of his own cronies. One of these, Simon Virkusis, a subordinate of Reddick at Eastern Shore, was appointed by Reddick as president and asked to sign 40 blank licenses to practice medicine. Reddick then wasted no time in issuing six of these to the initial applicants. Despite court proceedings over the next 3 years, either as plaintiff or defendant against the State of Maryland or its State Commissioner of Personnel, Reddick persisted in issuing licenses, including on one occasion to an automobile mechanic.

On June 4, 1956, Chepko's board met and invalidated Reddick's licenses. By this time, Reddick had resigned as secretary/treasurer of the official board, but ran his own shadow board and continued examining as many as 59 applicants. All this was occurring as the state filed suits in June 1956. While Reddick and cronies were in the midst of a meeting to process these 59 applications, sheriff and deputies broke in, but not before 50 candidates had received their licenses.

Seeing an opportunity for enrichment, Reddick essentially organized a *coup d'état* of the local homeopathic society and appointed himself at various times as its president, secretary, and treasurer. He sold licenses to anyone who had graduated from an "approved school of homeopathy teaching a resident course," and by 1956 there were 96 licensees practicing thanks to Reddick. Following investigation, the attorney-general warned one applicant that he would face criminal prosecution if he continued practice, and 1 year later Reddick was ordered to cease and desist issuing licenses. Simultaneously, he was fired from his position at Eastern Shore for "moral turpitude" [15, p. 414]. In this matter, Reddick filed a countersuit against the State Commissioner of Personnel, which proved to be unsuccessful.

Despite appeals and countersuits by Reddick, the court found against him and, in October 1957, sentenced him to 5 years in the penitentiary. The court's opinion was given as follows: "Reddick's conduct was reprehensible in the extreme. The evidence establishes beyond doubt a fixed, determined and inexorable disposition on his part to give the examinations under any guise or pretext whatsoever; that he had planned and was conducting the June examinations with the idea of making it impossible for legal process to reach members of his purported Board" [15, pp. 415–417, 16–19]. His appeal was rejected and before he could serve his sentence, he fled Maryland for California, where he continued his nefarious activities.

In December 1959, he was tried in a California court for selling Maryland homeopathic licenses, assuring holders that California offered reciprocity [20]. A Los Angeles County court convicted him of felony and sentenced him to probation, a move which failed to deter Reddick who, in 1975, was still selling Maryland licenses, and in 1976 proclaimed himself as a director of the American Coordinated Medical Society. Beyond that date, little is known of his activities. Reddick appears to have shown utter disregard for truth, for the law, and for failure to learn from experience in pursuing a course of action that not only debased the practice of medicine but put untold numbers of trusting patients at risk of harm. Many psychiatrists would be tempted to wonder about psychopathic personality traits in such a person. Reddick enjoyed his day of fame in the local and national press. *Time* Magazine, for example, carried an article on August 20, 1956, in which it referred to "Go-Getter Reddick" advertising for new members in his rejuvenated society [21]. It referred to opposition of his state society peers and of the American Medical Association, who in Reddick's opinion were "out to get homeopathy." While he was surely correct in this regard, this time other far more important issues were at stake.

Gregory Miller

Gregory Miller was yet another homeopath who sold fraudulent licenses. Miller apparently had received his medical and homeopathic training in Mexico and set up shop in New York in 1984, styling himself as an MD, which he probably could claim legitimately, as well as claiming fellowship of the American Academy of Homeopathic Medicine (FAAHM) as one of his achievements. The AAHM was his own creation and had no legitimacy, yet he proceeded to mail out letters inviting gullible individuals to activate their fellowship for a fee of $150. Shortly afterwards, another mailing was sent out, inviting recipients to be "grandfathered" as being board certified in homeopathic medicine through the rules of the AAHM. For this privilege, the cost was $500. Alternatively, for the lower sum of $300, candidates could sit an examination in July 1985, which would confer board certification if they passed, at which time another $200 came due.

The organization published one issue of its journal and advertised a national conference with prominent speakers. When the homeopath, Julian Winston, checked with two of the named individuals, they knew nothing about the conference. Further, the academy claimed to have 45 fellows, but again, when Winston checked with 11 of them, they were unaware of the organization or why their names had appeared [15, pp. 533–534]. By 1986, the academy had disappeared from visibility and Miller apparently had died within the year.

Power and Betrayal: George Simmons

George Simmons (1852–1937) was born in England, left home at an early age after the deaths of his parents, came to the United States, and enrolled as a theology student in Tabor, Iowa, after which he moved to Lincoln, Nebraska, to study agriculture. His choice of subjects was determined by the fact that they were offered free of charge. In Lincoln, he met the woman who was to become his first wife, and they moved to Chicago so that George could study medicine. In 1882, he received his degree from the Hahnemann Medical College, practiced in Nebraska as a homeopath for 10 years, encountered serious financial problems, and then repudiated all things homeopathic. He joined the allopathic community and became general manager for the Western Surgical Association. In this capacity, he came into close contact with leaders of the American Medical Association (AMA), who were impressed with Simmons' organizational abilities. In 1899, he accepted a position as general secretary and general manager of the AMA, as well as editor of its journal (*JAMA*). Over the next 25 years, he put AMA on a strong footing financially and politically. At the time of his appointment,

the AMA was a ragtag organization, and medical doctors as a whole were not held in high regard – they certainly did not command the status and salary that came their way later. Moreover, the incumbent secretary's performance had been an embarrassment to the AMA for a number of years [22], and he had been rebuked in public at the 1898 annual meeting. Simmons' appointment proved to be a good choice, for under his leadership the AMA prospered and the circulation of its journal increased from 10,000 to 80,000 weekly subscriptions; at the time of his retirement, *JAMA* had become the top general medical journal in the world and the source of considerable income to the AMA. Under Simmons' initiative, the AMA began to publish other specialty journals, starting with the *Archives of Internal Medicine* in 1909 and growing into a family of kindred publications, all of which remain among today's most *élite* medical journals. Meanwhile, the organization established a sound financial base, came together with greater unity and strength, and spoke effectively on behalf of American medicine. For this, Dr. Simmons has been given much credit [23, 24] and one might suppose that he would be well remembered for his services. However, Simmons cannot be whitewashed from the taint of scandal.

The early years of Simmons' career do not cast him in a good light. *JAMA* and other mainstream publications made virtually no mention of Simmons' homeopathic background and generally overlooked his qualification from the Chicago Hahnemann Medical College [25]. He then (supposedly) attended courses at the Rotunda Hospital in Dublin, Ireland, in 1884 and returned to Nebraska, where he practiced medicine until 1898 [26, p. 37]. He established the Lincoln Medical Institute and Water Cure (i.e., hydrotherapy), where he conducted homeopathic practice for several years (Fig. 17.10). During this period, he "occasionally attended classes" [26, p. 37] at Rush Medical College in Chicago and obtained an MD in 1892, "but just a conferred diploma," according to Fishbein. In the 1880 s, Rush was well known as a diploma mill, and the college withdrew from the American Medical College Association when that organization passed a resolution to tighten up training requirements [27]. According to a sworn affidavit by Simmons' first wife, Margaret E. Simmons, also an MD, he spent just 12 days at Rush, then arranged for a colleague to answer roll call in class, and said that he would return at the end to take the examination. Simmons made good on this pledge and obtained his regular MD degree from Rush on the basis of about 2 weeks' class attendance [28]. Simmons may have been conflicted about the provenance of his Rush degree, since it featured in his 1922 *Who's Who* profile, but not in the 1936 update [29]. Even if one accepts that Simmons earned a double qualification as homeopath and allopath, his allopathic training would appear to have been subsidiary [25]. Indeed, according to Fishbein, when the ethics committee of

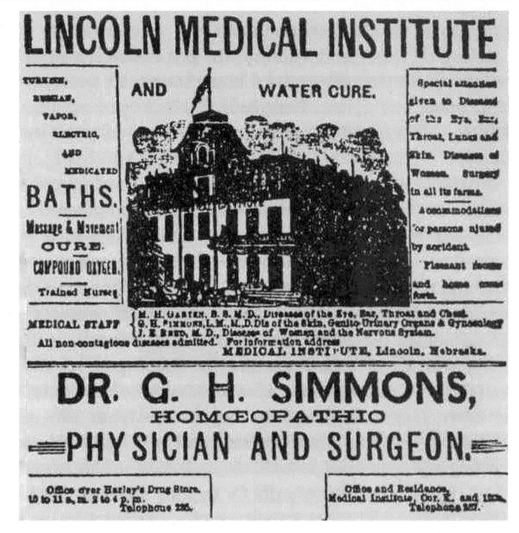

Fig. 17.10 Advertisement for Dr. Simmons' homeopathic medical practice in Lincoln, NE. Simmons was later to become secretary of the American Medical Association (Image in the public domain)

Simmons' local medical society questioned him about his training, he reported that Rush issued a diploma strictly on the basis of his having already completed full training as a homeopath, thus unwittingly endorsing a homeopathic MD degree. When Simmons was supposedly attending classes in Chicago, records showed that he was writing prescriptions and signing death certificates in Nebraska [30]. An advertisement of the time represents Simmons as being a specialist in women's diseases and a licentiate in obstetrics and gynecology from the abovementioned Rotunda Hospital, even though it is said that the hospital never issued diplomas of this kind. In the early days of his Nebraska practice, Simmons advertized himself as a "homeopathic physician and surgeon" who used treatments like "compound oxygen" and hydrotherapy – something that he later repudiated as a form of quackery. His professional announcement stated that he accommodated "a limited number of lady patients" at his residence. According to his wife's testimony, this was polite language indicating the performance of abortions, which were then illegal. Indeed, Margaret Simmons witnessed

evidence of this practice, when patients or their relatives visited the Simmons' home. Of personal significance to George and Margaret Simmons was their own conflict over having children: Margaret wanted to raise a family, whereas George was adamantly opposed, and whenever Margaret became pregnant, which occurred six times, her husband performed an abortion on her. The effect of these abortions was "terrible" and Mrs. Simmons stated that "No woman ever passed through such a hell as he made for me. He said he wanted me to get out of his life. Every morning he would say that he wished I was dead and out of the way, so that he could marry --------."

In the late 1880s, George Simmons encountered major financial problems: his institute failed and he was threatened with jail if he failed to pay a $1,200 debt. He made his wife find the money to bail him out of trouble. Subsequently, he forced her to give up teaching and to attend medical school so they could boost their income. Margaret said of George that "He was brutal to me in our private life, and treated me as his slave." To no one's surprise, Mrs. Simmons' health started to deteriorate and she developed troublesome head-aches, which her husband treated with morphine. Eventually she became addicted to the drug and "Dr. Simmons confessed to my mother that he was to blame for my forming the habit. I tried to keep from it, but in my poor health and my misery from the hell my husband's acts caused, I was helpless" [28]. She required psychiatric hospitalization in her home town of Mount Vernon, Ohio, and her husband would write ordering her to stay there at least 6 months. He said if she left sooner, she would be sorry about it.

In October 1892, George Simmons sued for, and was granted, divorce on grounds of cruelty. He married again in 1897. Many years later, in 1917, Margaret Simmons sought to have the decree annulled, encouraged by the manufacturers of nostrums which George Simmons' had refused to promote. According to his lawyer, Frank Loesch, one of these manufacturers remarked, "We expect a pile of money out of Dr. Simmons before we're through with him" [31]. The basis of Mrs. Simmons' case was that the original divorce was granted from documents that carried her forged signature, and she claimed that her husband was systematically drugging her with morphine so she would need prolonged hospitalization [32]. Dr. George Simmons however, asserted that his wife had first asked for a divorce and that he was unaware of her morphine problems until late in the day. The state district court upheld the 1892 divorce in 1917, a decision that was affirmed in 1919 by the state supreme court [33]. The surrounding publicity and scandal were believed to have played a part in Simmons' retirement, which was ostensibly on the grounds of poor health. Among other things, it has been claimed that the trial inspired Patrick Hamilton to write his successful play *Angel Street* (known in the United Kingdom as *Gaslight*), which enjoyed a long run on Broadway and was made into a film starring Ingrid Bergman [30, p. 363].

The divorce trial was not the only scandal to embroil Simmons. In 1909, the Chicago Medical Society investigated allegations of unethical conduct [29, 34]. Much of the trouble arose from the private investigations of his AMA rival, Dr. Frank Lydston, who assembled a dossier that revealed evidence of unethical practice by Simmons [35]. When Simmons explained that his apparently ill-gotten MD diploma from Rush was given on the basis of credit for his homeopathic training, he was able to escape the society's censure [32, pp. 50–51].

At one point, Simmons ran afoul of the Abbott pharmaceutical company for refusing to advertize its products, a situation that occurred because Abbott would not pay shakedown money demanded by Dr. Simmons in exchange for AMA's goodwill or "Seal of Approval" of a company's product. An unhappy Wallace Abbott, founder of the company, hired private detectives to gather evidence of Simmons' past indiscretions and then confronted him with the unsavory details, such as the aforementioned dubious diplomas,

patients allegedly dying from medical negligence, and charges of improper relations with female patients. In her affidavit, given under oath, Mrs. Simmons attested to the veracity of Abbott's statements. After these were presented to Simmons, the disputes with Abbott were quickly resolved.

Simmons incurred the wrath of Dr. Frank Lydston, who was upset at Simmons' disproportionate power in the AMA, which Lydston described as being run by an oligarchy. He was aggrieved that Simmons held three powerful offices in the organization which, Lydston claimed, represented the interests of those who ran the organization more than its members. Lydston argued in court that the board of directors was holding office illegally, contending they should have been elected in Illinois; because this had not happened, he demanded the removal of all AMA directors. After a 5-year legal battle, the Illinois Supreme Court upheld the decision of an appellate court ordering removal of the AMA's officers – a decision that was expected to bring about the reorganization of the AMA [36]. Despite this outcome, when writing his history of the AMA 32 years later, Fishbein saw it as a triumph for the association [37].

Beaten down by incessant attacks, in 1923, Simmons announced his retirement. According to Fishbein, his health was poor, with painful herpes causing him to miss more time from work than ever before. Fishbein maintained that the constant hostility of his opponents had turned Simmons into a social recluse [26, p. 93]. However, he made no mention of the personal problems and shady record described above. When Simmons retired, he took all his personal files home and burned them.

Obituaries in *JAMA* and the *British Medical Journal* hailed Simmons for his contributions as a journalist, administrator, and reformer. He clearly made the AMA into a powerful force, and he gave high priority to fighting quackery and unproven treatments, even though he had used these same treatments in his own practice. Homeopathy was counted by the AMA as a form of quackery, yet the archbishop of anti-quackery, George Simmons, not only was a one-time homeopath but had been awarded his regular medical degree on the basis of homeopathic training. Could then homeopathy be so terrible after all? For one who trained in homeopathy and spent 10 years making his living out of the practice, Simmons was disingenuous in stating that "Of all the medical systems of past or present times, there is none which in my opinion has a scantier basis of fact or reason, a poorer excuse for existence, or a more fantastic set of principles and methods, than homoeopathy" [15, p. 446].

Homeopaths in Nazi Germany

By the end of World War I, homeopathy was at its nadir in Germany. A small homeopathic community coexisted with a vastly greater allopathic profession, who took no notice of their cousins. Publications on homeopathy rarely appeared in allopathic journals. In 1925 however, homeopathy found itself revitalized by one of the country's most prominent surgeons, August Bier, whose stature made his pronouncements impossible to ignore. Bier's contributions to medicine are described in Chap. 5, and his influence on the revival of homeopathy in twentieth-century German medicine is well summarized by Ernst [38]. Therefore, orthodox medicine paid attention to Bier's surprising publication entitled *"Wie sollen wir uns zur Homöopathie stellen?"* (*"What shall be our attitude towards homoeopathy?"*) [39]. Bier's publication sparked interest in homeopathy, and he has been credited for its brief appearance as an academic discipline in German universities for promoting research and for the broader growth of *Neue Deutsche Heilkunde* (New German Medicine) over the next 10–15 years. *Neue Deutsche Heilkunde* represented a hybrid of standard and alternative medicine, in which homeopathy was given unaccustomed prominence [40].

When the Nazis seized power in 1933, *Neue Deutsche Heilkunde* was implemented as the official government health policy. Among the reasons Nazi leaders found it attractive were that it promoted "pure German" medicine and that homeopathy was inexpensive, natural, and in line with the personal beliefs of some leading Nazis such as Rudolf Hess and Julius Streicher. A forced alliance was thus created between allopathic and homeopathic leaders. However, these doctors were not simply chosen on meritorious professional distinction, for they had to be willing stooges who would implement the policy of racial medicine. As stated by Ernst, Nazi health policy was geared to enforce the aims of national socialism, in which needs of the state (*Vorsorge*) were placed before care of the individual (*Fürsorge*). Under such circumstances, professionals would often be confronted by major ethical challenges and in this respect homeopaths were no exception. While homeopaths were probably not guilty of the excessive ethical breaches or atrocities that occurred at the hands of some regular doctors, they were not above criticism for complicity with Nazi policy. Two major offenders will be described.

Karl Koetschau

Karl Koetschau (1892–1982) trained in allopathic medicine. Early in his career at the University of Jena, stimulated by Bier's paper, he decided to investigate homeopathy and subsequently devoted several years to homeopathic research at Jena and in New York. He focused on dose-response patterns and their relation to homeopathy, the main results of this work having been presented in Chap. 16.

In 1933, Emil Klein, the Jewish professor of alternative medicine, was forced to leave his position at Jena and was replaced by Koetschau, who remained there until 1937 before he too was fired, but for different reasons having to do with rivalry within the Nazi health administration. In 1935, he was appointed director of the Reich Association for New German Medicine, a conglomerate of alternative medicine groups tasked with coordinating the new "natural medicine" health policy. Although this commission was short lived, Koetschau's influence remained a factor throughout Nazi rule. After World War II, he was interned by American occupation forces, but later liberated. He then continued to preach the same political message in Communist East Germany, where he defended and wrote further about his beliefs in *Vorsorge*.

Koetschau has been described as "the most prominent and influential proponent of a medical philosophy of *Vorsorge*, manipulating the meaning and purpose of care within the Nazi political worldview" [41], in which the weak and chronically ill had no place [42].

Vorsorge may appear to resemble public health medicine, but under the Nazis, it became grossly distorted: it was in no way a form of preventive medicine to enhance the well-being of the citizenry. On the contrary, it was used to (a) submerge *Fürsorge* or the idea of caring for the individual and (b) to force health professions to execute government-based ideas of what was good for the country. Hitler had stated that "What is useful for the community has priority over what is useful for the individual" and "You are nothing, your nation is everything" [43]. It was now expected that the medical profession should follow these principles, which were introduced as official policy into the teaching curricula of German medical and nursing schools, as well as primary and secondary schools [44]. On this foundation, any medical practice could be justified if it was for the betterment of the *Volk*, including elimination of the unfit, and it was this policy that Koetschau tried his best to implement.

Koetschau advanced his views in two key publications [45, 46] which argued that doctors should be mainly concerned with keeping the healthy well, since this segment of the population had the most to offer society, while they were to diminish care for "the sick, the weakly, and the useless who are only preserved in an artificial world … such as a mental hospital" [41, 47, 48]. As Proctor points out, Koetschau played a leading role in re-casting the philosophy of medical care in a way that dovetailed with Nazi policies. It was the task of the medical profession, Koetschau said, to view medicine within the Nazi *Weltanschauung* (or worldview), and that anyone who proclaimed science to be "value-free" was unaware of their own allegiances. He characterized any non-Nazi "value-free" worldview as a "dogma of the Jewish-international conception of the world." His writings in the late 1930s were openly anti-Semitic, and Julius Streicher afforded him protection as head of the Paracelsus Institute after he had been removed from his position in Jena.

As quoted by Pross, Koetschau unambiguously advocated the extermination of invalids by means of a forced selection process in which they were trained for fitness and health. If they failed in this attempt, and their health worsened, they were to be eliminated [42].

Although there was no indication that Koetschau was directly responsible for medical crimes, and he was found not guilty in the postwar denazification courts, he clearly helped pave the way for the worst excesses of Nazi medical crimes and made no attempt to conceal his anti-Semitic views. After the end of World War II, Koetschau was imprisoned, although not charged with any crimes. It was at this time that a stroke of good fortune came his way. Otto Guttentag had known Koetschau since the 1930s, when Guttentag still lived in Germany. They shared an interest in homeopathy as well as a philosophical attraction to holistic medicine. As the clouds darkened in Germany, Koetschau intervened on behalf of his friend. As Guttentag wrote in a letter to Dr. Alan Sutherland, editor of the *Journal of the American Institute of Homeopathy*, "Were it not for his intervention on my behalf, I myself would not be here today" [49]. Guttentag left Germany for the United States in 1933. In 1947, Guttentag returned to Germany as part of a US military mission to reform German medicine and bring its transgressors to account. He took the opportunity to visit Koetschau, who was still interned, and persuaded the authorities to free him. In spite of Koetschau's open anti-Semitism, Guttentag saw him as neither anti-Semitic nor involved in any criminal acts.

Koetschau lived until 1982 and is still remembered for his work in natural medicine and his exploration of homeopathic remedy dose patterns. He continued to write books, including a text on natural medicine, *Naturmedizin, neue Wege* [50] and one on the ideology of healthcare, *Vorsorge oder Fürsorge? Auftakte einer Gesundheitslehre* [51]. While scholars make a strong case for Koetschau's anti-Semitic leanings, and for articulating a philosophy that was used to justify Nazi medical practice, he was a complex character, as evidenced by Guttentag's more favorable view of the man [52], as well as Boyd's admiration for his pharmacological research. Nevertheless, Koetschau's darker deeds remain.

Other Transgressors: Hans Wapler and Gerhard Madaus

While Koetschau was perhaps the most prominent homeopathic spokesman for government policy, others supported Nazi policies. Hans Wapler (1866–1951) trained in orthodox medicine and then adopted homeopathy, becoming director of the Leipzig homeopathic clinic and editor of the *Allgemeine Homöopathische Zeitung*. Juette has noted that,

during the Nazi years, Wapler "had seriously veered off course and straight into Nazi waters" [53], and in the same article, noted Wapler's opinion that "There can be no national socialist physician who – if made aware of it – would not recognize the crucial importance that Hitler's political evaluation of the Similia similibus has had for Germany," referring to this principle in connection with preserving German culture and values. Juette notes that when the *Allgemeine Homöopathische Zeitung* reappeared in 1948, it failed to mention its previous support for Nazi policies; the closest it came was an editorial that referred to the "unfortunate political circumstances of the past" and that the journal would henceforth be "unperturbed by any political currents, entirely neutral in the service of a pure and applied science" [54]. Not until 1988 did the journal publish a more forthright account of its orientation in the 1930s and 1940s.

Other inferences have been made concerning the abuse of homeopathy for medical experiments. These appear to have little substance and do not implicate homeopaths directly, even if homeopathic preparations may have been involved [53]. The homeopathic manufacturer and physician Gerhard Madaus (1890–1942) had conducted some experiments with the plant *Dieffenbachia seguine* (also known as *Caladium seguine*), which demonstrated its ability to cause sterility. These experiments took place for scientific and, perhaps, commercial purposes. However, Heinrich Himmler took an interest in the work, after being alerted to Madaus' two publications by Dr. Adolf Pokorny, a (non-homeopathic) dermatologist with connections to Himmler. The potential of *Dieffenbachia* to sterilize the three million Bolsheviks in German prisons, who could then be used as laborers but unable to reproduce, was an attractive one and opened "the most far-reaching perspective" [55]. An aide to Himmler regarded this as a top-secret project of national importance and arranged for representatives from the large industrial complex I.G. Farben to visit the Madaus company and obtain a supply of the plant. Madaus himself was instructed not to publish anything further on the topic, but was given the opportunity to continue work with criminals who would have been sterilized anyway under existing law. Madaus declined this offer and the project eventually died for lack of plant supplies.

At the Nuremberg Doctors' Trial, Dr. Pokorny was indicted for crimes against humanity, but was acquitted. Although the Madaus company supplied *Dieffenbachia* to the SS, Gerhard Madaus and his company were not implicated in human experimentation and no charges were pressed. Madaus did join the Nazi party, but his allegiance may have been weak, for he was imprisoned briefly on account of having a Jewish business associate [56]. Meanwhile, the potential of *Dieffenbachia* to modify sexual or reproductive function remains unexplored in medicine.

Other Events Relevant to Homeopathy in Nazi Germany

In the late 1930s, the German government coordinated with leaders of regular and homeopathic medicine in order to study the efficacy of homeopathy. This initiative focused on homeopathic remedy provings and on treating tuberculosis, pernicious anemia, and gonorrhea. The initial round of provings was negative and a decision was taken not to publish the findings. Neither the provings nor the clinical trials ever reached the light of day, although a subjective account was eventually provided by Fritz Donner, one of the chief homeopaths on the project, indicating the lack of any positive results [57, 58]. He believed that part of the problem in conducting this massive project was the existence of personality conflicts between strong egos, pursuit of self-interest, and other investigator-related issues.

While the emphasis here has been on how homeopathy strayed off course during the Nazi period, it should not be forgotten that several talented homeopaths were forced to leave the country because of their heritage. These included Otto Leeser, Edward Whitmont, Otto Guttentag, Martin Gumpert, and William Gutman.

Homeopathy and Murder

Hawley Crippen and James Munyon

Hawley Crippen (1862–1910) is one of the twentieth century's most notorious murderers, being the first person apprehended through the newly invented transcontinental wireless as he and his lover were escaping to America (Fig. 17.11). The drama of Dr. Crippen and the murder of his wife Cora (or "Belle") has been told many times, including in a recent book, *Thunderstruck*, which interwove the stories of Crippen and Guglielmo Marconi, inventor of the radio [59].

Crippen's peripatetic life, unhappy marriage, affair with Ethel LeNeve, and the murder of his wife have been recounted elsewhere. Here, the focus is placed on the medical career of an individual who unquestionably belongs in the homeopathic rogues' gallery. Hawley Crippen entered the University of Michigan's Homeopathic Medical School in 1882, but left the next year before completing his studies. He determined to continue his education in England, but the best he could achieve was a lowly position in the Bethlehem Hospital, now known as the Maudsley Hospital, which has evolved into the United Kingdom's premier psychiatric training facility. In the 1880s however, it was little more than a psychiatric holding facility, and there was no real competition for medical appointments there. The staff came to value Crippen's knowledge of drugs, while he enriched acquaintance with the drug hyoscine (or scopolamine), a derivative of the

henbane plant. As a commonly used sedative, hyoscine would have been used from time to time by Crippen in treating agitated or disturbed patients [60]. In higher doses, this drug is toxic.

It was not long before Crippen returned to the United States, and he enrolled again in medical school, this time at the Cleveland Homeopathic Medical College, from which he graduated in 1884. He entered private practice in Detroit, where he remained for 2 years before moving to New York for specialist training in ophthalmology at the New York Ophthalmic Hospital. He graduated in 1887 and then accepted an internship in the New York Hahnemann Hospital, where he met a nursing student, Charlotte Bell, who became his first wife. Together with Charlotte, they moved to San Diego, where Crippen started a practice. The couple had one son, Otto, but his wife died unexpectedly in her second pregnancy. Thereafter, Crippen left young Otto to be raised by his maternal grandparents and moved back to New York to join another doctor in practice. It was here that he met his second

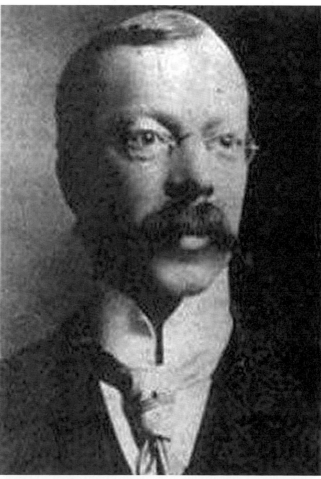

Fig. 17.11 Hawley Crippen. Homeopathic physician who was sentenced to death for murdering his wife (Image in the public domain)

and ill-fated wife, Cora, who later took the name of Belle as she pursued a career on the musical stage.

In the wake of a severe economic recession during 1893, fewer people were able to afford medical care, and many physicians, including Crippen, found it hard to make a living. He was thus obliged to seek other employment. Mail order businesses for patent medicines continued to prosper and Crippen was offered a job with Munyon's Homeopathic Home Remedies, where he took charge of formulating the company's products [61]. Munyon was impressed by Crippen's work ethics and noted how company sales had increased under Crippen's management. He was accordingly promoted to oversee the Philadelphia office in 1895. Munyon's expanded its business activities in England, and in 1897 Crippen was assigned to open offices in London and Liverpool. Accompanying this appointment was a handsome salary of around $220,000 in today's dollars [62]. The good times were not to last however, for Belle Crippen was very demanding of her husband's time and money as she tried to break into the London stage scene. His work deteriorated and Dr. Munyon became increasingly unhappy with Crippen's performance. Late in 1899, Crippen was recalled to run the Philadelphia office, but when he returned to London, he learned that he was no longer employed by Munyon. He took employment with the Sovereign Remedy Company at a reduced salary. Crippen's career and marriage were crumbling, and during his temporary absence in the United States, Belle took a lover. Crippen's work with Sovereign came to an end with the failure of that company, and he then accepted a position as consulting physician to Drouet's Institute for the Deaf [63], where he made the acquaintance of an employee by the name of Ethel LeNeve. In time, the two became close and romance blossomed. Meanwhile, Crippen's professional life continued to slide as Drouet failed. He next joined Aural Remedies as medical advisor, but this company also failed after 6 months, although not before Aural and Dr. Crippen had been exposed by a popular magazine, *Truth*, in a cautionary list of companies to avoid. Fortunately for Crippen, Munyon's was prepared to take him back, but only on a commission basis, so his income was far below what he had been paid previously. Around 1908, Crippen entered into partnership with a London dentist, Gilbert Rylance, who performed dental surgery, while Crippen administered anesthesia. Meanwhile, Crippen continued a side business designing and selling medicines. Both activities continued until he precipitously left Britain with his lover in 1910 (Figs. 17.12 and 17.13).

Early in 1910, Crippen placed an order for five grains of hyoscine at his customary London pharmacy. This large amount was about five times more than the pharmacy normally carried and would be enough to kill twenty people. Although he had to sign for the drug, the pharmacist still made it available to Crippen, who said it was to be used for

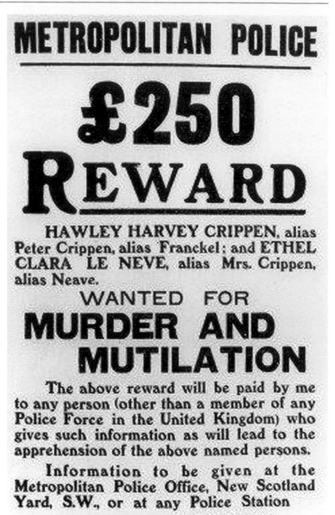

Fig. 17.12 Metropolitan Police Reward Poster for Dr. Crippen (Image by permission of Murderpedia.org)

homeopathic purposes by Munyon's (with whom Crippen had only a loose connection by that time). It is impossible to see how one person needed so much hyoscine for homeopathic purposes, and Crippen's ultimate intentions became clear several months later at Belle Crippen's autopsy, where the famous London forensic chemist, Dr. William Willcox, isolated 0.4 grains of hyoscine from her gastrointestinal tract [64]. Even this small dose would be sufficient to kill a person, and many consider that Crippen administered all five grains to his wife.

So an initially promising career lead nowhere: brief periods of medical practice in Detroit, San Diego, and New York, then work as area manager for Munyon's mail order remedy company and others like it in the United States and the United Kingdom, all of which failed for one reason or another.

Fig. 17.13 Crippen and LeNeve in court, 1910 (Image in the public domain. Source: Library of Congress Prints and Photographs Division Washington, DC)

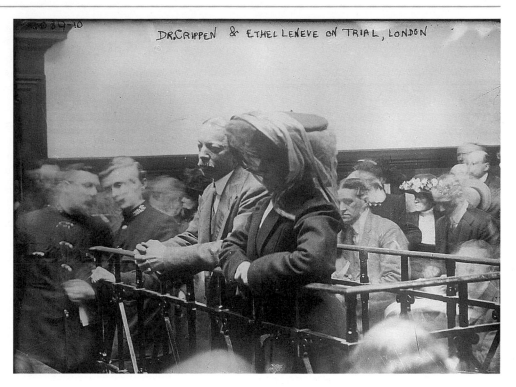

We may not know if Crippen's remedies at Munyon's contained any active substance, but it should be said that Munyon himself was something of an imposter, and many of his company's remedies contained nothing more than sugar and alcohol (Fig. 17.14). An investigation by the British Medical Association in 1908 [65] found that Munyon's Pile Ointment only contained paraffin and <0.2 % ichthyol to add slight odor, yet an unwarranted guarantee of permanent cure was made for the ointment. For those who were not helped by this nostrum, Munyon invited customers to submit a written medical history, in response to which they would be mailed "in a plain envelope" a careful diagnostic evaluation at no cost from one of the consultants, although there was no guarantee that this would be a medically qualified and licensed practitioner. In Britain, the company had come into disrepute by 1908 and at least one of its consulting doctors lost his medical license for activities related to working there. Yet Munyon's was still in business as late as the 1940s, when their products were seized by the government; one brand called Paw Paw Tonic was found to contain strychnine [66]. Munyon not only provided home remedies but ran a "permanent palace of homeopathy" at his New York office, which he called the New School of Homeopathy, where demonstrations were offered for doctors and patients. He also arranged for doctors to make house calls to diagnose and prescribe at no cost to the patient. When Munyon died in March 10, 1918, the New York Times published an obituary, which noted that he was styled "Doctor" but was not a physician [67].

His name now completely forgotten, it is hard to imagine the fame that Munyon enjoyed during his lifetime. For example, in *Men of the Century* [68], he is described as attracting wide attention and that "Certainly no other man has made such strides as he in revolutionizing the practice of medicine." The article quoted the *Philadelphia Times* which stated that "Professor Munyon is to medicine what Thomas Edison is to electricity." It was said that he "formulated a specific for each disease, so labeled that anyone can be his own doctor, and adapted to the cure of that disease alone." He built up what was believed at the time to be the largest medical mail order business in the world and amassed great personal wealth. To Munyon's credit, the essay noted that he made it a working principle to give away ten percent of his annual income to charities. Although Munyon was awarded an honorary doctor of laws degree from the American University of Tennessee, this by no means entitled him to further his medical and homeopathic work as "Professor Munyon." More apt were the monikers "Money Munyon" and "The Papa of Pawpaw" [69]. Testimonials suggest that lack of medical training did not prevent Munyon from diagnosing and treating some patients. For example, an impressed US government official who visited Munyon's office wrote: "Under Prof. Munyon's skillful treatment I noticed an immediate improvement, and, although I was under his care but a few weeks, my hearing has been restored, and I can pronounce myself radically cured" [70].

In his association with Munyon, Crippen hitched his wagon to a dubious star, and the possibility that he consciously or unconsciously deceived the public with inert nostrums has to be strongly considered. Regardless of the ingredients in Crippen's remedies, his marital problems took

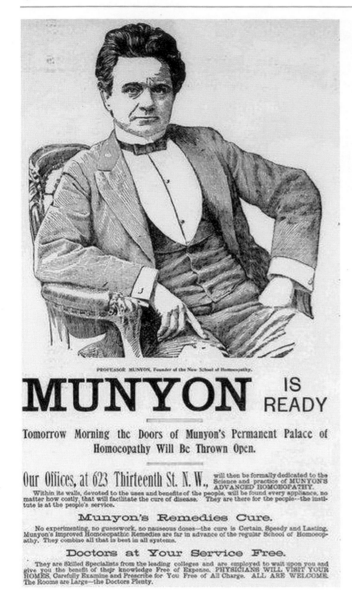

PROFESSOR MUNYON, Founder of the New School of Homeopathy.

MUNYON IS READY

Tomorrow Morning the Doors of Munyon's Permanent Palace of Homeopathy Will Be Thrown Open.

Our Offices, at 623 Thirteenth St. N. W., will then be formally dedicated to the Science and practice of MUNYON'S ADVANCED HOMEOPATHY. Within its walls, devoted to the uses and benefits of the people, will be found every appliance, no matter how costly, that will facilitate the cure of disease. They are there for the people—the institute is at the people's service.

Munyon's Remedies Cure.

No experimenting, no guesswork, no nauseous doses—the cure is Certain, Speedy and Lasting. Munyon's Improved Homeopathic Remedies are far in advance of the regular School of Homeopathy. They combine all that is best in all systems.

Doctors at Your Service Free.

They are Skilled Specialists from the leading colleges and are employed to wait upon you and give you the benefit of their knowledge Free of Expense. PHYSICIANS WILL VISIT YOUR HOMES, Carefully Examine and Prescribe for You Free of All Charge. ALL ARE WELCOME. The Rooms are Large—the Doctors Plenty.

Fig. 17.14 James Munyon, self-styled homeopath, manufacturer, and one-time employer of Dr. Crippen (Source: Morning Times, Washington, DC. December 13, 1896. Image in the public domain)

him down a disastrous path, accompanied by serial failures in his professional life and culminating in the very un-Hippocratic use of a medicine explicitly for the purposes of doing harm. With regard to Munyon, as one might expect, none of his therapeutic contributions have withstood the test of time, but he undoubtedly serves as a reminder of how fraud can pay, and that few could have been more successful at self-promotion than James Monroe Munyon.

Luc Jouret

The mass murder orchestrated in 1994 by Luc Jouret [71, p. 121–123, 72–74] marks him as one of the darkest of all homeopaths. Luc Jouret was born to Belgian parents in 1947. He completed medical training at the Free University of Brussels in 1974. Thereafter, he joined the Belgian army, serving as a paratrooper and taking part in a daring rescue of European hostages in Zaire. Once discharged from the military, Jouret returned to Belgium, where he practiced family medicine for 2 years, before embarking on a worldwide quest to learn about other systems of medicine. It was during a visit to India that he encountered and developed an interest in homeopathy. In the late 1970s and early 1980s, he conducted a homeopathic practice near Geneva, Switzerland. In his public life, he was "strongly centered on homeopathic medical philosophy," which he saw as connecting closely to the unity of all energies [71, p. 121].

Jouret did not limit his activities to medicine. While in Switzerland, he came in contact with Joseph di Mambro, ordained priest of an occult order known as the Renewed Order of the Temple. In due course, Jouret became a priest in this order and later rose to its leadership. In 1984, Jouret founded the Solar Temple and for the rest of his life invested his energies in this new order. The charismatic Jouret was described as follows: "With his deep, soothing, voice and dark penetrating eyes, Jouret was, by all accounts, a riveting speaker" [71, p. 122]. He gave lectures and wrote articles and books that sold widely in New Age circles, where Jouret became a renowned figure, particularly in French-speaking Europe, Martinique, and Canada. He believed that the mission of the Solar Temple was to bring humanity into a new era of enlightenment.

Money was raised by large donations, including $500,000 from one benefactor and over $1,000,000 from another, who had been told by Jouret that he was dying of cancer before Jouret intervened with a miraculous treatment. Other sources of money came from the steep fees paid by initiates into the order. Recruits came largely from Jouret's lectures and writings, but he also persuaded several of his patients into joining the order and, ultimately, led them to their deaths.

As the Temple grew, so did financial and other problems. By the 1990s, Jouret and his inner circle had grown disenchanted with the Temple's ability to achieve its goals; they felt that people were unable to evolve to the new state of enlightenment. Meanwhile, Jouret was being pursued in Canada for money laundering and arms trafficking; he was arrested for attempting to purchase handguns with silencers in Quebec and then fled the country. Jouret and his colleagues assembled plans for a final act by which he and his followers were to escape from earthly life to a higher plane. As part of the plan, Jouret urged his followers to stockpile a weapons arsenal in preparation for Armageddon. The plan culminated on October 3–5, 1994, with a simultaneous mass murder/suicide in Quebec and two villages in Switzerland. All told, 53 followers died, along with Jouret and di Mambro. Many of the deaths probably were by suicide, but in some cases there was evidence of execution-style slaying and bludgeoning. For his actions, Jouret must be counted with the ranks of other cult mass murderers like David Koresh and Jim Jones.

References

1. Rutkow IM. Seeking the cure. New York: Scribner; 2010.
2. Gollaher DJ. From ritual to science: the medical transformation of circumcision in America. J Soc Sci. 1994;28:5–36.
3. Rutkow IM. Edwin Hartley Pratt and orificial surgery. Surgery. 1993;114:558–63.
4. Wilson JL. Stanford University School of Medicine and the Predecessor Schools: an historical perspective [Internet]. [Cited 2012 May 22]. Available from: http://elane.stanford.edu/wilson/index.html.
5. Huff D. Abrams, Boyd, and the emanometer [Internet]. Adapted from list messages by Julian Winston 2003 [Cited 2012 Nov 18]. Available from: http://homeoinfo.com/08_non-classical_topics/dowsing/abrams_boyd_emanometer.php.
6. van Vleck R. The electronic reactions of Albert Abrams [Internet]. American Artifacts; 1999. [Cited 2012 May 22]. Available from: http://www.americanartifacts.com/smma/abrams/abrams.htm.
7. "Albert Abrams". J Am Med Assoc. 1922;78:1072.
8. "Further information regarding Dr. Abrams." Boston Med Surg J. 1922;187:677.
9. Humphris FH. The "electronic reactions" of Abrams (E.R.A.). Lancet. 1924;207:176–8.
10. Haller Jr JS. The history of American homeopathy: from rational medicine to holistic health care. New Brunswick: Rutgers University Press; 2009. p. 55–7.
11. Horder Sir T. The "Electronic Reactions of Abrams". Nature. 1925;115(2899): 789–90.
12. Young JH, McFadyen RE. The Koch cancer treatment. J Hist Med. 1998;53:254–84.
13. Ferrell V. Dr. William F. Koch. [Internet]. Simple health solutions 2011. [Cited 2012 May 23]. Available from: http://simplehealthsolutions.info/hall-of-fame/main-hall/dr-william-koch/.
14. The Koch Family. Scientific therapy and practical research: a biography of William F. Koch, PhD, MD [Cited 2013 Mar 8]. William F. Koch, PhD, MD Official Research Site. Available from: http://www.williamfkoch.com/web/version2/biography.php.
15. Winston J. The faces of homoeopathy. Tawa: Great Auk Publishing; 1999.
16. Reddick v. State Commissioner of Personnel [Internet]. Court of Appeals of Maryland. 3 May 1957. [Cited 2012 Aug 4]. Available from: http://md.findacase.com/research/wfrmDocViewer.aspx/xq/fac.19570503_0040192.MD.htm/qx.
17. Reddick v. State [Internet]. Court of Appeals of Maryland 16 Feb 1959. [Cited 2012 Aug 4]. Available from: http://md.findacase.com/research/wfrmDocViewer.aspx/xq/fac.19590216_0040259.MD.htm/qx.
18. Willard D. A history of homeopathy in Baltimore [Internet]. Baltimore Homeopathic Study Group. Undated [Cited 2012 Aug 4]. Available from: http://homeopathy.inbaltimore.org/history.html.
19. Reddick v. State. Court of Appeals of Maryland [Internet]. 9 Apr 1957 [Cited 2012 Aug 4]. Available from: http://md.findacase.com/research/wfrmDocViewer.aspx/xq/fac.19570409_0040217.MD.htm/qx.
20. People v. Reddick. 176 Cal. App. 2d 806 [Internet]. 31 Dec 1959 [Cited 2012 Aug 4]. Available from: http://law.justia.com/cases/california/calapp2d/176/806.html.
21. Medicine: homeopathic Hassle [Internet]. Time. 20 Aug 1956 [Cited 2012 Aug 4]. Available from: www.time.com.
22. Riley RW. A century of editors. J Am Med Assoc. 1983;250:230–7.
23. Deaths. George H. Simmons. J Am Med Assoc. 1937;109:807–8.
24. Obituary. George H. Simmons, MD. BMJ. 1937;ii:602–3.
25. An Interview with Morris Fishbein, MD [Internet]. 12 Mar 1968. [Cited 2012 May 19]. Available from: http://www.fda.gov/downloads/AboutFDA/WhatWeDo/History/OralHistories/SelectedOralHistoryTranscripts/UCM264166.pdf.
26. Fishbein M. Morris Fishbein, MD An Autobiography. Garden City: Doubleday & Company; 1969. p. 37.
27. Editorial. Diploma mills, St. Louis Clinical Record. 1880:277.
28. McCormick C. A system of mature medicine as taught in McCormick Medical College, vol. II. Chicago: McCormick Medical College; 1922. p. 207–302.
29. Mullins E. Murder by injection: the story of the medical conspiracy against America. Staunton: The National Council for Medical Research; 1988.
30. Ullman D. The homeopathic revolution. Berkeley: North Atlantic Books; 2007. p. 362.
31. "Ex-wife's suit against doctor called a plot". The Chicago Daily Tribune. 28 Jun 1917. ProQuest Historical Newspapers: Chicago Tribune (1849–1988).
32. Ausubel K. When healing becomes a crime. Rochester: Healing Arts Press; 2000. p. 51.
33. "Decree granted Chicago doctor in 1892 is upheld". The Chicago Daily Tribune. 24 June 1919. ProQuest Historical Newspapers: Chicago Tribune (1849–1988). p. 1.
34. George H. Simmons, letter to Ethical Relations Committee, Chicago Medical Society, University of Chicago Library, April 29, 1909.
35. Lydston Would Have Whites and Negroes Marry. Texas State Med J. 1910;5:284.
36. Lydston Wins A.M.A Suit [Internet]. The North Platte Semi-Weekly Tribune. 31 Dec 1915 [Cited 2012 Jul 25]. Available from: www.chronicling.loc.gov/.
37. Fishbein M. History of the American Medical Association. J Am Med Assoc. 1947;133:836–49.
38. Ernst E. August Bier and German homoeopathy in the early 20th century. Br Homeopath J. 1996;85:49–52.
39. Bier A. Wie sollen wir uns zur Homöopathie stellen? Münch Med Wochenschr. 1925;72:713–7 and 773–6.
40. Ernst E. "Neue Deutsche Heilkunde": complementary/alternative medicine in the Third Reich. Complement Ther Med. 2001;9:45–51.
41. Reich WT. The care-based ethic of Nazi medicine and the moral importance of what we care about. Am J Bioeth. 2001;1:64–74.
42. Pross C. The attitude of German émigré doctors towards medicine under National Socialism. Soc Hist Med. 2009;22:531–52.
43. Alschner R. Lebensvolle Sprachübungen in Sachgruppen des Alltags. 11th ed. Leipzig: Dürr; 1940. Reprinted 1982 in Volk und Gesundheit: Heilen und Vernichten im Nationalsozialismus, editor. Projektgruppe "Volk und Gesundheit." Tübingen: Tübinger Vereinigung fur Volkskunde.
44. Ramm R. Ärztliche Rechts- und Standeskunde: der Arzt als Gesundheitserzieher. Berlin: Gruyter; 1942.
45. Koetschau K. Vorsorge und Fürsorge im Rahmen einer neuen Deutsche Heilkunde. Ziel und Weg. 1936;6:240–6.
46. Koetschau K. Gesundheitshege durch Bbung und Vororge. Stuttgart: Hippokrates Verlag Marquhardt & Cie; 1941.
47. Harrington A. Reenchanted science: holism in German culture from Wilhelm II to Hitler. Princeton: Princeton University Press; 1966. p. 187.
48. Proctor R. Racial hygiene: medicine under the Nazis. Cambridge: Harvard University Press; 1988. p. 164–5. and 231–7.
49. Unpublished letter, January 3, 1962. Otto Guttentag Collection. San Francisco: University of California.
50. Koetschau K. Naturmedizin, neue Wege. Ostfreideland: Verlag Grundlagen u. Praxis in Leer; 1978.

51. Koetschau K. Vorsorge oder Fürsorge? Auftakte einer Gesundheitslehre. Stuttgart: Hippokrates; 1954.

52. Guttentag O. Professor Karl Koetschau on his seventieth birthday. Submission to Alan Sutherland, editor. Journal American Institute of Homeopathy. 3 Jan 1962. Otto Guttentag Collection, University of California, San Francisco

53. Juette R. The role of homoeopathy in Nazi Germany – a historical expertise (as of June 2008) [Internet]. Robert Juette 2008 [Cited 2012 May 29]. Available from: http://www.igm-bosch.de/content/language2/downloads/HomoeopathyNaziGermany.pdf.

54. Schoeler H. Editorial. Allgemeine Homoopathische Zeitung. 1948;193:1.

55. Kenny MG. A darker shade of green: medical botany, homeopathy, and cultural politics in interwar Germany. Soc Hist Med. 2002;15:481–504.

56. Timmerman C. Rationalizing "Folk Medicine" in interwar Germany: faith, business, and science at "Dr. Madaus & Co". Soc Hist Med. 2001;14:459–82.

57. Ernst E. Evaluation of homoeopathy in Nazi Germany. Br Homeopath J. 1995;84:229.

58. Donner F. Bemerkungen zu-der Uberprufung der Homoopathie durch das Reichgesundheitsamt 1936–1939. Perfusion 1995;8:3–7 (part 1), 35–40 (part 2), 84–8 (part 3), 124–9 (part 4), 164–6 (part 5).

59. Larson E. Thunderstruck. New York: Crown Publishers; 2006.

60. Larson E. Thunderstruck. New York: Crown Publishers; 2006. p. 33–4.

61. Larson E. Thunderstruck. New York: Crown Publishers; 2006. p. 47–9.

62. Larson E. Thunderstruck. New York: Crown Publishers; 2006. p. 51.

63. Larson E. Thunderstruck. New York: Crown Publishers; 2006. p. 135–42.

64. Larson E. Thunderstruck. New York: Crown Publishers; 2006. p. 367.

65. Anonymous. The composition of certain secret remedies. BMJ. 1908;2:86–9.

66. Caro. The Quack Doctor. Munyon is Ready [Internet]. 17 July 2010 [Cited 2012 May 15]. Available from: http://thequackdoctor.com/index.php/munyon-is-ready/.

67. Dr. Munyon dies in Florida [Internet]. The New York Times. 11 Mar 1918 [Cited 2012 May 16]. Available from: http://query.nytimes.com/gst/abstract.html?res=F60712F73E5C1B728DDDA80994DB405B888DF1D3.

68. Charles Morris. Men of the century: an historical work giving portraits and sketches of eminent citizens of the United States. Philadelphia: L.R. Hamersly & Co; 1896. p. 193.

69. Priest G. Mingo springs hotel: The early days [Internet]. North Reading: Gary Priest Publisher; 2009. [Cited 2012 May 18]. Available from: www.garypriestrnageley.com.

70. All eyes on Munyon [Internet]. The New York Times. 30 Sept 1894 [Cited 2012 May 16]. Available from: http://query.nytimes.com/gst/abstract.html?res=F70A14FB3A5515738DDDA90B94D1405B8485F0D3.

71. Hall JR, Schuyler PD, Trinh S. Apocalypse observed: religious movements and the state in North America, Europe and Japan. New York: Routledge; 2000.

72. Riding A. Cult leader in Swiss case still missing. The New York Times. 11 Oct 1994. [Cited 2012 Aug 6]. Available from: http://www.nytimes.com/1994/10/11/world/cult-leader-in-swiss-case-still-missing.html?pagewanted=print&src=pm.

73. Lacayo R. In the reign of fire. TIME [Internet]. Monday, 17 Oct 1994 [Cited 2012 Aug 6]. Available from: http://www.time.com/time/magazine/article/0,9171,981616,00.html.

74. Luc Jouret [Internet]. 5 May 2012 [Cited 2012 Aug 6]. Available from: http://en.wikipedia.org/w/index,php?oldid=492513429.

Concluding Thoughts

Samuel Hahnemann has been characterized as a "sower of seed …[which] fell on widening circles" [1]. Some of these seeds have grown into veritable trees and others perhaps into healthy shrubs, as shown by the many individuals described in the previous pages. Some seeds, too, fell on stony ground. On balance, however, medicine has undoubtedly benefited from the homeopathic impulse and in a variety of unexpected ways.

Not only did Hahnemann bring about a new system of therapeutics, but through the industry of his followers in the United States, his system gave rise to a number of progressive medical schools, which were among the first to admit women, minorities, and the disabled. They pioneered in other ways too, for example, by introducing longer curricula, courses in public health and radiology, formal anesthesia training, and advances in surgical practice. Some outstanding research was also stimulated, and one of the first endowed academic research units in the United States was established at a homeopathic school as the direct result of a benefactor who was pleased with the care given to her husband. Hahnemann's concern for public health and medicine's societal responsibilities was translated into action by the several homeopathic physicians who entered politics and public health. The collective impact of these homeopaths will be summarized.

Perhaps what stands out above all else is the moral force that homeopathy expressed through its female practitioners (and some of its male practitioners), who devoted themselves to reform, social justice, and care of the poor and oppressed in a manner that calls to mind the healing legacy of medieval monastic orders and the Knights Hospitaller [2, 3]. It is difficult to imagine any group of physicians that has come closer to fulfilling the core mission of medicine: to relieve suffering for all human beings, no matter what their station in life. By their actions, these homeopaths embodied Mahatma Gandhi's maxim of "Be the change you want to see in the world."

For much of the nineteenth and early twentieth centuries, homeopathy attracted physicians with reformist inclinations.

Among the large number of women described in Chap. 3, Clemence Lozier is the most notable in US medicine, while Emily Stowe in Canada and Maria Estrella in Brazil stand out in their respective countries. Harriet Clisby's name lives on today through the WEIU/Crittenton Women's Union. Laura Towne is considered to have been a primary force in keeping the Gullah culture alive, and several women homeopaths led the fight for women's suffrage, such as Anna Shaw, Leila Bedell, and Mary Safford Blake. Other homeopaths who battled for healthcare among minority groups included the first Native American medical graduate, Charles Eastman, who attempted to bridge the divide between Native and white American cultures and improve the welfare of the Indian population; similarly, Solomon Fuller, Walter Crump, and Geraldine Burton-Branch led trailblazing efforts on behalf of healthcare and medical training opportunity for African-Americans. Bayard Holmes was yet another pioneering homeopath. James Cocke, blind from infancy, graduated first in his class and serves to inspire that that no barrier could stand in the way of fulfilling one's ambition.

Homeopaths have played a crucial role in advancing the growth of medical specialties, most notably anesthesiology, cardiac surgery, urology, and ophthalmic surgery, particularly through individuals at Hahnemann Medical College, Philadelphia, and the New York Homeopathic Medical College between the 1890s and 1940s. The disciplines of pathology and physiology were also indebted to the efforts of certain individuals working in Boston and New York schools during their homeopathic eras, while the work of Robert Dudgeon and Edward Cronin Lowe in Britain should not be discounted. The growth of allergy as a medical specialty was stimulated by the careful studies of Charles Blackley in England and later by Grant Selfridge in the United States, who organized one of the earliest professional allergy societies; Charles Millspaugh was the first to treat hay fever by desensitization with grass pollen.

Homeopathically trained physicians left an enduring mark in psychiatry, notably Charles Menninger, founder of the Menninger Clinic, Solomon Fuller for his work on dementia,

Winfred Overholser as an administrative and forensic psychiatrist, Clara Barrus for her studies on mental illness in women, and the teaching and administration in Boston by Emmons Paine, Frank Richardson, and Henry Pollock. Two homeopathic asylum doctors (Selden Talcott and Samuel Worcester) were regarded highly enough to appear as expert witnesses at the trial of a presidential assassin.

Surgery has been enriched by the original work of many physicians who trained at homeopathic medical schools. These include the pioneers Charles Bailey (cardiac surgeon), Ralph Lloyd (ophthalmologist), William Helmuth, and Israel Talbot (general surgeons).

In the realm of education and academic administration, three homeopathic graduates stand out: Ira Remsen as president of Johns Hopkins University, Marcus Kogel as dean of New York Medical College, and Charles Cameron as dean of the reinvented Hahnemann Medical College.

In the politico-legislative arena, measures to protect patient rights and improve safety in drug development were undertaken by two homeopathic senators, and in England, an important resource for complementary medicine was preserved through the intervention of a senior member of parliament, who was a homeopathic physician. In the public health sector, health departments in San Francisco, Los Angeles, Washington, New York State and City, and Puerto Rico communities were all led at various times by homeopaths. John Hayward and John Drysdale, who were part of the domestic sanitation movement in England, concerned themselves with the question of home design and improved ventilation as factors to reduce disease.

Otto Guttentag put bioethics on the medical map shortly after World War II; William Dieffenbach, Francis Benson, John Mallory Lee, and Emil Grubbé were prominent innovators in radiology; Oscar Auerbach and Charles Cameron conducted groundbreaking work in cancer research; Matthias Roth and George Taylor introduced massage into medicine, and Diocletian Lewis developed a system of gymnastics which was widely adopted.

Finally, homeopaths have produced their share of villains. Although George Simmons put the AMA on a strong footing, his professional and personal life was tarnished by scandal. Other ne'er-do-wells included murderers (Luc Jouret and Hawley Crippen), perpetrators of license scams (Robert Reddick), promoters of dubious treatments (Edwin Pratt, Albert Abrams, William Koch), and some who aligned themselves with Nazi policies which attempted to subordinate personal health needs to those of the state (Karl Koetschau and Hans Wapler).

In appraising the legacy of many of these physicians, it is not difficult to accept that they contributed to medical progress, but in very few cases was it under the banner of homeopathy. Any search for traces of homeopathy in the practice of modern medicine would disappoint those hoping to find it – there are few, but they are not altogether absent. The concept of sensitization is rooted in homeopathic thought, which stressed from the early days that diseased patients were often more sensitive to treatment effects than were healthy subjects. The unanswered question, even today, is how sensitive can a diseased individual, body tissue, or organ be? And related to that question, we may ask how low can the dose be taken while preserving a therapeutic effect? There are recent studies showing that picogram and nanogram doses of some medicines can be effective. These units correspond, respectively, to milligram dilutions of 10^{-9} and 10^{-6}, doses common in homeopathy, but which orthodox medicine has so much difficulty accepting, yet on occasion has embraced them as though homeopathy had never existed [4]. Nicholls [5] has pointed out that, for several decades, British medicine actually incorporated many homeopathic remedies into its pharmacopeia, as, for example, in Ringer's authoritative *Handbook of Therapeutics*, which in its first edition acknowledged medicine's debt to homeopathy, but subsequently deleted any reference to this provenance.

Persecution Against Homeopaths

The reason why homeopathy has failed to make overt inroads to medicine is obvious – it has forever been met with resistance and prejudice – allopathy has not made room for it. Examples of persecution are legion, although it is beyond the scope of this book to go into detail on that matter. However, such persecution should be regarded as one of medicine's more shameful chapters – in some other walks of life, such behavior would be illegal. Even when distinguished and decorated scientists, such as Luc Montagnier and Jacques Benveniste, have turned their sights towards homeopathy or kindred concepts, the scientific community accuses them of being unhinged, and it is not long before the witch-hunt begins. In the 1990s, a bizarre scenario unfolded in the case of George Guess, a competent and well-qualified family physician in North Carolina who chose to practice homeopathy. For no sound reason, the state licensing board awakened long-dormant ghosts of the past by unaccountably pursuing him and ordering that he either relinquish his license or give up practicing homeopathy and revert to orthodox medicine. This occurred in spite of the board's acknowledgement that Dr. Guess was a competent practitioner whose only "crime" was that of using homeopathy. After long and costly litigation with appeals and counter-appeals, Dr. Guess left North Carolina for Virginia, where he still practices. One local consequence of the Guess affair was that public opinion became so stirred up that legislation followed which made it possible to practice homeopathy and other forms of alternative medicine without fear of persecution by the state licensing authority simply on the grounds that such practice was not customary. Curiously, about 20 years after the Dr. Guess ruckus, the same state licensing board elected a doctor of osteopathy

(D.O.) as its president, and one of the tasks he placed on his presidential agenda was to chip away at discrimination against osteopaths [6]. He noted that, even as of 2009, one large hospital system refused to recognize osteopathic board certification as equivalent to the allopathic certification.

The medical legacy of homeopaths is broadly based, as described in the preceding chapters. There are the few instructive cases of distinguished academic homeopaths practicing in the mid-twentieth century, at a time when it had become impossible to conduct homeopathic practice and research in medical schools. The experience of these individuals seemed to be that modern medicine with its magic bullets had rendered homeopathy irrelevant, although with the growth of antibiotic resistance, some of these wonder drugs are beginning to lose their luster.

In the case of Conrad Wesselhoeft, his later writings on infectious disease make no mention of homeopathy. The exact reasons are open to conjecture: unwillingness by mainstream journals to countenance it, or ambivalence about Wesselhoeft's homeopathic past and the need to downplay it in order to prosper in the changing world of medicine. It is therefore possible that such homeopathic allegiance went underground and never truly disappeared, as we have seen with Fuller and Menninger. As to Thomas McGavack and Linn Boyd, although they were active in homeopathy until around 1940, their later writings also made very little mention of homeopathic treatment. Boyd was probably the last to conduct substantial homeopathic research and practice in a medical school, which he continued well into the 1930s with drug provings on NYMC medical students and animal model experiments.

The homeopathic impulse was more evident in the humanitarian side of medicine – patient rights, bioethics, disparities on healthcare, and healthcare legislation, all aspects of medicine that are as important as the scientific. These humanitarian values were upheld by the founder of homeopathy, which may explain why progressive people were attracted to the specialty. Although homeopathic medical schools were often slighted and regarded as inferior, they produced many high achievers. One has to regret the passing of these schools; the presence of an "alternative" system of medicine perhaps proved more a boon than a bane to medical progress. Even though therapeutic innovations were comparatively few in the narrow sense of homeopathic remedies, a vigorous homeopathic community provided a constant stimulus to think out of the box and challenge established prejudices.

The Evidence for Efficacy: Does Homeopathy Work?

Although this is not a book on homeopathic research, failure to touch on the subject could be seen as an important omission, so a brief overview will be presented. Firstly, the general topic of evidence will be discussed.

Basic Rules of Medical Evidence: Some Brief Considerations

In the preface, I shared a personal anecdote about Dr. Ernest Hawkes and his family of Liverpool homeopaths. Let us revisit this family to illustrate a fundamental point about medical evidence. In 1906, Ernest Hawkes' father, Alfred Hawkes, compared death rates from measles in four regular Liverpool hospitals to the number of deaths in the outpatient homeopathic practices of Hawkes' two sons. The author observed a combined death rate of 6.7 % from conventional treatment in the four hospitals and a death rate of 4 % from 466 outpatients managed homeopathically [7]. While one might be tempted to conclude that deaths from the homeopathic sample were about 40 % lower, such a conclusion would be unwarranted for the following reasons: (1) the samples differed and it is possible that those admitted to hospital were more severely ill than those in the homeopathic group, (2) it is unclear whether patients who were treated homeopathically by other doctors would have done so well (i.e., a "doctor" effect), (3) it is not stated how the four regular hospitals were chosen and whether they were representative of all city hospitals, and (4) the demographic characteristics may have differed, for example, the homeopathic outpatients may have been from a higher socioeconomic group and contained more private patients.

In order to show if homeopathy truly reduced the mortality of measles, it would have been necessary to balance the two groups beforehand so that they were as identical as possible, apart from the method of treatment. Another modification would have been to compare inpatients treated each way, or to compare outpatients, but not to mix them up, as was done by Hawkes, whose report could be construed as a comparison of inpatient vs. outpatient management as much as one of homeopathy vs. allopathy.

Such principles were not understood at the time, but today any claims made for a treatment must be supported by means of randomized, double-blind, controlled trials. In the following paragraphs, the results of such trials for homeopathy will be summarized.

Major Reviews of Homeopathy

Between 1991 and 2005, three research groups published comprehensive reviews of homeopathy in major medical journals. These reviews all examined whether homeopathy was superior to placebo in randomized, placebo-controlled, double-blind trials, a method that has been the bread and butter of drug testing in medicine for over 50 years. Homeopathy was evaluated as a general method of treatment for a wide range of conditions, which obscures the possibility that its efficacy could be more effective for some diseases than for others, or that certain types of homeopathy could be better than others, but it still answers an important question about the general method of homeopathy. Leaving that reservation aside, it is salutary that all the reviews found superiority for homeopathy, although they did not reach the same conclusions.

In the first review, Kleijnen et al. concluded positively that they would be prepared to accept that homeopathy was effective "if only the mechanism of action was more plausible" [8]. Such a conclusion conflates two different questions of *whether* a treatment works and *how* it works. While medicine has not generally had a problem accepting uncontroversial treatment even when its mechanism of action was unknown (e.g., aspirin, nitroglycerin, and digitalis), this seems to have become an issue in the case of homeopathy, which has been expected by opponents to deliver stronger proof of efficacy than other types of treatment. In other words, the standards of proof were arbitrarily expected to be higher. Anti-homeopathic critics have consistently failed to recognize that much homeopathy is practiced with material doses of drug (e.g., picogram and nanogram amounts), and, as such, there is no sound reason to adopt a higher set of research standards.

Six years after the Kleijnen review, Linde et al. [9] analyzed a different series of studies and found that their results were incompatible with the hypothesis that homeopathy and placebo did not differ. Homeopathy was more effective, including in the better quality trials, which was an important observation since low quality studies often favor a treatment over placebo because other influences (sources of bias) have not been adequately controlled. If higher quality trials demonstrate efficacy, then one has greater confidence that this is due to differences between treatments rather than to other factors, such as unblinding of assessors during the trial. Adding further support were two later analyses of the same data by Linde's group, which showed that good quality studies of any homeopathy [10] and of individualized homeopathy [11] exerted greater effect than placebo, although they did show that magnitude of difference diminished as study quality increased and that in one subgroup of the best studies, the treatments were equivalent: they accepted that their 1997 report may have overestimated the effect of homeopathy [12].

The third study will be described in more detail, since it has gained wide visibility. Shang and colleagues [13] compared the funnel plots in 110 studies of homeopathy vs. placebo to those of 110 conventional medicine vs. placebo. (A funnel plot shows the relation between treatment effect and study size. Larger trials are more likely to have effects that cluster near to the average effect, while small samples spread further away from the mean. Under ideal circumstances, the resulting pattern shows a distribution of effects that visually resembles an inverted funnel. Any asymmetry suggests the possibility that large effects from small sample trials are exerting undue influence on the conclusions and/or that neg-

ative studies have not been included in the analysis.) In the Shang report, there was no difference in the funnel patterns for the two kinds of study, with homeopathic and allopathic treatments both being superior to placebo. Moreover, study quality was assessed as good in 19 % of homeopathic trials, compared to only 8 % in allopathic ones, a finding that was glossed over in the paper. Rather than concluding, as did Kleijnen and Linde, that homeopathy was effective, Shang's group then picked eight top quality homeopathic studies and compared them to six conventional trials of comparable quality. But in this small subsample, the authors reportedly altered their criteria of high quality and also compared different diseases in the two groups. For example, the homeopathy group contained six conditions that were absent in the conventional group, and, vice versa, three conditions appeared in the conventional group that did not appear in the homeopathy sample [14]. In this subsample, homeopathy did not fare so well, leading the authors to opine that, in the best studies, allopathic treatments remained superior, while homeopathy failed to outperform placebo. Readers could have been further puzzled by Shang's finding that a sample of eight homeopathic trials for upper respiratory infection significantly favored remedy over placebo. Following on this particular finding, a later report by Lüdtke and Rutten showed that if Shang had analyzed their 21 allopathic respiratory infection studies, they would have found no conclusive evidence in favor of conventional treatment. So it is far from clear that Shang's results spelled "the end of homeopathy," as the editor of *Lancet* claimed [15].

Subsequent to the reviews by Kleijnen, Linde, and Shang, a health technology assessment (HTA) report was published by Bornhoft and Mattiesen, as part of the Swiss government's Complementary Medicine Evaluation Program (PEK). This report found that homeopathy was effective, safe, and most probably cost-efficient [16]. The methods used in this report (e.g., its selective inclusion of reports) have come under some valid criticism, however [17], although the editorial critical of the report has itself been criticized for inaccuracies [18]. A similar assessment by the Belgian authorities in 2011 found no evidence for efficacy of homeopathy.

While reviews such as those described above have become the cement in all evidence-based medicine, we should adopt a cautious approach and not regard them as infallible pronouncements. Ezzo and colleagues have noted that it is common for such reviews to give conflicting results, to show no effect or insufficient evidence for a treatment, and for their results to be influenced by subjective factors on the part of reviewers [19].

So what does the evidence say? Does homeopathy work? The time has not yet arrived to dismiss the practice, and even from a skeptic's point of view, it must be admitted that light still flickers. While there is room for disagreement [20], the evidence against homeopathy is not robust enough to warrant its defenestration: for that, one would need to see serial and unambiguously negative results. As Lüdtke and Rutten [21] have stated, conclusions on the effectiveness of homeopathy depend substantially on the set of trials analyzed and decisions underlying study selection; the choice of outcome parameters and their interpretation is much determined by subjective factors. Many of the same arguments that have taken place about homeopathy have been raised against other types of treatment including, for example, the effect of antidepressants. Although it is beyond argument that antidepressants are superior to placebo, positions pro and con have often been staked out in advance based on personal prejudices, and what are termed "evidence-based" treatment guidelines can be influenced by the composition of review committees and the rules they establish to organize and interpret the data.

For homeopathy, the door is not yet closed. In respect of the therapeutic contest, perhaps the Dodo-bird's words in Lewis Carroll's (real name: Charles Lutwidge Dodgson) *Alice's Adventures in Wonderland* are apposite. When the Dodo was asked who had won the Caucus race, it had trouble making up its mind and concluded that "everybody has won and all must have prizes." Such could be the verdict for homeopathy in comparison to other forms of treatment at this time.

There is also a portfolio of indirect evidence from animal and plant models that supports its activity, although of course not proving that homeopathy works as a treatment for medical disorders. Some of this secondary evidence has been replicated, including histamine H_2-receptor-mediated inhibition of basophil activation from high dilutions (10^{-32} M) of histamine, actions of aspirin as inhibitor of COX-2-mediated PGI_2 production in blood vessel endothelium, and effects of thyroxine dilutions on frog metamorphosis. This body of science has been reviewed elsewhere and will not be discussed in detail here.

The level of prejudice that exists for and against homeopathy may be insurmountable unless conscious efforts are made to examine the effect of such prejudice on rational scientific discourse. Wisdom consists, among other things, of the ability to deal with uncertainty, tolerate different perspectives, regulate emotion, develop self-understanding, and set prejudice aside [22]. A bit more sagacity on all sides of the debate would benefit everyone and help advance a more constructive, participatory, investigation of homeopathy and its place in medicine.

How Might Homeopathy Work?

Besides the question of whether homeopathy works, we may look for possible mechanisms of action, of which three offer particular appeal.

1. The first possibility is that remedies work according to usual pharmacological principles. For this to be the case, measurable amounts of drug would be required. If a diseased organism shows enhanced sensitivity to a drug, it is plausible that extremely low doses may have an effect. One way to demonstrate this would be to assess whether low but measurable doses are more effective than the higher dilutions that supposedly contain no drug. While the literature is sparse, one revealing analysis of the 21 best-quality trials in the Shang et al. data has shown that low molecular dose (i.e., a measurable amount of drug) was the only one of seven variables to emerge as a significant factor [21, p. 2004]. In other words, homeopathy was superior to placebo in the group of studies where material dose was used, while in those studies that used dilutions with no presumed drug content, homeopathy failed to show an effect. Other variables that could potentially have affected outcome, such as type of analysis, country of study, use of single remedy, or combination remedy, made no difference. Although the number of studies was small, this intriguing finding supports low dose homeopathy.

2. The above argument does not entirely dispense with high dilution homeopathy, as there have been a number of studies showing efficacy, including some good quality trials. Either this type of homeopathy works by non-pharmacological mechanisms, as has been proposed by Bell, for example [23], or a trace level of the mother tincture (original drug) remains in the dilution, which gives enough of a pharmacological stimulus to produce an effect, as was discussed in Chap. 16. At the present time, neither of these mechanisms can be discounted, and both need to be investigated further.

3. A third explanation concerns the possibility that homeopathy of all kinds is nothing more than a good placebo. Considering that a thorough homeopathic interview takes time and can result in the patient feeling understood, there is every reason to believe that the encounter would be therapeutic – perhaps homeopathy could be classified as a form of psychotherapy with presently undetermined active ingredients. To demonstrate this third possibility, a study design would need to include the following groups: a homeopathic consultation with and without the remedy and a standard non-homeopathic consultation with and without the remedy. Such a study was conducted by Brien et al. in 56 patients with rheumatoid arthritis (RA), who had been stabilized on conventional medicine, which they continued in the trial. It was found that the homeopathic consultation produced a clinically meaningful effect on a composite RA scale and global assessment. No difference was found between the remedy and placebo groups, leading the authors to conclude that the active ingredient of homeopathy was to be found in the consultation process [24].

This study provides a clear finding but is limited by its small size and the need for replication. However, even if the result was to be repeated many times, rather than suggesting that homeopathy is "only placebo," it suggests that whatever occurs in a homeopathic consultation – empathy, infusion of hope, enablement, narrative competency, and so forth – can augment the effect of regular treatments, at least in some chronic diseases. In the Brien study, the magnitude of benefit for homeopathy was greater than what has been found for cognitive behavioral therapy. Brien's findings also suggest that the curriculum which was emphasized in homeopathic medical schools may have enhanced therapy in general.

In the last 20 years, there has been an accumulation of good quality research in homeopathy, much of which was summarized in two issues of the journal *Homeopathy* (October 2009 and January 2010). Research continues unabated, and it is hoped that in due course we will achieve a better grasp on the important questions about homeopathy, including its efficacy, mechanisms, indications, and method of delivery. We still cannot entirely escape from the question whether (1) Hahnemann promoted one of the biggest hoaxes in medicine; if, (2) ahead of his time, he revealed truths that show us the way to better medicine, but which we still do not yet fully comprehend; or if (3) it was a mixture of both. Meanwhile, as this book has tried to show, regardless of these questions, apart from some notable villains, homeopathically trained physicians have given medicine much to be grateful for.

References

1. Cameron CS. Homeopathy in retrospect. Trans Stud Coll Physicians Phila. 1959;27:28–33.
2. Bagwell CE. Nosokomia to sacred infirmary: legacy of the Knights Hospitaller and Chimbarazo Hospital in the evolution of hospitals from medieval to modern. J Am Coll Surg. 2013;216:e35–42. http://dx.doi.org/10.1016/j.jamcollsurg.2013.01.001.
3. Bagwell CE. "Respectful image": revenge of the barber-surgeon. Ann Surg. 2005;241:872–88.
4. Watters WH. A pathologist's view of homeopathy. N Engl Med Gazette. 1909;43:407–18.
5. Nicholls PA. Homoeopathy and the medical profession. New York: Croom Helm; 1988. p. 170–1.
6. Jablonski D. A milestone for osteopathic medicine – and the NCSB. Forum: North Carolina Medical Board. 2009;Winter:1–2.
7. Hawkes AE. Homeopathy in England – a letter from Alfred Edward Hawkes. Trans Am Inst Homeopath, 62nd Session. 1906;62:94–7.
8. Kleijnen J, Knipschild P, ter Riet G. Clinical trials of homeopathy. BMJ. 1991;302:316–23.
9. Linde K, Clausius N, Ramirez G, Melchart F, Eitel F, Hedges LV, et al. Are the clinical effects of homeopathy placebo effects? A meta-analysis of placebo-controlled trials. Lancet. 1997;350:834–43.
10. Linde K, Scholz M, Ramirez G, Clausius N, Melchart D, Jonas WB. Impact of study quality on outcome in placebo-controlled trials of homeopathy. J Clin Epidemiol. 1999;52:631–6.
11. Linde K, Melchart D. Randomized controlled trials of individualized homeopathy: a state-of-the-art review. J Altern Complement Med. 1998;4:371–88.
12. Singh S, Ernst E. Trick or treatment: the undeniable facts about alternative medicine. New York: W.W. Norton & Company; 2008. p. 135.
13. Shang A, Huwiler-Müntener D, Nartey L, Jüni P, Dörig S, Sterne JAC, et al. Are the clinical effects of homeopathy placebo effects? Comparative study of placebo-controlled trials of homeopathy and allopathy. Lancet. 2005;366:726–32.
14. Rutten L, Mathie RT, Fisher P, Goossens M, van Vassenhoven M. Plausibility and evidence: the case of homeopathy. Med Health Care Philos. 2013;16(3):525–32. doi:10.1007/s11019-012-9413-9.
15. Editorial. The end of homeopathy. Lancet. 2005;336:690.
16. Bornhoft G, Matthiesen PF, editors. Homeopathy in healthcare – effectiveness, appropriateness, safety, costs. Berlin: Springer-Verlag GmbH; 2011.
17. Shaw DM. The Swiss report on homeopathy: a case study of research misconduct. Swiss Med Wkly. 2012;142:W13594. doi:10.4414/smw.2012.13594.
18. Gurtner F. The report "Homeopathy in healthcare: effectiveness, appropriateness, safety and costs" is not a "Swiss report". Counterstatement to Shaw D.M. The Swiss report on homeopathy: a case study of research misconduct. Swiss Med Wkly. 2012;142:w13594. doi:10.4414/smw.2012.13723.
19. Ezzo J, Bauzell B, Moerman DE, Berman B, Hadhazy V. Reviewing the reviews. How strong is the evidence? How clear are the conclusions? Int J Technol Assess Health Care. 2001;17:457–66.
20. Ernst E. A systematic review of systematic reviews of homeopathy. Br J Clin Pharmacol. 2002;54:577–82.
21. Lüdtke R, Rutten ALB. The conclusions on the homeopathy highly depend on the set of analyzed trials. J Clin Epidemiol. 2008;61:1197–2004.
22. Meeks TW, Jeste DV. Neurobiology of wisdom. Arch Gen Psychiatry. 2009;66:355–65.
23. Bell IR. Nanoparticles, adaptation and network medicine: an integrative theoretical framework for homeopathy [Internet] [Cited 2012 Dec 4]. HRI Research Article. 2012;17:1–2. Available from: www.homeoinst.org.
24. Brien S, Lachance L, Prescott P, McDermott C, Lewith G. Homeopathy has clinical benefits in rheumatoid arthritis patients that are attributable to the consultation process but not the homeopathic remedy: a randomized controlled clinical trial. Rheumatology. 2011;50:1070–82.

Index

A

Abrams, Albert, 180–184
Allergy and allergic disorders, 3
    Blackley, Charles Harrison, 115–118
    Millspaugh, Charles Frederick, 120
    Reilly studies, 120–121
    Selfridge, Grant L., 118–119
    von Behring, Emil, 119–120
Alzheimer's disease, 3, 78–79
American Association for the Study of Allergy (AASA), 118
American Association of Orificial Surgeons, 179–180
American Institute of Homeopathy (AIH), 29
American Institute of Instruction (AII), 144
American Medical Association (AMA), 29, 159, 186, 187, 188
American Psychiatric Association (APA), 77
Anesthesiology, 3, 197
    Bier, August, 59–60
    Boothby, Walter M., 50
    Buchanan, Thomas Drysdale, 49–50
    Griffith, Harold Randall, 52–54
    Keown, Kenneth K., 56–57
    Matthews, Caleb, 57–58
    modern anesthetic era, 47
    morbidity and mortality, 48
    Neff, William, 55–56
    Northrop, Herbert Leo, 48–49
    professionalism, 48
    risk factors, 47
    Ruth, Henry, 51–52
    Sankey, Brant Burdell, 56
    Skinner, Thomas, 58–59
    Tyler, Everett A., 50–51
    Whitacre, Rolland, 54–55
Anthroposophical medicine (AM), 141
Apologia, 59
Arndt, Rudolf, 66, 170–171
Arndt-Schulz law, 174–175
Auerbach, Oscar, 137–138

B

Barrus, Clara, 23–24, 74
Bedell, Leila Gertrude, 20–21
Beinfield, William, 111
Benson, Francis Colgate, 101
Bier, August, 59–60
Bioethics, 3
Blackley, Charles Harrison, 3, 115–118, 197
Blackwell, Elizabeth, 11–12
Blake, Mary Safford, 14–15
Boltz, Oswald, 84–85

Boone, Joel, 154–157
Boothby, Walter M., 50
Boston University School of Medicine (BUSM), 112
Boyd, Linn J., 130–132
British Journal of Homeopathy, 97
British Medical Journal (BMJ), 59, 99
Buchanan, Thomas Drysdale, 49–50
Burton-Branch, Geraldine, 17–18, 34–35, 96

C

Cameron, Charles S., 138–139
Campbell, Alice Boole, 15
Cardiac surgery, 43–44
Cardiology, 3
    Dudgeon, Robert Ellis, 111–112
    Geckeler, George, 109–110
    Hering, Constantine, 107–109
    Likoff, William, 109, 110
    Raisbeck, Milton, 110–111
    Weysse, Arthur, 112
Cardiovascular Institute (CVI), 109–110
Carleton, Bukk, 35
Carleton, Sprague, 35
Chapin, Charles V., 93
Charles Bailey, 43–44
Chemistry and administration, 147–148
Clisby, Harriet, 12
Cocke, James Richard, 85
Cole, Hills, 94
Constipation, 125–126
Copeland, Royal S., 3, 40–41, 94, 159–161
Crippen, Hawley, 191–194
Crumpler, Rebecca Lee, 9, 19
Crump, Walter, 33–34
Cyclopropane anesthesia, 55–56

D

Danforth, Willis, 157
Dieffenbachia, 190
Dieffenbach, William Hermann, 102–104
Domestic sanitation movement, 97
Donner, Fritz, 191
Dorsey, Rebecca Lee, 22–23, 32, 93
Dowling, Joseph Ivimey, 42–43
Drug dosage
    actual dose *vs.* labeled dose, 177
    Arndt-Schulz law, 174–175
    daily usage, 175–176
    intermittent administration, 175

J. Davidson, *A Century of Homeopaths,*
DOI 10.1007/978-1-4939-0527-0, © Springer Science+Business Media New York 2014

Drug dosage (*cont.*)
  "inverted U-shaped" dose-response curve, 169
  linear model, 169
  Time dependent sensitivity (TDS), 176
  threshold model, 169
  "U-shaped" dose-response curve, 169
Drysdale, John James, 97
Dudgeon, Robert Ellis, 111–112, 197

E
Eastman, Charles, 149–150
Edson, Susan, 26
Electroconvulsive therapy (ECT), 175–176
Electronic Reactions of Abrams (ERA), 182–184
Elliotson, John, 116
Estrella, Maria Augusta Generoso, 17
Evans Memorial Institution, 126
*Experimental Researches on the Cause and Nature
    of Catarrhus Aestivus,* 116, 117

F
Fellowship of the American Academy of Homeopathic
    Medicine (FAAHM), 186
Field, Alfred, 108
Finsen, Niels, 103
Fischer, Carl, 148–149
Flagg, Josiah Foster, 30–32
The Fleuro-O-Scope, 96
Fobes, Joseph, 30
Franklin, Edward C., 35–36
Fuller, Solomon Carter, 3
  academic career, 79–80
  African-American psychiatry, 80–81
  Alzheimer's disease, 78–79
  autopsy work, 79
  education, 78
  and homeopathy, 81–82
  psychiatry and psychoanalysis, 79

G
Gallinger, Jacob H., 158–159
Geckeler, George, 109–110
General surgery
  Franklin, Edward C., 35–36
  Helmuth, William Tod, 37
  Lee, John Mallory, 39
  Talbot, Israel Tisdale, 37–39
Gregory, Samuel, 10
Griffith, Harold Randall, 3, 52–54
Grubbé, Emil, 4, 99–101
Guiteau, Charles, 69
Guttentag, Otto Ernest, 198
  academic career, 166
  bioethics and medical humanities, 167–168
  double-blind-controlled trials, 166
  personal life and training, 165–166
  teachings of homeopathy, 166
  UCSF Library, 166–167
Gymnastics, 143–146
Gynecology and obstetrics
  Burton-Branch, Geraldine, 34–35
  Crump, Walter, 33–34

Dorsey, Rebecca Lee, 32
Southwick, George, 32
Taylor, George, 32
Waite, Lucy, 33
Ward, Florence Nightingale, 32–33
Ward, James, 32–33
Wood, James, 32

H
Hahnemann Cardiovascular Institute, 109–110
Hahnemann, Samuel, 4, 63, 197
  as medical pioneer, 7–8
  personality and relationships, 5–7
Hawks, Esther Hill, 19–20
Hay fever, 115–120
Hayward, John William, 97
Health technology assessment (HTA) report, 200
Helmuth, William Tod, 37
Hering, Constantine
  Hering's law of cure, 109
  nitroglycerin, 107–108
  snake venoms, 108–109
A History of Medicine, 119
Holmes, Bayard, 3
  education, 70
  medical library, 70
  schizophrenia, 71–72
  surgical and bacteriological career, 70
Homeopaths
  anesthesiology (*see* Anesthesiology)
  definition, 2–3
  role of, 29
  women homeopaths, 3–4, 9–27
Homeopathy
  allergic disease (*see* Allergy and allergic disorders)
  anesthesiology (*see* Anesthesiology)
  antidepressants, 201
  anti-homeopathic critics, 200
  bioethics (*see* Bioethics)
  cardiology (*see* Cardiology)
  "evidence-based" treatment guidelines, 201
  Fuller, Solomon Carter, 81–82
  history of, 1–2
  homeopathy *vs.* placebo, 200
  HTA report, 200
  mechanisms of action, 201
  medical evidence, rules of, 199
  persecution, 198–199
  pharmacology (*see* Pharmacology)
  and psychiatry
    body's adaptation process, 63
    diagnosis, 64
    drug dose, 64
    at Fergus Falls State Hospital, 76–77
    patient visit, 64
    self-correction/self-healing principle, 63
    symptom appear and disappearance, 64
Homeopathy and Gynecology, 59
Horder Committee report, 183, 184
Hormesis, 173–174
Hueppé, Ferdinand, 173–174
Hydrotherapy, 103
Hypericum, 158
Hyperthyroidism, 166

I

Ignatia, 158

J

Jackson, Mercy B., 18
Jouret, Luc, 194–195

K

Keown, Kenneth K., 56–57
Klopp, Henry I., 74–76
Koch, William Frederick, 184
Koetschau, Karl, 189–190
Kogel, Marcus, 95–96

L

Lee, John Mallory, 39, 104–105
Lewis, Aubrey, 64
Lewis, Diocletian, 143–146
License fraud, 184–188
Likoff, William, 109, 110
Ling, Per, 146
Lloyd, Ralph, 41–42
Lowe, Edward Cronin, 141, 150–151, 197
Lozier, Clemence, 10–11
Lung cancer, 137, 139

M

Mabon, Dickson, 3
Mabon, Jesse Dickson, 161–162
Madaus, Gerhard, 190
Malaria, 126
Mariano, Connie, 156
Mary Thompson, 9
Matthews, Caleb, 57–58
McGavack, Thomas H., 3, 132–133
McLean, William, 42
Menninger, Charles Frederick, 65–66, 197
Mental Diseases and Their Modern Treatment, 67
Miller, Gregory, 186
Millspaugh, Charles Frederick, 120, 197
Missionary School of Medicine (MSM), 162
Mixed catarrhal vaccine (MCV), 151
Munson, Edwin Sterling, 40
Munyon, James Monroe, 192–194

N

Nagamatsu, George, 35
Nazi Germany, 188–191
Neff, William, 55–56
Neuroscientists
    Arndt, Rudolf, 66
    Barrus, Clara, 74
    Boltz, Oswald, 84–85
    Cocke, James Richard, 85
    Fuller, Solomon Carter
        academic career, 79–80
        African-American psychiatry, 80–81
        Alzheimer's disease, 78–79
        autopsy work, 79
        education, 78

        and homeopathy, 81–82
        psychiatry and psychoanalysis, 79
    Guiteau, Charles, 69
    Hahnemann, Samuel, 63
    Holmes, Bayard
        education, 70
        medical library, 70
        schizophrenia, 71–72
        social activism, 70–71
        surgical and bacteriological career, 70
    Klopp, Henry I., 74–76
    Menninger, Charles Frederick, 65–66
    Overholser, Winfred
        education, 82
        Ezra Pound and CIA, 83
        forensic psychiatry, 84
        homeopathic community, 83
        hyperthyroidism, 83
        religion, 84
    Paine, Emmons, 72
    Pollock, Henry M., 73–74
    Richardson, Frank C., 72–73
    Talcott, Selden
        administrator and educator, 68–69
        baseball therapy, 67–68
        education, 66
        healthy diet, rest, and exercise, 68
        Mental Diseases and Their Modern Treatment, 67
        sleep-wake cycle rhythms, 67
    Worcester, Samuel, 69–70
New Concepts in Diagnosis and Treatment, 182
New England Female Medical College (NEFMC), 9
Nitroglycerin, 107–108
Nobel, Alfred, 108
Non-monotonic dose-response curves (NMDRC), 169, 170, 174, 175
Northrop, Herbert Leo, 48–49
Nowell, Howard Wilbert, 140

O

Oncology
    Auerbach, Oscar, 137–138
    Cameron, Charles S., 138–139
    Lowe, Edward Cronin, 141
    Nowell, Howard Wilbert, 140
    Wegman, Ita, 141
Ophthalmology and otolaryngology
    Copeland, Royal S., 40–41
    Dowling, Joseph Ivimey, 42–43
    Lloyd, Ralph, 41–42
    McLean, William, 42
    Munson, Edwin Sterling, 40–43
    Selfridge, L. Grant, 43
Orificial surgery, 179–181
*Orificial Surgery and its Application to the Treatment
    of Chronic Diseases,* 180
Ortiz, Pedro, 94–95
Oscilloclast, 182, 183
Overholser, Winfred, 3, 198
    education, 82
    Ezra Pound and CIA, 83
    forensic psychiatry, 84
    homeopathic community, 83
    hyperthyroidism, 83
    religion, 84

P

Paine, Emmons, 72
Pathology, 150–151
Pediatrics, 148–149
Pharmacology, 3
Pollock, Henry M., 73–74
Porter, Eugene, 91–93
Pratt, Edwin Hartley, 179–181
professionalism, 48
Psoriasis, 104
Psychiatry
    body's adaptation process, 63
    diagnosis, 64
    drug dose, 64
    at Fergus Falls State Hospital, 76–77
    patient visit, 64
    self-correction/self-healing principle, 63
    symptom appear and disappearance, 64
Public health physicians
    Burton-Branch, Geraldine, 96
    Chapin, Charles V., 93
    Cole, Hills, 94
    Copeland, Royal, 94
    domestic sanitation movement, 97
    Dorsey, Rebecca Lee, 93
    Drysdale, John James, 97
    Hayward, John William, 97
    Kogel, Marcus, 95–96
    Ortiz, Pedro, 94–95
    Porter, Eugene, 91–93
    Sumner, Charles, 91
    Verdi, Tullio S., 89–91
    Ward, James W., 94
Pure Food and Drugs Act, 159

R

Radiation
    Benson, Francis Colgate, 101
    Dieffenbach, William Hermann, 102–104
    Grubbé, Emil, 99–101
    Lee, John Mallory, 104–105
Raisbeck, Milton, 110–111
Ransom, Eliza Taylor, 25
Rectal cancer, 102
Reddick, Robert, 184–185
Remsen, Ira, 147–148
Richardson, Frank C., 72–73
Ripley, Martha George, 21–22
Roth, Matthias, 146
Royal London Homeopathic Hospital (RLHH), 161, 162
Royal London Hospital for Integrated Medicine (RLHIM). *See* Royal
    London Homeopathic Hospital (RLHH)
Ruth, Henry, 51–52
Rutkow, 29–30

S

Sankey, Brant Burdell, 56
Sawyer, Charles E., 153–154
Scarlet fever, 126, 128
Schizophrenia, 71–72
Schulz, Hugo, 171–173
Selfridge, Grant L., 118–119
Selfridge, L. Grant, 43
Shaw, Anna Howard, 22

Simmons, George, 186–188
Simpson, James Young, 47
Skinner, Thomas, 58–59
Smith, Julia Holmes, 20
Snake venoms, 108–109
Sobrero, Ascanio, 108
Society for Health and Human Values (SHHV), 167
Sphygmograph, 112
Steward, Susan Smith McKinney, 15–16
Stowe, Emily, 12–14
Stowe, Harriet Beecher, 9
A Study of the Simile in Medicine, 130
Sumner, Charles, 91
Swedish massage
    Roth, Matthias, 146
    Taylor, Charles, 146–147
    Taylor, George, 146

T

Talbot, Israel Tisdale, 37–39
Talcott, Selden
    administrator and educator, 68–69
    baseball therapy, 67–68
    education, 66
    healthy diet, rest, and exercise, 68
    Mental Diseases and Their Modern Treatment, 67
    sleep-wake cycle rhythms, 67
Taylor, Charles, 146–147
Taylor, George, 32, 146
Thayer, David, 9
Thompson, Mary H.
    abdominal and pelvic surgery, 18
    achievements, 18
    eclectic training, 19
    medical training, 18
Thyrotropin-releasing hormone (TRH), 64
Time-dependent sensitization (TDS), 176
Towne, Laura Matilda, 26–27
Tyler, Everett A., 50–51

U

University of California San Francisco (UCSF), 165–167
Upham, Roy, 123
Urology
    Carleton, Bukk, 35
    Carleton, Sprague, 35
    Nagamatsu, George, 35
    Wershub, Leonard P., 35

V

Verdi, Tullio S., 89–91
Vitamin B, 119
von Behring, Emil, 119–120

W

Waite, Lucy, 19, 33
Wapler, Hans, 190
Ward, Florence Nightingale, 16–17, 32–33
Ward, James W., 32–33, 94
Weaver, Rufus, 44
Wegman, Ita, 141
Weir, John, 157–158

Wershub, Leonard P., 35
Wesselhoeft, Conrad, 3, 123–125, 128–130
    constipation, 125–126
    Hahnemann's contributions, 127
    heart disease, digitalis for, 127
    mumps orchitis, 127
    quinine for malaria, 126
    scarlet fever, 126, 128
    whooping cough, 126–127

Wesselhoeft, Hadwig, 124
Wesselhoeft, Robert, 124
Wesselhoeft, Walter, 125
Weysse, Arthur, 112
Whitacre, Rolland, 54–55
Winslow, Caroline Brown, 25–26
Women's Christian Temperance Union (WCTU),
    144, 146
Wood, James, 32

Printed by Printforce, the Netherlands